Learning Disabilities Sourcebook, 3rd Edition

Leukemia Sourcebook

Liver Disorders Sourcebook

Lung Disorders Sourcebook

Medical Tests Sourcebook, 3rd Edition

Men's Health Concerns Sourcebook, 2nd Edition

Mental Health Disorders Sourcebook, 4th Edition

Mental Retardation Sourcebook

Movement Disorders Sourcebook, 2nd Edition

Multiple Sclerosis Sourcebook

Muscular Dystrophy Sourcebook

Obesity Sourcebook

Osteoporosis Sourcebook

Muhlenberg Coun
117 South
Greenville,

D1168523

Teen Health Series

Abuse & Violence Information for
Teens

Accident & Safety Information for
Teens

Alcohol Information for Teens, 2nd
Edition

Allergy Information for Teens

Asthma Information for Teens, 2nd
Edition

Body Information for Teens

nformation for Teens

nentary & Alternative
icine Information for Teens

Information for Teens

ormation for Teens, 2nd Edition

formation for Teens, 3rd Edition

Disorders Information for Teens,
Edition

information for Teens, 2nd
ion

g Disabilities Information for
is

Health Information for Teens,
Edition

cy Information for Teens

Health Information for Teens,
Edition

alth Information for Teens, 2nd
ion

formation for Teens

njuries Information for Teens,
Edition

information for Teens

Information for Teens, 2nd
ion

Information for Teens, 2nd
ion

DATE DUE

GAYLORD   PRINTED IN U.S.A.

Cardiovascular Disorders

Disorders

SOURCEBOOK

Fourth Edition

Health Reference Series

Fourth Edition

Cardiovascular Disorders SOURCEBOOK

Basic Consumer Health Information about Heart and Blood Vessel Diseases and Disorders, Such as Angina, Heart Attack, Heart Failure, Cardiomyopathy, Arrhythmias, Valve Disease, Atherosclerosis, Aneurysms, and Congenital Heart Defects, Including Information about Cardiovascular Disease in Women, Men, Children, Adolescents, and Minorities

Along with Facts about Diagnosing, Managing, and Preventing Cardiovascular Disease, a Glossary of Related Medical Terms, and a Directory of Resources for Additional Information

HM 4352
Ref.
$85.00
9/2010

Edited by
Amy L. Sutton

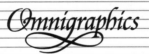

P.O. Box 31-1640, Detroit, MI 48231

Bibliographic Note

Because this page cannot legibly accommodate all the copyright notices, the Bibliographic Note portion of the Preface constitutes an extension of the copyright notice.

Edited by Amy L. Sutton

Health Reference Series

Karen Bellenir, *Managing Editor*
David A. Cooke, MD, FACP, *Medical Consultant*
Elizabeth Collins, *Research and Permissions Coordinator*
Cherry Edwards, *Permissions Assistant*
EdIndex, Services for Publishers, *Indexers*

* * *

Omnigraphics, Inc.

Matthew P. Barbour, *Senior Vice President*
Kevin M. Hayes, *Operations Manager*

* * *

Peter E. Ruffner, *Publisher*

Copyright © 2010 Omnigraphics, Inc.

ISBN 978-0-7808-1080-8

Library of Congress Cataloging-in-Publication Data

Cardiovascular disorders sourcebook : basic consumer health information about heart and blood vessel diseases and disorders, such as angina, heart attack, heart failure, cardiomyopathy, arrhythmias, valve disease, atherosclerosis, aneurysms, and congenital heart defects, including information about cardiovascular disease in women, men, children, adolescents, and minorities along with facts about diagnosing, managing, and preventing cardiovascular disease, a glossary of related medical terms, and a directory of resources for additional information / Edited by Amy L. Sutton. -- 4th ed.
    p. cm.
  Includes bibliographical references and index.
  Summary: "Provides basic consumer health information about risk factors, diagnosis, and treatment of heart and vascular diseases and disorders, along with prevention strategies and tips for maintaining heart health. Includes index, glossary of related terms, and other resources"--Provided by publisher.
  ISBN 978-0-7808-1080-8 (hardcover : alk. paper) 1. Cardiovascular system--Diseases--Popular works. I. Sutton, Amy L.
  RC672.C35 2010
  616.1--dc22
                                                                      2010000749

This book is printed on acid-free paper meeting the ANSI Z39.48 Standard. The infinity symbol that appears above indicates that the paper in this book meets that standard.

Printed in the United States

Table of Contents

Visit www.healthreferenceseries.com to view *A Contents Guide to the Health Reference Series*, a listing of more than 15,000 topics and the volumes in which they are covered.

Part II: Heart Disease

Part III: Blood Vessel Disease

Part IV: Cardiovascular Disorders in Specific Populations

Part V: Identifying Cardiovascular Disorders

Part VI: Managing Cardiovascular Disorders

Preface

About This Book

Statistics indicate that cardiovascular diseases account for more than one third of all deaths in the United States. In addition, more than 80 million Americans live with one or more forms of cardiovascular disease, including heart disease, high blood pressure, heart failure, and stroke. Although cardiovascular disorders may sometimes produce sudden symptoms, such as chest or head pain, they may also develop silently, providing no warning of the heart and blood vessel damage being done. Fortunately, advances in disease detection, recommendations regarding lifestyle choices, new medications, and innovative treatments now make it possible to reduce—or even prevent—the disabling health consequences frequently associated with many common cardiovascular disorders.

Cardiovascular Disorders Sourcebook, Fourth Edition provides updated information about disorders of the heart and blood vessels. It offers anatomical facts, presents statistics, and identifies risk factors for cardiovascular diseases. It describes the treatment of common disorders, including angina, heart attack, heart failure, cardiomyopathy, arrhythmias, valve disease, atherosclerosis, aneurysms, and congenital heart defects. In addition, it discusses diagnostic tests and concerns related to managing cardiovascular diseases with medicines, surgery, and lifestyle changes. The book concludes with a glossary and a directory of resources for further help and information.

How to Use This Book

This book is divided into parts and chapters. Parts focus on broad areas of interest. Chapters are devoted to single topics within a part.

Part I: Introduction to Cardiovascular Disorders provides an overview of the function and structures of the heart. It identifies conditions that increase the risk of cardiovascular disorders, including high blood pressure, high blood cholesterol, and diabetes. Information on how stress, genetics, and aging influence the development of cardiovascular disease is also included, along with warning signs of heart attack and stroke and guidelines for responding to cardiovascular emergencies.

Part II: Heart Disease details the symptoms, diagnosis, and treatments for common heart problems, including coronary artery disease, angina, heart attack, cardiac arrest, and heart failure. Details about heart rhythm abnormalities (such as atrial fibrillation, heart block, and long QT syndrome) and heart valve disease are also presented.

Part III: Blood Vessel Disease gives readers comprehensive information about atherosclerosis and stroke, two of the most common disorders affecting blood vessels. Facts about other forms of vascular disease (including carotid artery disease, aneurysms, peripheral arterial disease, venous disorders, and vasculitis) are also included.

Part IV: Cardiovascular Disorders in Specific Populations discusses the impact of heart and blood vessel disease on women, men, and minorities. In addition, parents will find information about cardiac disorders, heart murmurs, and other defects sometimes diagnosed during childhood or adolescence.

Part V: Identifying Cardiovascular Disorders describes common blood and imaging tests used to diagnose the presence and extent of heart and blood vessel disease, including echocardiography, electrocardiogram, exercise stress tests, cardiac angiography, computed tomography, magnetic resonance imaging, and ultrasound.

Part VI: Managing Cardiovascular Disorders provides details on drugs often prescribed for cardiovascular disease, including blood thinners, statins, blood pressure medications, and stroke treatments. Patients with heart and blood vessel disease will also find information on common procedures and devices used to improve blood flow, regulate heart rhythm, and strengthen artery walls, such as catheterization, ablation, pacemakers, stents, and heart surgery and transplantation. Tips on adjusting to rehabilitation regimens are also provided.

Part VII: Preventing Disease and Regaining Cardiovascular Health suggests strategies for reducing the risk of heart and blood vessel disorders. Information is offered about weight management, physical activity, and good nutrition. Recent research on the influence of dietary supplements on cardiovascular health is discussed, and facts about quitting smoking, limiting alcohol intake, and managing stress—all of which are typically recommended to reduce cardiovascular disease risk—are also included.

Part VIII: Additional Help and Information offers a glossary of important terms related to cardiovascular diseases. A directory of organizations that help people with cardiovascular disorders is also included.

Bibliographic Note

This volume contains documents and excerpts from publications issued by the following U.S. government agencies: Agency for Healthcare Research and Quality (AHRQ); Centers for Disease Control and Prevention (CDC); National Cancer Institute (NCI); National Center for Complementary and Alternative Medicine (NCCAM); National Heart, Lung, and Blood Institute (NHLBI); National Human Genome Research Institute (NHGRI); National Institute of Diabetes and Digestive and Kidney Diseases (NIDDK); National Institute of Neurological Disorders and Stroke (NINDS); National Institute on Aging (NIA); National Institutes of Health (NIH); Office of Dietary Supplements (ODS); Office of Minority Health Resource Center (OMHRC); Office of Women's Health (OWH); and the U.S. Food and Drug Administration (FDA).

In addition, this volume contains copyrighted documents from the following organizations: A.D.A.M., Inc.; American Academy of Family Physicians; American College of Cardiology; American College of Sports Medicine; American Heart Association, Inc.; American Psychological Association; American Society of Health-System Pharmacists, Inc.; The Endocrine Society; University of Michigan Health System; University of Pittsburgh Medical Center; and the Women's Heart Foundation.

Full citation information is provided on the first page of each chapter or section. Every effort has been made to secure all necessary rights to reprint the copyrighted material. If any omissions have been made, please contact Omnigraphics to make corrections for future editions.

Acknowledgements

Thanks go to the many organizations, agencies, and individuals who have contributed materials for this *Sourcebook* and to medical consultant Dr. David Cooke and document engineer Bruce Bellenir. Special thanks go to managing editor Karen Bellenir and research and permissions coordinator Liz Collins for their help and support.

About the Health Reference Series

The *Health Reference Series* is designed to provide basic medical information for patients, families, caregivers, and the general public. Each volume takes a particular topic and provides comprehensive coverage. This is especially important for people who may be dealing with a newly diagnosed disease or a chronic disorder in themselves or in a family member. People looking for preventive guidance, information about disease warning signs, medical statistics, and risk factors for health problems will also find answers to their questions in the *Health Reference Series*. The *Series*, however, is not intended to serve as a tool for diagnosing illness, in prescribing treatments, or as a substitute for the physician/patient relationship. All people concerned about medical symptoms or the possibility of disease are encouraged to seek professional care from an appropriate health care provider.

A Note about Spelling and Style

Health Reference Series editors use *Stedman's Medical Dictionary* as an authority for questions related to the spelling of medical terms and the *Chicago Manual of Style* for questions related to grammatical structures, punctuation, and other editorial concerns. Consistent adherence is not always possible, however, because the individual volumes within the *Series* include many documents from a wide variety of different producers and copyright holders, and the editor's primary goal is to present material from each source as accurately as is possible following the terms specified by each document's producer. This sometimes means that information in different chapters or sections may follow other guidelines and alternate spelling authorities. For example, occasionally a copyright holder may require that eponymous terms be shown in possessive forms (Crohn's disease *vs.* Crohn disease) or that British spelling norms be retained (leukaemia *vs.* leukemia).

Locating Information within the Health Reference Series

The *Health Reference Series* contains a wealth of information about a wide variety of medical topics. Ensuring easy access to all the fact sheets, research reports, in-depth discussions, and other material contained within the individual books of the *Series* remains one of our highest priorities. As the *Series* continues to grow in size and scope, however, locating the precise information needed by a reader may become more challenging.

A Contents Guide to the Health Reference Series was developed to direct readers to the specific volumes that address their concerns. It presents an extensive list of diseases, treatments, and other topics of general interest compiled from the Tables of Contents and major index headings. To access *A Contents Guide to the Health Reference Series*, visit www.healthreferenceseries.com.

Medical Consultant

Medical consultation services are provided to the *Health Reference Series* editors by David A. Cooke, MD, FACP. Dr. Cooke is a graduate of Brandeis University, and he received his M.D. degree from the University of Michigan. He completed residency training at the University of Wisconsin Hospital and Clinics. He is board-certified in Internal Medicine. Dr. Cooke currently works as part of the University of Michigan Health System and practices in Ann Arbor, MI. In his free time, he enjoys writing, science fiction, and spending time with his family.

Our Advisory Board

We would like to thank the following board members for providing guidance to the development of this *Series*:

- Dr. Lynda Baker, Associate Professor of Library and Information Science, Wayne State University, Detroit, MI

- Nancy Bulgarelli, William Beaumont Hospital Library, Royal Oak, MI

- Karen Imarisio, Bloomfield Township Public Library, Bloomfield Township, MI

- Karen Morgan, Mardigian Library, University of Michigan-Dearborn, Dearborn, MI

- Rosemary Orlando, St. Clair Shores Public Library, St. Clair Shores, MI

Health Reference Series *Update Policy*

The inaugural book in the *Health Reference Series* was the first edition of *Cancer Sourcebook* published in 1989. Since then, the *Series* has been enthusiastically received by librarians and in the medical community. In order to maintain the standard of providing high-quality health information for the layperson the editorial staff at Omnigraphics felt it was necessary to implement a policy of updating volumes when warranted.

Medical researchers have been making tremendous strides, and it is the purpose of the *Health Reference Series* to stay current with the most recent advances. Each decision to update a volume is made on an individual basis. Some of the considerations include how much new information is available and the feedback we receive from people who use the books. If there is a topic you would like to see added to the update list, or an area of medical concern you feel has not been adequately addressed, please write to:

Editor
Health Reference Series
Omnigraphics, Inc.
P.O. Box 31-1640
Detroit, MI 48231
E-mail: editorial@omnigraphics.com

Part One

Introduction to Cardiovascular Disorders

Chapter 1

How the Heart Works

What Is the Heart?

Your heart is a muscular organ that acts like a pump to continuously send blood throughout your body.

Your heart is at the center of your circulatory system. This system consists of a network of blood vessels, such as arteries, veins, and capillaries. These blood vessels carry blood to and from all areas of your body.

An electrical system regulates your heart and uses electrical signals to contract the heart's walls. When the walls contract, blood is pumped into your circulatory system. A system of inlet and outlet valves in your heart chambers work to ensure that blood flows in the right direction.

Your heart is vital to your health and nearly everything that goes on in your body. Without the heart's pumping action, blood can't circulate within your body.

Your blood carries the oxygen and nutrients that your organs need to work normally. Blood also carries carbon dioxide, a waste product, to your lungs to be passed out of your body and into the air.

A healthy heart supplies the areas of your body with the right amount of blood at the rate needed to work normally. If disease or

Excerpted from "How the Heart Works," by the National Heart, Lung, and Blood Institute (NHLBI, www.nhlbi.nih.gov), part of the National Institutes of Health, January 2007.

3

injury weakens your heart, your body's organs won't receive enough blood to work normally.

Anatomy of the Heart

Your heart is located under the ribcage in the center of your chest between your right and left lungs. Its muscular walls beat, or contract, pumping blood continuously to all parts of your body.

The size of your heart can vary depending on your age, size, and the condition of your heart. A normal, healthy, adult heart most often is the size of an average clenched adult fist. Some diseases of the heart can cause it to become larger.

The Exterior of the Heart

The heart has four chambers: the right and left atria and the right and left ventricles.

Some of the main blood vessels—arteries and veins—that make up your blood circulatory system are directly connected to the heart.

The ventricle on the right side of your heart pumps blood from your heart to your lungs. When you breathe air in, oxygen passes from your lungs through your blood vessels and into your blood. Carbon dioxide, a waste product, is passed from your blood through blood vessels to your lungs and is removed from your body when you breathe out.

The left atrium receives oxygen-rich blood from your lungs. The pumping action of your left ventricle sends this oxygen-rich blood through the aorta (a main artery) to the rest of your body.

The right side of your heart: The superior and inferior vena cavae are to the left of the heart muscle. These veins are the largest veins in your body.

After your body's organs and tissues have used the oxygen in your blood, the vena cavae carry the oxygen-poor blood back to the right atrium of your heart.

The superior vena cava carries oxygen-poor blood from the upper parts of your body, including your head, chest, arms, and neck. The inferior vena cava carries oxygen-poor blood from the lower parts of your body.

The oxygen-poor blood from the vena cavae flows into your heart's right atrium and then on to the right ventricle. From the right ventricle, the blood is pumped through the pulmonary arteries to your lungs. There, through many small, thin blood vessels called capillaries, the blood picks up more oxygen.

The oxygen-rich blood passes from your lungs back to your heart through the pulmonary veins.

The left side of your heart: Oxygen-rich blood from your lungs passes through the pulmonary veins. It enters the left atrium and is pumped into the left ventricle. From the left ventricle, the oxygen-rich blood is pumped to the rest of your body through the aorta.

Like all of your organs, your heart needs blood rich with oxygen. This oxygen is supplied through the coronary arteries as blood is pumped out of your heart's left ventricle.

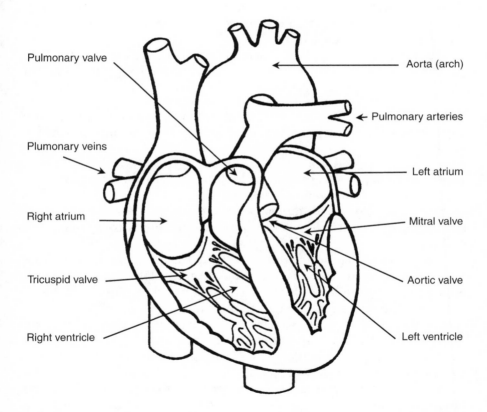

Figure 1.1. Anatomy of the heart. (Image source: From "Introduction to the Cardiovascular System," Surveillance, Epidemiology and End Results (SEER) Program, National Cancer Institute; redrawn by Alison DeKleine.)

Your coronary arteries are located on your heart's surface at the beginning of the aorta. Your coronary arteries carry oxygen-rich blood to all parts of your heart.

The Interior of the Heart

The septum: The right and left sides of your heart are divided by an internal wall of tissue called the septum. The area of the septum that divides the atria (the two upper chambers of your heart) is called the atrial or interatrial septum.

The area of the septum that divides the ventricles (the two lower chambers of your heart) is called the ventricular or interventricular septum.

Heart chambers: The inside of your heart is divided into four chambers. The two upper chambers of your heart are called atria. The atria receive and collect blood.

The two lower chambers of your heart are called ventricles. The ventricles pump blood out of your heart into the circulatory system to other parts of your body.

Heart valves: Your heart has four valves. The valves include the aortic valve, the tricuspid valve, the pulmonary valve, and the mitral valve.

Blood flow: Blood enters the right atrium of your heart from the superior and inferior vena cavae.

From the right atrium, blood is pumped into the right ventricle. From the right ventricle, blood is pumped to your lungs through the pulmonary arteries.

Oxygen-rich blood comes in from your lungs through the pulmonary veins into your heart's left atrium. From the left atrium, the blood is pumped into the left ventricle. The left ventricle pumps the blood to the rest of your body through the aorta.

For the heart to work properly, your blood must flow in only one direction. Your heart's valves make this possible. Both of your heart's ventricles have an "in" (inlet) valve from the atria and an "out" (outlet) valve leading to your arteries.

Healthy valves open and close in very exact coordination with the pumping action of your heart's atria and ventricles. Each valve has a set of flaps called leaflets or cusps that seal or open the valves. This allows pumped blood to pass through the chambers and into your arteries without backing up or flowing backward.

Heart Contraction and Blood Flow

Heartbeat

Almost everyone has heard the real or recorded sound of a heartbeat. When your heart beats, it makes a "lub-DUB" sound. Between the time you hear "lub" and "DUB," blood is pumped through your heart and circulatory system.

A heartbeat may seem like a simple, repeated event, but it's a complex series of very precise and coordinated events that take place inside and around your heart.

Each side of your heart uses an inlet valve to help move blood between the atrium and ventricle. The tricuspid valve does this between the right atrium and ventricle. The mitral valve does this between the left atrium and ventricle. The "lub" is the sound of the tricuspid and mitral valves closing.

Each of your heart's ventricles has an outlet valve. The right ventricle uses the pulmonary valve to help move blood into the pulmonary arteries. The left ventricle uses the aortic valve to do the same for the aorta. The "DUB" is the sound of the aortic and pulmonary valves closing.

Each heartbeat has two basic parts: diastole, or relaxation, and atrial and ventricular systole, or contraction.

During diastole, the atria and ventricles of your heart relax and begin to fill with blood. At the end of diastole, your heart's atria contract (atrial systole) and pump blood into the ventricles. The atria then begin to relax. Next, your heart's ventricles contract (ventricular systole) and pump blood out of your heart.

Pumping Action

Your heart uses its four valves to ensure your blood flows only in one direction. Healthy valves open and close in coordination with the pumping action of your heart's atria and ventricles.

Each valve has a set of flaps called leaflets or cusps. These seal or open the valves. This allows pumped blood to pass through the chambers and into your blood vessels without backing up or flowing backward.

Oxygen-poor blood from the vena cavae fills your heart's right atrium. The atrium contracts (atrial systole). The tricuspid valve located between the right atrium and ventricle opens for a short time and then shuts. This allows blood to enter into the right ventricle without flowing back into the right atrium.

7

When your heart's right ventricle fills with blood, it contracts (ventricular systole). The pulmonary valve located between your right ventricle and pulmonary artery opens and closes quickly.

This allows blood to enter into your pulmonary arteries without flowing back into the right ventricle. This is important because the right ventricle begins to refill with more blood through the tricuspid valve. Blood travels through the pulmonary arteries to your lungs to pick up oxygen.

Oxygen-rich blood returns from the lungs to your heart's left atrium through the pulmonary veins. As your heart's left atrium fills with blood, it contracts. This event also is called atrial systole.

The mitral valve located between the left atrium and left ventricle opens and closes quickly. This allows blood to pass from the left atrium into the left ventricle without flowing backward.

As the left ventricle fills with blood, it contracts. This event also is called ventricular systole. The aortic valve located between the left ventricle and aorta opens and closes quickly. This allows blood to flow into the aorta. The aorta is the main artery that carries blood from your heart to the rest of your body.

The aortic valve closes quickly to prevent blood from flowing back into the left ventricle, which is already filling up with new blood.

Taking Your Pulse

When your heart pumps blood through your arteries, it creates a pulse that you can feel on the arteries close to the skin's surface. For example, you can feel the pulse on the artery inside of your wrist, below your thumb.

You can count how many times your heart beats by taking your pulse. You will need a watch with a second hand.

To find your pulse, gently place your index and middle fingers on the artery located on the inner wrist of either arm, below your thumb. You should feel a pulsing or tapping against your fingers.

Watch the second hand and count the number of pulses you feel in 30 seconds. Double that number to find out your heart rate or pulse for 1 minute.

The usual resting pulse for an adult is 60 to 100 beats per minute. To find your resting pulse, count your pulse after you have been sitting or resting quietly for at least 10 minutes.

Circulation and Blood Vessels

Your heart and blood vessels make up your overall blood circulatory system. Your blood circulatory system is made up of four subsystems.

Arterial Circulation

Arterial circulation is the part of your overall blood circulatory system that involves arteries, like the aorta and pulmonary arteries.

Arteries are blood vessels that carry blood away from your heart. Healthy arteries are strong and elastic. They become narrow between beats of the heart, and they help keep your blood pressure consistent. This helps blood circulate efficiently through your body.

Arteries branch into smaller blood vessels called arterioles. Arteries and arterioles have strong, flexible walls that allow them to adjust the amount and rate of blood flowing to various parts of your body.

Venous Circulation

Venous circulation is the part of your overall blood circulatory system that involves veins, like the vena cavae and pulmonary veins. Veins are blood vessels that carry blood to your heart.

Veins have thinner walls than arteries. Veins can widen as the amount of blood passing through them increases.

Capillary Circulation

Capillary circulation is the part of your overall blood circulatory system where oxygen, nutrients, and waste pass between your blood and parts of your body.

Capillaries connect the arterial and venous circulatory subsystems. Capillaries are very small blood vessels.

The importance of capillaries lies in their very thin walls. Unlike arteries and veins, capillary walls are thin enough that oxygen and nutrients in your blood can pass through the walls to the parts of your body that need them to work normally.

Capillaries' thin walls also allow waste products like carbon dioxide to pass from your body's organs and tissues into the blood, where it's taken away to your lungs.

Pulmonary Circulation

Pulmonary circulation is the movement of blood from the heart to the lungs and back to the heart again. Pulmonary circulation includes both arterial and venous circulation.

Blood without oxygen is pumped to the lungs from the heart (arterial circulation). Oxygen-rich blood moves from the lungs to the heart through the pulmonary veins (venous circulation).

Pulmonary circulation also includes capillary circulation. Oxygen you breathe in from the air passes through your lungs into your blood through the many capillaries in the lungs. Oxygen-rich blood moves through your pulmonary veins to the left side of your heart and out of the aorta to the rest of your body.

Capillaries in the lungs also remove carbon dioxide from your blood so that your lungs can breathe the carbon dioxide out into the air.

Your Heart's Electrical System

Your heart's electrical system controls all the events that occur when your heart pumps blood. The electrical system also is called the cardiac conduction system. If you've ever seen the heart test called an EKG (electrocardiogram), you've seen a graphical picture of the heart's electrical activity.

Your heart's electrical system is made up of three main parts:

- The sinoatrial (SA) node, located in the right atrium of your heart

- The atrioventricular (AV) node, located on the interatrial septum close to the tricuspid valve

- The His-Purkinje system, located along the walls of your heart's ventricles

A heartbeat is a complex series of events that take place in your heart. A heartbeat is a single cycle in which your heart's chambers relax and contract to pump blood. This cycle includes the opening and closing of the inlet and outlet valves of the right and left ventricles of your heart.

Each heartbeat has two basic parts: diastole and atrial and ventricular systole. During diastole, the atria and ventricles of your heart relax and begin to fill with blood.

At the end of diastole, your heart's atria contract (atrial systole) and pump blood into the ventricles. The atria then begin to relax. Your heart's ventricles then contract (ventricular systole), pumping blood out of your heart.

Each beat of your heart is set in motion by an electrical signal from within your heart muscle. In a normal, healthy heart, each beat begins with a signal from the SA node. This is why the SA node is sometimes called your heart's natural pacemaker. Your pulse, or heart rate, is the number of signals the SA node produces per minute.

The signal is generated as the two vena cavae fill your heart's right atrium with blood from other parts of your body. The signal spreads across the cells of your heart's right and left atria. This signal causes the atria to contract. This action pushes blood through the open valves from the atria into both ventricles.

The signal arrives at the AV node near the ventricles. It slows for an instant to allow your heart's right and left ventricles to fill with blood. The signal is released and moves along a pathway called the bundle of His, which is located in the walls of your heart's ventricles.

From the bundle of His, the signal fibers divide into left and right bundle branches through the Purkinje fibers that connect directly to the cells in the walls of your heart's left and right ventricles.

The signal spreads across the cells of your ventricle walls, and both ventricles contract. However, this doesn't happen at exactly the same moment.

The left ventricle contracts an instant before the right ventricle. This pushes blood through the pulmonary valve (for the right ventricle) to your lungs, and through the aortic valve (for the left ventricle) to the rest of your body.

As the signal passes, the walls of the ventricles relax and await the next signal.

This process continues over and over as the atria refill with blood and other electrical signals come from the SA node.

Chapter 2

Cardiovascular Disorders Statistics

Chapter Contents

Section 2.1

Heart Disease Statistics

From "Heart Disease Facts," by the Centers for Disease
Control and Prevention (CDC, www.cdc.gov), February 12, 2009.

- Heart disease is the leading cause of death for both women and men in the United States.[1]

- In 2005, 652,091 people died of heart disease (50.5% of them women). This was 27.1% of all U.S. deaths. The age-adjusted death rate was 222 per 100,000 population.[1]

- Heart disease is the leading cause of death for American Indians and Alaska Natives, blacks, Hispanics, and whites. For Asians and Pacific Islanders, cancer is the leading cause of death (accounting for 27.5% of all deaths); heart disease is a close second (25.0%).[2]

- Heart disease crude death rates per 100,000 population for the five largest U.S. racial/ethnic groups are as follows: Hispanics, 69.2; Asians and Pacific Islanders, 73; American Indians, 82.5; blacks, 189.8; and whites, 235.5.[2]

- In 2005, the age-adjusted death rates for diseases of the heart was 211.1 deaths per 100,000 for all Americans. The age-adjusted death rate for whites was 207.8, and 271.3 for African Americans. Age adjusted rates are used to compare populations with differing age distributions.[2]

- By state, age-adjusted death rates per 100,000 for diseases of the heart ranged from 141.1 (Minnesota) to 306.8 (Mississippi) in 2005.[1]

- Coronary heart disease is the principal type of heart disease. In 2005, 445,687 people that died from coronary heart disease. That is about 68.3% of all heart disease deaths.[5]

- It is estimated that about 47% of cardiac deaths occur before emergency services or transport to a hospital.[4]

- In 2009, heart disease is projected to cost more than $304.6 billion, including health care services, medications, and lost productivity.[5]

- Worldwide, coronary heart disease killed more than 7.6 million people in 2005.[6]

- Risk factors for heart disease among adults (for years 2003–2004 unless noted, age-adjusted) include the following:[3]

  - Percentage of persons aged 20 years and older with hypertension or taking hypertension medications: 32.1%.

  - Percentage of persons aged 20 years and older with high blood cholesterol: 16.9%.

  - Percentage of persons aged 20 years and older with physician-diagnosed diabetes: 10.0%.

  - Percentage of persons aged 20 years and older who are obese: 32.0%.

  - Percentage of adults aged 18 years and older who are current cigarette smokers (2004–2006): 18.4%.

  - Percentage of adults aged 18 years and older who engage in no leisure-time physical activity (2006): 39.5%.

- In 2003, approximately 37% of adults reported having two or more of six risk factors for heart disease and stroke (high blood pressure, high cholesterol, diabetes, current smoking, physical inactivity, and obesity).[7]

- Timely access to emergency cardiac care and survival is partly dependent on early recognition of heart attack symptoms and immediate action by calling emergency services. In a 2005 survey, most persons (92%) recognized chest pain as a heart attack symptom, but only 27% correctly classified all symptoms and knew to call 911 when someone was having a heart attack.[8]

- Studies among people with heart disease have shown that lowering high blood cholesterol and high blood pressure can reduce the risk of dying of heart disease, having a nonfatal heart attack, and needing heart bypass surgery or angioplasty.

- Studies among people without heart disease have shown that lowering high blood cholesterol and high blood pressure can reduce the risk of developing heart disease.

References

1. Kung HC, Hoyert DL, Xu J, Murphy SL. Deaths: final data for 2005. National Vital Statistics Reports. 2008;56(10).

2. CDC. Deaths: leading causes for 2004. National Vital Statistics Reports. 2007;56(5).

3. CDC. Health, United States, 2007 with chartbook on trends in the health of Americans. Hyattsville; National Center for Health Statistics: 2007.

4. Zheng ZJ, Croft JB, Giles WH, Ayala C, Greenlund K, Keenan NL, Neff L, Wattigney WA, Mensah GA. State specific mortality from sudden cardiac death: United States, 1999. *MMWR.* 2002;51:123–126.

5. American Heart Association. *Heart Disease and Stroke Statistics—2009 Update.* Dallas; AHA:2009. Statistics Committee and Stroke Statistics Subcommittee. *Circulation.* 2008 Dec 15.

6. World Health Organization. The Global Burden of Disease: 2004 Update. Geneva; WHO:2008.

7. Hayes DK, Greenlund KJ, Denny CH, Keenan NL, Croft JB. Disparities in multiple risk factors for heart disease and stroke, 2003. *MMWR.* 2005;54:113–116.

8. Fang J, Kennan NL, Dai S, Denny C. Disparities in adult awareness of heart attack warning signs and symptoms—14 states, 2005. *MMWR.* 2008:57(7):175–179.

Section 2.2

Stroke Statistics

From "Stroke Facts," by the Centers for Disease Control and Prevention (CDC, www.cdc.gov), February 12, 2009.

- Stroke is the third leading cause of death in the United States. Over 143,579 people die each year from stroke in the United States.

- Stroke is a leading cause of serious long-term disability.

- About 795,000 strokes occur in the United States each year. About 610,000 of these are first or new strokes. About 185,000 occur in people who have already had a stroke before.

- Nearly three quarters of all strokes occur in people over the age of 65. The risk of having a stroke more than doubles each decade after the age of 55.

- Strokes can—and do—occur at **any** age. Nearly one quarter of strokes occur in people under the age of 65.

- Stroke death rates are higher for African Americans than for whites, even at younger ages.

- According to the American Heart Association, stroke will cost almost $68.9 billion in both direct and indirect costs in 2009. (American Heart Association. *Heart Disease and Stroke Statistics—2009 Update*. American Heart Association; 2009)

- It has been noted for several decades that the southeastern United States has the highest stroke mortality rates in the country. It is not completely clear what factors might contribute to the higher incidence of and mortality from stroke in this region.

Chapter 3

Overview of Cardiovascular Disorder Risk Factors

What Are Heart Disease Risk Factors?

Heart disease risk factors are conditions or habits that raise your risk for coronary heart disease (CHD; also called coronary artery disease) and heart attack. These risk factors also increase the chance that existing heart disease will worsen.

CHD is a condition in which a fatty material called plaque builds up on the inner walls of the coronary arteries.

These arteries carry oxygen-rich blood to your heart muscle. Plaque narrows the arteries and reduces blood flow to your heart muscle. This can cause chest pain, especially when you're active. Eventually, an area of plaque can rupture, causing a blood clot to form on the plaque's surface.

If the clot becomes large enough, it can mostly or completely block the flow of oxygen-rich blood to the part of the heart muscle fed by the artery. This causes a heart attack.

Overview

There are a number of known heart disease risk factors. You can control some risk factors, and others you can't. Risk factors you can control include the following:

Excerpted from "Heart Disease Risk Factors," by the National Heart, Lung, and Blood Institute (NHLBI, www.nhlbi.nih.gov), part of the National Institutes of Health, March 2009.

19

- High blood cholesterol and high triglyceride levels
- High blood pressure
- Diabetes and prediabetes
- Overweight and obesity
- Smoking
- Lack of physical activity
- Unhealthy diet
- Stress

The risk factors you can't control are age, gender, and family history.

Many people have at least one heart disease risk factor. Your risk for heart disease and heart attack increases with the number of risk factors you have and their severity. Also, some risk factors, such as smoking and diabetes, put you at greater risk for heart disease and heart attack than others.

Many heart disease risk factors start during childhood. This occurs even more now because many children are overweight and don't get enough physical activity. Some heart disease risk factors can even develop within the first 10 years of life.

Researchers continue to study and learn more about heart disease risk factors.

Outlook

Heart disease is the number-one killer of both women and men in the United States. Following a healthy lifestyle can help you and your children prevent or control many heart disease risk factors.

Because many lifestyle habits begin during childhood, parents and families should encourage their children to make heart-healthy choices. For example, if you maintain a healthy weight, follow a healthy diet, do physical activity regularly, and don't smoke, you can reduce your heart disease risk.

On average, people who have a low risk for heart disease live up to 10 years longer than people at high risk for heart disease.

If you already have heart disease, lifestyle changes can help you control your risk factors. This may prevent heart disease from worsening. Even if you're in your seventies or eighties, a healthy lifestyle can lower your risk of dying from heart disease by nearly two thirds.

If lifestyle changes aren't enough, your doctor may recommend other treatments to help control your risk factors.

Your doctor can help you find out whether you have heart disease risk factors. He or she also can help you create a plan for lowering your risk for heart disease, heart attack, and other heart problems. If you have children, talk to their doctor about their heart health and whether they have heart disease risk factors.

Heart Disease Risk Factors

High Blood Cholesterol and High Triglyceride Levels

Cholesterol: High blood cholesterol is a condition in which there's too much cholesterol—a waxy, fat-like substance—in your blood. The higher your blood cholesterol level, the greater your risk for heart disease and heart attack.

Cholesterol travels in the bloodstream in small packages called lipoproteins. Two major kinds of lipoproteins carry cholesterol throughout your body:

- Low-density lipoproteins (LDL): LDL cholesterol is sometimes called "bad" cholesterol. This is because it carries cholesterol to tissues, including your heart arteries. The higher the level of LDL cholesterol in your blood, the greater your risk for heart disease.

- High-density lipoproteins (HDL): HDL cholesterol is sometimes called "good" cholesterol. This is because it helps remove cholesterol from your arteries. A low HDL cholesterol level raises your risk for heart disease.

A number of factors affect your blood cholesterol levels. For example, after menopause, women's LDL cholesterol levels tend to rise and their HDL cholesterol levels tends to fall. Other factors, such as age, gender, and diet, also affect your cholesterol levels.

Healthy levels of both LDL and HDL cholesterol will prevent plaque from building up in your arteries. Routine blood tests can show whether your blood cholesterol levels are healthy. Talk to your doctor about having your cholesterol tested and what the results mean.

Children also can have high blood cholesterol, especially if they're overweight. Talk to your child's doctor about testing your child's cholesterol levels.

Triglycerides: Triglycerides are another type of fat found in the blood. Some studies suggest that a high level of triglycerides in the blood also may raise the risk for heart disease, particularly in women.

High Blood Pressure

"Blood pressure" is the force of blood pushing against the walls of your arteries as your heart pumps out blood. If this pressure rises and stays high over time, it can damage your heart and lead to plaque buildup.

Often, high blood pressure (HBP) has no signs or symptoms. However, the condition can be detected using a simple test that involves placing a blood pressure cuff around your arm.

Most adults should have their blood pressure checked at least once a year. Talk to your doctor about how often you should have your blood pressure checked. If you have HBP, you will likely need to have your blood pressure checked more often.

Children also can develop HBP, especially if they're overweight. Your child's doctor should check your child's blood pressure at each routine checkup.

Blood pressure numbers consist of systolic and diastolic pressures. Systolic blood pressure is the pressure when your heart beats. Diastolic blood pressure is the pressure when your heart is at rest between beats.

You will most often see blood pressure numbers written with the systolic number above or before the diastolic number, such as 120/80 mmHg. (The mmHg is millimeters of mercury—the units used to measure blood pressure.)

All levels above 120/80 mmHg raise your risk for heart disease. This risk grows as blood pressure levels rise. Only one of the two blood pressure numbers has to be above normal to put you at greater risk for heart disease and heart attack.

Blood pressure normally rises with age and body size. Newborns often have very low blood pressure numbers, while older teens have numbers similar to adults.

The ranges for normal blood pressure and HBP are generally lower for youth than for adults. These ranges are based on the average blood pressure numbers for age, gender, and height.

Your child should have routine blood pressure checks starting at 3 years of age. To find out whether a child has HBP, a doctor will compare the child's blood pressure numbers to average numbers for his or her age, height, and gender.

Both children and adults are more likely to develop HBP if they're overweight or have diabetes.

Diabetes and Prediabetes

Diabetes is a disease in which the body's blood sugar level is too high. The two types of diabetes are type 1 and type 2.

In type 1 diabetes, the body's blood sugar level is high because the body doesn't make enough insulin. Insulin is a hormone that helps move blood sugar into cells, where it's used for fuel. In type 2 diabetes, the body's blood sugar level is high mainly because the body doesn't use its insulin properly.

Over time, a high blood sugar level can lead to increased plaque buildup in your arteries. Having diabetes doubles your risk for heart disease.

Prediabetes is a condition in which your blood sugar level is higher than normal, but not as high as it is in diabetes. If you have prediabetes and don't take steps to manage it, you're likely to develop type 2 diabetes within 10 years. You're also at higher risk for heart disease.

Being overweight or obese raises your risk for type 2 diabetes. With modest weight loss and moderate physical activity, people who have prediabetes may be able to delay or prevent type 2 diabetes. They also may be able to lower their risk for heart disease and heart attack. Weight loss and physical activity also can help control diabetes.

Even children can develop type 2 diabetes. Most children who have type 2 diabetes are overweight.

Type 2 diabetes develops over time and sometimes has no symptoms. Go to your doctor or local clinic to have your blood sugar levels tested regularly to check for diabetes and prediabetes.

Overweight and Obesity

The terms "overweight" and "obesity" refer to a person's overall body weight and whether it's too high. Overweight is having extra body weight from muscle, bone, fat, and/or water. Obesity is having a high amount of extra body fat.

The most commonly used measure of overweight and obesity is body mass index (BMI). BMI is calculated from your height and weight.

In adults, a BMI of 18.5 to 24.9 is considered normal. A BMI of 25 to 29.9 is considered overweight. A BMI of 30 or above is considered obese. Over two thirds of American adults are overweight, and almost one third of these adults are obese.

Overweight is defined differently for children and teens than it is for adults. Children are still growing, and boys and girls mature at different rates. Thus, BMIs for children and teens compare their heights and weights against growth charts that take age and gender into account. This is called BMI-for-age percentile.

Being overweight or obese can raise your risk for heart disease and heart attack. This is mainly because overweight and obesity are linked to other heart disease risk factors, such as high blood cholesterol and triglyceride levels, high blood pressure, and diabetes.

Smoking

Smoking tobacco or long-term exposure to secondhand smoke raises your risk for heart disease and heart attack.

Smoking triggers a buildup of plaque in your arteries. Smoking also increases the risk of blood clots forming in your arteries. Blood clots can block plaque-narrowed arteries and cause a heart attack.

Some research shows that smoking raises your risk for heart disease in part by lowering HDL cholesterol levels.

The more you smoke, the greater your risk for heart attack. Studies show that if you quit smoking, you cut your risk for heart attack in half within a year. The benefits of quitting smoking occur no matter how long or how much you've smoked.

Most people who smoke start when they're teens. Parents can help prevent their children from smoking by not smoking themselves. Talk to your child about the health dangers of smoking and ways to overcome peer pressure to smoke.

Lack of Physical Activity

Inactive people are nearly twice as likely to develop heart disease as those who are active. A lack of physical activity can worsen other heart disease risk factors, such as high blood cholesterol and high triglyceride levels, high blood pressure, diabetes and prediabetes, and overweight and obesity.

It's important for children and adults to make physical activity part of their daily routines. One reason many Americans aren't active enough is because of hours spent in front of TVs and computers doing work, schoolwork, and leisure activities.

Some experts advise that children and youth reduce screen time because it limits time for physical activity. They recommend that children aged 2 and older should spend no more than 2 hours a day watching television or using a computer (except for school work).

Being physically active is one of the most important things you can do to keep your heart healthy. The good news is that even modest amounts of physical activity are good for your health. The more active you are, the more you will benefit.

Unhealthy Diet

An unhealthy diet can raise your risk for heart disease. For example, foods that are high in saturated and trans fats and cholesterol raise LDL cholesterol. Thus, you should try to limit these foods.

Saturated fats are found in some meats, dairy products, chocolate, baked goods, and deep-fried and processed foods. Trans fats are found in some fried and processed foods. Cholesterol is found in eggs, many meats, dairy products, commercial baked goods, and certain types of shellfish.

It's also important to limit foods that are high in sodium (salt) and added sugars. A high-salt diet can raise your risk for high blood pressure.

Added sugars will give you extra calories without nutrients like vitamins and minerals. This can cause you to gain weight, which raises your risk for heart disease. Added sugars are found in many desserts, canned fruits packed in syrup, fruit drinks, and nondiet sodas.

You also should try to limit how much alcohol you drink. Too much alcohol will raise your blood pressure. It also will add calories, which can cause weight gain.

Stress

Stress and anxiety may contribute to the development of heart disease. Stress and anxiety also can trigger your arteries to tighten. This can raise your blood pressure and your risk for heart attack.

The most commonly reported trigger for a heart attack is an emotionally upsetting event, especially one involving anger. Stress also may indirectly raise your risk for heart disease if it makes you more likely to smoke or overeat foods high in fat and sugar.

Age

As you get older, your risk for heart disease and heart attack rises. This is in part due to the slow buildup of plaque inside your heart arteries, which can start during childhood.

In men, the risk for heart disease increases after age 45. In women, the risk increases after age 55.

Most people have some plaque buildup in their heart arteries by the time they're in their seventies. However, only about 25 percent of those people have chest pain, heart attacks, or other signs of heart disease.

Gender

Before age 55, women have a lower risk for heart disease than men. After age 55, however, the risk for heart disease increases similarly in both women and men. This is because before menopause, estrogen provides some protection against heart disease for women.

Some risk factors may affect heart disease risk differently in women than in men. For example, diabetes raises the risk for heart disease more in women.

Family History

Family history plays a role in heart disease risk. Your risk increases if your father or brother was diagnosed with heart disease before 55 years of age, or if your mother or sister was diagnosed with the disease before 65 years of age.

However, having a family history of heart disease doesn't mean that you will have it, too. This is especially true if your affected family member smoked or had other heart disease risk factors that were not well treated.

Making lifestyle changes and taking medicines to treat other risk factors often can lessen genetic influences and stop or slow the progress of heart disease.

Chapter 4

High Blood Pressure

High blood pressure (HBP) is a serious condition that can lead to coronary heart disease, heart failure, stroke, kidney failure, and other health problems.

"Blood pressure" is the force of blood pushing against the walls of the arteries as the heart pumps out blood. If this pressure rises and stays high over time, it can damage the body in many ways.

Overview

About one in three adults in the United States has HBP. HBP itself usually has no symptoms. You can have it for years without knowing it. During this time, though, it can damage the heart, blood vessels, kidneys, and other parts of your body.

This is why knowing your blood pressure numbers is important, even when you're feeling fine. If your blood pressure is normal, you can work with your health care team to keep it that way. If your blood pressure is too high, you need treatment to prevent damage to your body's organs.

Blood Pressure Numbers

Blood pressure numbers include systolic and diastolic pressures. Systolic blood pressure is the pressure when the heart beats while

Excerpted from text by the National Heart, Lung, and Blood Institute (NHLBI, www.nhlbi.nih.gov), part of the National Institutes of Health, November 2008.

pumping blood. Diastolic blood pressure is the pressure when the heart is at rest between beats.

You will most often see blood pressure numbers written with the systolic number above or before the diastolic, such as 120/80 mmHg. (The mmHg is millimeters of mercury—the units used to measure blood pressure.)

Table 4.1 shows normal numbers for adults. It also shows which numbers put you at greater risk for health problems. Blood pressure tends to goes up and down, even in people who have normal blood pressure. If your numbers stay above normal most of the time, you're at risk.

The blood pressure ranges are measured in millimeters of mercury. The ranges in Table 4.1 apply to most adults (aged 18 and older) who don't have short-term serious illnesses.

All levels above 120/80 mmHg raise your risk, and the risk grows as blood pressure levels rise. "Prehypertension" means you're likely to end up with HBP, unless you take steps to prevent it.

If you're being treated for HBP and have repeat readings in the normal range, your blood pressure is under control. However, you still have the condition. You should see your doctor and stay on treatment to keep you blood pressure under control.

Your systolic and diastolic numbers may not be in the same blood pressure category. In this case, the more severe category is the one you're in. For example, if your systolic number is 160 and your diastolic number is 80, you have stage 2 HBP. If your systolic number is 120 and your diastolic number is 95, you have stage 1 HBP.

If you have diabetes or chronic kidney disease, HBP is defined as 130/80 mmHg or higher. HBP numbers also differ for children and teens.

Outlook

Blood pressure tends to rise with age. Following a healthy lifestyle helps some people delay or prevent this rise in blood pressure.

People who have HBP can take steps to control it and reduce their risks for related health problems. Key steps include following a healthy lifestyle, having ongoing medical care, and following the treatment plan that your doctor prescribes.

Other Names for High Blood Pressure

High blood pressure (HBP) also is called hypertension.

Table 4.1. Categories for Blood Pressure Levels in Adults

Category	Systolic (top number)		Diastolic (bottom number)
Normal	Less than 120	And	Less than 80
Prehypertension	120–139	Or	80–89
High blood pressure			
Stage 1	140–159	Or	90–99
Stage 2	160 or higher	Or	100 or higher

When HBP has no known cause, it may be called essential hypertension, primary hypertension, or idiopathic hypertension.

When another condition causes HBP, it's sometimes called secondary high blood pressure or secondary hypertension.

In some cases of HBP, only the systolic blood pressure number is high. This condition is called isolated systolic hypertension (ISH). Many older adults have this condition. ISH can cause as much harm as HBP in which both numbers are too high.

Causes of High Blood Pressure

Blood pressure tends to rise with age, unless you take steps to prevent or control it.

Certain medical problems, such as chronic kidney disease, thyroid disease, and sleep apnea, may cause blood pressure to rise. Certain medicines, such as asthma medicines (for example, corticosteroids) and cold-relief products, also may raise blood pressure.

In some women, blood pressure can go up if they use birth control pills, become pregnant, or take hormone replacement therapy.

Women taking birth control pills usually have a small rise in both systolic and diastolic blood pressures. If you already have high blood pressure (HBP) and want to use birth control pills, make sure your doctor knows about your HBP. Talk to him or her about how often you should have your blood pressure checked and how to control it while taking the pill.

Taking hormones to reduce the symptoms of menopause can cause a small rise in systolic blood pressure. If you already have HBP and want to start using hormones, talk to your doctor about the risks and benefits. If you decide to take hormones, find out how to control your blood pressure and how often you should have it checked.

Children younger than 10 years who have HBP often have another condition that's causing it (such as kidney disease). Treating the underlying condition may resolve the HBP.

The older a child is when HBP is diagnosed, the more likely he or she is to have essential hypertension. This means that doctors don't know what's causing the HBP.

Risk for High Blood Pressure

Certain traits, conditions, or habits are known to raise the risk for HBP. These conditions are called risk factors. This portion of text describes the major risk factors for HBP.

Older Age

Blood pressure tends to rise with age. If you're a male older than 45 or a female older than 55, your risk for HBP is higher. Over half of all Americans aged 60 and older have HBP.

Isolated systolic hypertension (ISH) is the most common form of HBP in older adults. ISH occurs when only systolic blood pressure (the top number) is high. About two out of three people over age 60 who have HBP have ISH.

HBP doesn't have to be a routine part of aging. You can take steps to keep your blood pressure at a normal level.

Race/Ethnicity

HBP can affect anyone. However, it occurs more often in African American adults than in Caucasian or Hispanic American adults. In relation to these groups, the following is true of African Americans:

- Tend to get HBP earlier in life
- Often have more severe HBP
- Are more likely to be aware that they have HBP and to get treatment
- Are less likely than Caucasians and about as likely as Hispanic Americans to achieve target control levels with HBP treatment
- Have higher rates than Caucasians of premature death from HBP-related complications, such as coronary heart disease, stroke, and kidney failure

HBP risks vary among different groups of Hispanic-American adults. For instance, Puerto Rican-American adults have higher rates of HBP-related death than all other Hispanic groups and Caucasians. But, Cuban Americans have lower rates than Caucasians.

Overweight or Obesity

You're more likely to develop prehypertension or HBP if you're overweight or obese. Overweight is having extra body weight from muscle, bone, fat, and/or water. Obesity is having a high amount of extra body fat.

Gender

Fewer adult women than men have HBP. But, younger women (aged 18–59) are more likely than men to be aware of and get treatment for HBP.

Women aged 60 and older are as likely as men to be aware of and treated for HBP. However, among treated women aged 60 and older, blood pressure control is lower than it is in men in the same age group.

Unhealthy Lifestyle Habits

A number of lifestyle habits can raise your risk for HBP, including the following:

- Eating too much sodium (salt)
- Drinking too much alcohol
- Not getting enough potassium in your diet
- Not doing enough physical activity
- Smoking

Other Risk Factors

A family history of HBP raises your risk for the condition. Long-lasting stress also can put you at risk for HBP.

You're also more likely to develop HBP if you have prehypertension. Prehypertension means that your blood pressure is in the 120–139/80–89 mmHg range.

Signs and Symptoms of High Blood Pressure

High blood pressure (HBP) itself usually has no symptoms. Rarely, headaches may occur.

You can have HBP for years without knowing it. During this time, HBP can damage the heart, blood vessels, kidneys, and other parts of the body.

Some people only learn that they have HBP after the damage has caused problems, such as coronary heart disease, stroke, or kidney failure.

Knowing your blood pressure numbers is important, even when you're feeling fine. If your blood pressure is normal, you can work with your health care team to keep it that way. If your numbers are too high, you can take steps to lower them and control your blood pressure. This helps reduce your risk for complications.

Complications of High Blood Pressure

When blood pressure stays high over time, it can damage the body. HBP can cause the following to occur:

- The heart can get larger or weaker, which may lead to heart failure. Heart failure is a condition in which the heart can't pump enough blood throughout the body.

- Aneurysms may form in blood vessels. An aneurysm is an abnormal bulge or "ballooning" in the wall of an artery. Common spots for aneurysms are the main artery that carries blood from the heart to the body; the arteries in the brain, legs, and intestines; and the artery leading to the spleen.

- Blood vessels in the kidney may narrow. This may cause kidney failure.

- Arteries throughout the body may narrow in some places, which limits blood flow (especially to the heart, brain, kidneys, and legs). This can cause a heart attack, stroke, kidney failure, or amputation of part of the leg.

- Blood vessels in the eyes may burst or bleed. This may lead to vision changes or blindness.

Diagnosing High Blood Pressure

Your doctor will diagnose high blood pressure (HBP) using the results of blood pressure tests. These tests will be done several times to make sure the results are correct. If your numbers are high, your doctor may have you return for more tests to check your blood pressure over time.

If your blood pressure is 140/90 mmHg or higher over time, your doctor will likely diagnose you with HBP. If you have diabetes or chronic kidney disease, a blood pressure of 130/80 mmHg or higher is considered HBP.

The HBP ranges in children are different.

How Is Blood Pressure Tested?

A blood pressure test is easy and painless. This test is done at a doctor's office or clinic.

To prepare for the test, take the following steps:

- Don't drink coffee or smoke cigarettes for 30 minutes prior to the test. These actions may cause a short-term rise in your blood pressure.

- Go to the bathroom before the test. Having a full bladder can change your blood pressure reading.

- Sit for 5 minutes before the test. Movement can cause short-term rises in blood pressure.

- To measure your blood pressure, your doctor or nurse will use some type of a gauge, a stethoscope (or electronic sensor), and a blood pressure cuff.

- Most often, you will sit or lie down with the cuff around your arm as your doctor or nurse checks your blood pressure. If he or she doesn't tell you what your blood pressure numbers are, you should ask.

What Does a Diagnosis of High Blood Pressure Mean?

If you're diagnosed with HBP, you will need treatment. You also will need to have your blood pressure tested again to see how treatment affects it.

Once your blood pressure is under control, you will need to stay on treatment. "Under control" means that your blood pressure numbers are normal. You also will need regular blood pressure tests. Your doctor can tell you how often you should be tested.

The sooner you find out about HBP and treat it, the better your chances to avoid problems like heart attack, stroke, and kidney failure.

Treating High Blood Pressure

High blood pressure (HBP) is treated with lifestyle changes and medicines.

Most people who have HBP will need lifelong treatment.

Sticking to your treatment plan is important. It can prevent or delay the problems linked to HBP and help you live and stay active longer.

Goals of Treatment

The treatment goal for most adults is to get and keep blood pressure below 140/90 mmHg. For adults who have diabetes or chronic kidney disease, the goal is to get and keep blood pressure below 130/80 mmHg.

Lifestyle Changes

Healthy habits can help you control HBP. Healthy habits include the following:

- Following a healthy eating plan
- Doing enough physical activity
- Maintaining a healthy weight
- Quitting smoking
- Managing your stress and learning to cope with stress

If you combine these measures, you can achieve even better results than taking single steps. Making lifestyle changes can be hard. Start by making one healthy lifestyle change and then adopt others.

Some people can control their blood pressures with lifestyle changes alone, but many people can't. Keep in mind that the main goal is blood pressure control. If your doctor prescribes medicines as a part of your treatment plan, keep up your healthy habits. This will help you better control your blood pressure.

High Blood Pressure and Pregnancy

Many pregnant women who have HBP have healthy babies. However, HBP can cause problems for both the mother and the fetus. It can harm the mother's kidneys and other organs. It also can cause the baby to be born early and with a low birth weight.

If you're thinking about having a baby and you have HBP, talk to your health care team. You can take steps to control your blood pressure before and while you're pregnant.

Some women get HBP for the first time while they're pregnant. In the most serious cases, the mother has a condition called preeclampsia. This condition can threaten the lives of both the mother and the unborn child. You will need special care to reduce your risks. With such care, most women and babies have good outcomes.

Chapter 5

High Blood Cholesterol

To understand high blood cholesterol, it is important to know more about cholesterol.

- Cholesterol is a waxy, fat-like substance that is found in all cells of the body. Your body needs some cholesterol to work the right way. Your body makes all the cholesterol it needs.

- Cholesterol is also found in some of the foods you eat.

- Your body uses cholesterol to make hormones, vitamin D, and substances that help you digest foods.

Blood is watery, and cholesterol is fatty. Just like oil and water, the two do not mix. To travel in the bloodstream, cholesterol is carried in small packages called lipoproteins. The small packages are made of fat (lipid) on the inside and proteins on the outside. Two kinds of lipoproteins carry cholesterol throughout your body. It is important to have healthy levels of both:

- Low-density lipoprotein (LDL) cholesterol is sometimes called bad cholesterol.

  - High LDL cholesterol leads to a buildup of cholesterol in arteries. The higher the LDL level in your blood, the greater chance you have of getting heart disease.

Excerpted from text by the National Heart, Lung, and Blood Institute (NHLBI, www.nhlbi.nih.gov), part of the National Institutes of Health, September 2008.

- High-density lipoprotein (HDL) cholesterol is sometimes called good cholesterol.

  - HDL carries cholesterol from other parts of your body back to your liver. The liver removes the cholesterol from your body. The higher your HDL cholesterol level, the lower your chance of getting heart disease.

Understanding High Blood Cholesterol

Too much cholesterol in the blood, or high blood cholesterol, can be serious. People with high blood cholesterol have a greater chance of getting heart disease. High blood cholesterol on its own does not cause symptoms, so many people are unaware that their cholesterol level is too high.

Cholesterol can build up in the walls of your arteries (blood vessels that carry blood from the heart to other parts of the body). This buildup of cholesterol is called plaque. Over time, plaque can cause narrowing of the arteries. This is called atherosclerosis or hardening of the arteries.

Special arteries, called coronary arteries, bring blood to the heart. Narrowing of your coronary arteries due to plaque can stop or slow down the flow of blood to your heart. When the arteries narrow, the amount of oxygen-rich blood is decreased. This is called coronary heart disease (CHD). Large plaque areas can lead to chest pain called angina. Angina happens when the heart does not receive enough oxygen-rich blood. Angina is a common symptom of CHD.

Some plaques have a thin covering and can burst (rupture), releasing cholesterol and fat into the bloodstream. The release of cholesterol and fat may cause your blood to clot. A clot can block the flow of blood. This blockage can cause angina or a heart attack.

Lowering your cholesterol level decreases your chance for having a plaque burst and cause a heart attack. Lowering cholesterol may also slow down, reduce, or even stop plaque from building up.

Plaque and resulting health problems can also occur in arteries elsewhere in the body.

Other Names for High Blood Cholesterol

- Hypercholesterolemia
- Hyperlipidemia

Causes of High Blood Cholesterol

A variety of things can affect the cholesterol levels in your blood. Some of these things you can control and others you cannot.

You can control:

- **What you eat:** Certain foods have types of fat that raise your cholesterol level.

  - Saturated fat raises your low-density lipoprotein (LDL) cholesterol level more than anything else in your diet.

  - Trans fatty acids (trans fats) are made when vegetable oil is hydrogenated to harden it. Trans fatty acids also raise cholesterol levels.

  - Cholesterol is found in foods that come from animal sources, for example, egg yolks, meat, and cheese.

- **Your weight:** Being overweight tends to increase your LDL level, lower your high-density lipoprotein (HDL) level, and increase your total cholesterol level.

- **Your activity:** Lack of regular exercise can lead to weight gain, which could raise your LDL cholesterol level. Regular exercise can help you lose weight and lower your LDL level. It can also help you raise your HDL level.

You cannot control:

- **Heredity:** High blood cholesterol can run in families. An inherited genetic condition (familial hypercholesterolemia) results in very high LDL cholesterol levels. It begins at birth, and may result in a heart attack at an early age.

- **Age and sex:** Starting at puberty, men have lower levels of HDL than women. As women and men get older, their LDL cholesterol levels rise. Younger women have lower LDL cholesterol levels than men, but after age 55, women have higher levels than men.

Signs and Symptoms of High Blood Cholesterol

There are usually no signs or symptoms of high blood cholesterol. Many people don't know that their cholesterol level is too high.

Everyone age 20 and older should have their cholesterol levels checked at least once every 5 years. You and your doctor can discuss how often you should be tested.

Diagnosing High Blood Cholesterol

High blood cholesterol is diagnosed by checking levels of cholesterol in your blood. It is best to have a blood test called a lipoprotein profile to measure your cholesterol levels. You will need to not eat or drink anything (fast) for 9 to 12 hours before taking the test.

The lipoprotein profile will give information about the following:

- Total cholesterol

- Low-density lipoprotein (LDL) bad cholesterol, the main source of cholesterol buildup and blockage in the arteries

- High-density lipoprotein (HDL) good cholesterol, the good cholesterol that helps keep cholesterol from building up in arteries

- Triglycerides, another form of fat in your blood

If it is not possible to get a lipoprotein profile done, knowing your total cholesterol and HDL cholesterol can give you a general idea about your cholesterol levels. Testing for total and HDL cholesterol does not require fasting. If your total cholesterol is 200 mg/dL or more, or if your HDL is less than 40 mg/dL, you will need to have a lipoprotein profile done.

Cholesterol levels are measured in milligrams (mg) of cholesterol per deciliter (dL) of blood. See how your cholesterol numbers compares to Table 5.1.

Triglycerides can also raise your risk for heart disease. If you have levels that are borderline high (150–199 mg/dL) or high (200 mg/dL or more), you may need treatment. Things that can increase triglyceride levels include the following:

- Being overweight
- Physical inactivity
- Cigarette smoking
- Excessive alcohol use
- Very high carbohydrate diet
- Certain diseases and drugs
- Genetic disorders

Table 5.1. Understanding Cholesterol Levels

Total Cholesterol Level	Total Cholesterol Category
Less than 200 mg/dL	Desirable
200–239 mg/dL	Borderline high
240 mg/dL and above	High

LDL Cholesterol Level	LDL Cholesterol Category
Less than 100 mg/dL	Optimal
100–129 mg/dL	Near optimal/above optimal
130–159 mg/dL	Borderline high
160–189 mg/dL	High
190 mg/dL and above	Very high

HDL Cholesterol Level	HDL Cholesterol Category
Less than 40 mg/dL	A major risk factor for heart disease
40–59 mg/dL	The higher, the better
60 mg/dL and above	Considered protective against heart disease

Treating High Blood Cholesterol

The main goal of cholesterol-lowering treatment is to lower your low-density lipoprotein (LDL) level enough to reduce your risk for having a heart attack or diseases caused by hardening of the arteries. In general, the higher your LDL level and the more risk factors you have, the greater your chances of developing heart disease or having a heart attack. (A risk factor is a condition that increases your chance of getting a disease.)

Some people are at high risk for heart attack because they already have heart disease. Other people are at high risk for developing heart disease because they have diabetes or a combination of risk factors for heart disease. Follow the steps in the following text to find out your risk for getting heart disease. Talk with your doctor about lowering your risk.

Check the list to see how many of the risk factors you have. These are the risk factors that affect your LDL goal:

- Cigarette smoking

- High blood pressure (140/90 mg/dL or higher), or if you are on blood pressure medicine

- Low high-density lipoprotein (HDL) cholesterol (less than 40 mg/dL)

- Family history of early heart disease (heart disease in father or brother before age 55; heart disease in mother or sister before age 65)

- Age (men 45 years or older; women 55 years or older)

If you have two or more of the risk factors in the list above, use the NHLBI 10-Year Risk Calculator [http://hp2010.nhlbihin.net/atpiii/calculator.asp?usertype=pub] to find your risk score. Risk scores refer to the chance of having a heart attack in the next 10 years, given as a percentage.

Use your medical history, number of risk factors, and risk score to find your risk for developing heart disease or having a heart attack according to Table 5.2.

Table 5.2. Cholesterol Goals

If You Have	You Are in Category	And Your LDL Goal Is
Heart disease, diabetes, or a risk score higher than 20%	I. High risk	Less than 100 mg/dL*
Two or more risk factors and a risk score 10–20%	II. Moderately high risk	Less than 130 mg/dL
Two or more risk factors and a risk score lower than 10%	III. Moderate risk	Less than 130 mg/dL
One or no risk factors	IV. Low to moderate risk	Less than 160 mg/dL

*Note: Some people in this category are at very high risk because they have just had a heart attack or because they have a combination of heart disease together with diabetes, risk factors that are severe, or metabolic syndrome. If you are at very high risk, your doctor may set your LDL goal even lower, to less than 70 mg/dL. Your doctor may also set the LDL goal at this lower level if you have heart disease alone.

After following the above steps, you should have an idea about your risk for getting heart disease or having a heart attack. There are two main ways to lower your cholesterol in order to lower your risk:

- Therapeutic Lifestyle Changes (TLC) includes a cholesterol-lowering diet (called the TLC Diet), physical activity, and weight management. TLC is for anyone whose LDL is above goal.

- Drug treatment may also be used. If cholesterol-lowering drugs are needed, they are used together with TLC treatment to help lower your LDL.

Your doctor will set your LDL goal. The higher your risk for heart disease, the lower your LDL goal will be.

Lowering Cholesterol with TLC

TLC is a set of lifestyle changes you can make to help lower your LDL cholesterol. The main parts of TLC are the following:

- **The TLC Diet:** This diet recommends you do the following:

  - Limit the amount of saturated fat, trans fat, and cholesterol you eat.

  - Eat only enough calories to achieve or maintain a healthy weight.

  - Increase the soluble fiber in your diet. For example, oatmeal, kidney beans, and apples are good sources of soluble fiber.

  - Add cholesterol-lowering foods, such as margarines that contain plant sterol or stanol esters that can help lower cholesterol.

- **Weight management:** Losing weight if you are overweight can help lower LDL. Weight management is especially important for those with a group of risk factors that includes raised triglyceride and/or reduced HDL levels and being overweight with a large waist measurement (40 inches or more for men and 35 inches or more for women). This is called metabolic syndrome and it raises your risk for getting heart disease.

- **Physical activity:** Regular physical activity is recommended for everyone. It can help raise HDL levels and lower LDL levels, and is especially important for those with raised triglyceride and/or reduced HDL levels who are overweight with a large waist measurement. Aim for at least 30 minutes of moderate-intensity activity, such as brisk walking, on most, and preferably all, days of the week.

Cholesterol-Lowering Medicines

Along with suggesting that you change the way you eat and exercise regularly, your doctor may prescribe medicines to help lower your cholesterol. Even if you begin drug treatment, you will need to continue TLC. TLC lowers your risk not only by lowering LDL but also in other ways and helps keep down the dose of LDL-lowering medication you have to take. Drug treatment controls but does not "cure" high blood cholesterol. Therefore, you must continue taking your medicine to keep your cholesterol level in the recommended range.

The five major types of cholesterol-lowering medicines include the following:

- Statins
  - Very effective in lowering LDL (bad) cholesterol levels
  - Safe for most people
  - Rare side effects to watch for are muscle and liver problems
- Bile acid sequestrants
  - Help lower LDL cholesterol levels
  - Sometimes prescribed with statins
  - Not usually prescribed as the only medicine to lower cholesterol
- Nicotinic acid
  - Lowers LDL cholesterol and triglycerides and raises HDL (good) cholesterol
  - Should only be used under a doctor's supervision
- Fibrates
  - Lower triglycerides
  - May increase HDL (good) cholesterol levels
  - When used with a statin, may increase the chance of muscle problems
- Ezetimibe
  - Lowers LDL cholesterol
  - Acts within the intestine to block cholesterol absorption

When you are under treatment, you will be checked regularly to make sure your cholesterol level is controlled and check for other health problems.

You may take medicines for other health problems. It is important that you take **all** medicines as your doctor prescribes. The combination of medicines may lower your risk for heart disease or heart attack.

When trying to lower your cholesterol or keep it low, it is important to remember to follow your treatments for other conditions you may have, such as high blood pressure. Get help with quitting smoking and losing weight if they are risk factors for you.

Chapter 6

Conditions That Influence Cardiovascular Disorder Risk

Chapter Contents

Section 6.1

Depression and Heart Disease

You might think heart disease is linked only with physical activities—a lack of exercise, poor diet, smoking, and excessive drinking. While these habits do heighten the risk of high blood pressure, heart attacks, strokes, and other cardiovascular problems, your thoughts, attitudes, and emotions are just as important. They can not only accelerate the onset of heart disease, but also get in the way of taking positive steps to improve your health or that of a loved one.

Practicing Prevention

A healthy lifestyle can go a long way toward reducing the risk of heart disease or managing a diagnosed condition, even if you face a higher risk due to uncontrollable factors such as age, sex, or family history. But making changes in your daily life is not always easy. You may sense a loss of control over your life in having to give up favorite foods, make time for exercise in a busy schedule, or take regular medication.

It also takes personal discipline to ingrain these new habits into your lifestyle. Deviating from a prescribed diet or sneaking a cigarette when no one is looking may satisfy an immediate craving, but it won't achieve the long-term goal of improved health.

Coping with Life's Pressures

Heart disease has many other mind-body connections that you should consider. Prolonged stress due to the pressures at home, on the job, or from other sources can contribute to abnormally high blood pressure and circulation problems. As with many other diseases, the effects vary from person to person. Some people use stress as a motivator while others may "snap" at the slightest issue.

How you handle stress also influences how your cardiovascular system responds. Studies have shown that if stress makes you angry or irritable, you're more likely to have heart disease or a heart attack. In fact, the way you respond to stress may be a greater risk factor for heart problems than smoking, high blood pressure, and high cholesterol.

A Downward Spiral

Then there's depression, the persistent feeling of sadness and despair that can isolate you from the rest of the world. In its severest form, clinical depression, this condition can not only increase the risk of heart disease but also worsen an existing condition.

Research shows that while approximately 20 percent of us experience an episode of depression in our lifetimes, the figure climbs to 50 percent among people with heart disease. Long-term studies reveal that men and women diagnosed with clinical depression are more than twice as likely to develop coronary artery disease or suffer a heart attack. In addition, heart patients are three times as likely to be depressed at any given time than the population as a whole.

And happy people have healthier levels of fibrinogen and cortisol in their blood, making them less vulnerable to cardiovascular disease and other ailments.

Left untreated, depression can put you at substantially greater risk of suffering a heart attack or stroke. In fact, clinically depressed people are twice as likely to suffer a heart attack as long as 10 years after the initial depressive episode.

The Struggle to Rebound

Depression can also complicate the aftermath of a heart attack, stroke, or invasive procedure such as open-heart surgery. The immediate shock of coming so close to death is compounded by the prospect of a long recuperation, as well as the fear that another, potentially more serious event could occur without warning.

The result is often feelings of depression, anxiety, isolation, and diminished self-esteem. According to the National Institutes of Mental Health (NIMH), up to 65 percent of coronary heart disease patients with a history of heart attack experience various forms of depression.

Though such emotions are not unusual, they should be addressed as quickly as possible. Major depression can complicate the recovery process and actually worsen your condition. Prolonged depression in patients with cardiovascular disease has been shown to contribute to subsequent heart attacks and strokes.

What You Can Do

Although heart disease is a serious condition that requires constant monitoring, there are many things you can do to reduce your risk for cardiovascular problems and live a full, active life, even if you should suffer a heart attack.

- **Talk to your doctor.** No two people are alike, and some treatment or risk reduction strategies may be inappropriate or even harmful if you attempt to do too much too quickly.

- **Avoid trying to fix every problem at once, if possible.** Focus instead on changing one existing habit (e.g., eating habits, inactive lifestyle). Set a reasonable initial goal and work toward meeting it.

- **Don't ignore the symptoms of depression.** Feelings of sadness or emptiness, loss of interest in ordinary or pleasurable activities, reduced energy, and eating and sleep disorders are just a few of depression's many warning signs. If they persist for more than two weeks, discuss these issues with your heart doctor. It may be that a psychologist working in collaboration with your physician would be beneficial.

- **Identify the sources of stress in your life and look for ways to reduce and manage them.** Seeing a professional like a psychologist to learn to manage stress is helpful not only for preventing heart disease, but also for speeding recovery from heart attacks when used along with structured exercise programs and other intensive lifestyle changes.

- **Enlist the support of friends, family, and work associates.** Talk with them about your condition and what they can do to help. Social support is particularly critical for overcoming feelings of depression and isolation during recovery from a heart attack.

- **If you feel overwhelmed by the challenge of managing the behaviors associated with heart disease, consult a qualified psychologist.** He or she can help develop personal strategies for setting and achieving reasonable health improvement goals, as well as building on these successes to accomplish other more ambitious objectives. A psychologist can also help clarify the diagnosis of depression and work with the physician to devise a suitable treatment program.

The American Psychological Association Practice Directorate gratefully acknowledges the assistance of Sara Weiss, PhD, and Nancy Molitor, PhD, in developing this text.

Section 6.2

Diabetes, Heart Disease, and Stroke

Excerpted from text by the National Institute of Diabetes and Digestive and Kidney Diseases (NIDDK, www.niddk.nih.gov), part of the National Institutes of Health, December 2005.

Having diabetes or prediabetes puts you at increased risk for heart disease and stroke.

If you have already had a heart attack or a stroke, taking care of yourself can help prevent future health problems.

What is diabetes?

Diabetes is a disorder of metabolism—the way our bodies use digested food for energy. Most of the food we eat is broken down into glucose, the form of sugar in the blood. Glucose is the body's main source of fuel.

After digestion, glucose enters the bloodstream. Then glucose goes to cells throughout the body where it is used for energy. However, a hormone called insulin must be present to allow glucose to enter the cells. Insulin is a hormone produced by the pancreas, a large gland behind the stomach.

In people who do not have diabetes, the pancreas automatically produces the right amount of insulin to move glucose from blood into the cells. However, diabetes develops when the pancreas does not

51

make enough insulin, or the cells in the muscles, liver, and fat do not use insulin properly, or both. As a result, the amount of glucose in the blood increases while the cells are starved of energy.

Over time, high blood glucose levels damage nerves and blood vessels, leading to complications such as heart disease and stroke, the leading causes of death among people with diabetes. Uncontrolled diabetes can eventually lead to other health problems as well, such as vision loss, kidney failure, and amputations.

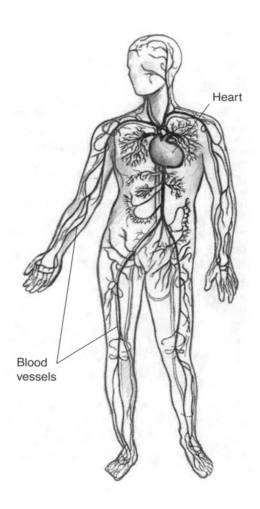

Figure 6.1. Diabetes can lead to heart and blood vessel disease.

What is prediabetes?

Prediabetes is a condition in which blood glucose levels are higher than normal but not high enough for a diagnosis of diabetes. Prediabetes is also called impaired fasting glucose or impaired glucose tolerance. Many people with prediabetes develop type 2 diabetes within 10 years. In addition, they are at risk for heart disease and stroke. With modest weight loss and moderate physical activity, people with prediabetes can delay or prevent type 2 diabetes and lower their risk of heart disease and stroke.

What is the connection between diabetes, heart disease, and stroke?

If you have diabetes, you are at least twice as likely as someone who does not have diabetes to have heart disease or a stroke. People with diabetes also tend to develop heart disease or have strokes at an earlier age than other people. If you are middle-aged and have type 2 diabetes, some studies suggest that your chance of having a heart

Cross section of a healthy blood vessel

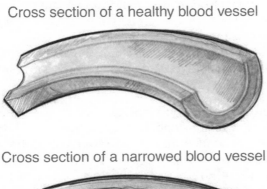

Cross section of a narrowed blood vessel

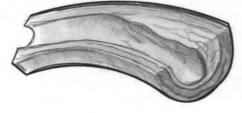

Figure 6.2. Atherosclerosis and the blood vessels.

attack is as high as someone without diabetes who has already had one heart attack.

Women who have not gone through menopause usually have less risk of heart disease than men of the same age. But women of all ages with diabetes have an increased risk of heart disease because diabetes cancels out the protective effects of being a woman in her child-bearing years.

People with diabetes who have already had one heart attack run an even greater risk of having a second one. In addition, heart attacks in people with diabetes are more serious and more likely to result in death. High blood glucose levels over time can lead to increased deposits of fatty materials on the insides of the blood vessel walls. These deposits may affect blood flow, increasing the chance of clogging and hardening of blood vessels (atherosclerosis).

What are the risk factors for heart disease and stroke in people with diabetes?

Diabetes itself is a risk factor for heart disease and stroke. Also, many people with diabetes have other conditions that increase their chance of developing heart disease and stroke. These conditions are called risk factors. One risk factor for heart disease and stroke is having a family history of heart disease. If one or more members of your family had a heart attack at an early age (before age 55 for men or 65 for women), you may be at increased risk.

You can't change whether heart disease runs in your family, but you can take steps to control the other risk factors for heart disease listed in the following text.

Having central obesity: Central obesity means carrying extra weight around the waist, as opposed to the hips. A waist measurement of more than 40 inches for men and more than 35 inches for women means you have central obesity. Your risk of heart disease is higher because abdominal fat can increase the production of LDL (low-density lipoprotein; or bad) cholesterol, the type of blood fat that can be deposited on the inside of blood vessel walls.

Having abnormal blood fat (cholesterol) levels: LDL cholesterol can build up inside your blood vessels, leading to narrowing and hardening of your arteries—the blood vessels that carry blood from the heart to the rest of the body. Arteries can then become blocked. Therefore, high levels of LDL cholesterol raise your risk of getting heart disease.

Triglycerides are another type of blood fat that can raise your risk of heart disease when the levels are high.

HDL (high-density lipoprotein; or good) cholesterol removes deposits from inside your blood vessels and takes them to the liver for removal. Low levels of HDL cholesterol increase your risk for heart disease.

Having high blood pressure: If you have high blood pressure, also called hypertension, your heart must work harder to pump blood. High blood pressure can strain the heart, damage blood vessels, and increase your risk of heart attack, stroke, eye problems, and kidney problems.

Smoking: Smoking doubles your risk of getting heart disease. Stopping smoking is especially important for people with diabetes because both smoking and diabetes narrow blood vessels. Smoking also increases the risk of other long-term complications, such as eye problems. In addition, smoking can damage the blood vessels in your legs and increase the risk of amputation.

Section 6.3

Metabolic Syndrome and Heart Disease

Excerpted from "Metabolic Syndrome," by the National Heart, Lung, and Blood Institute (NHLBI, www.nhlbi.nih.gov), part of the National Institutes of Health, April 2007.

Metabolic syndrome is the name for a group of risk factors linked to overweight and obesity that increase your chance for heart disease and other health problems such as diabetes and stroke. The term "metabolic" refers to the biochemical processes involved in the body's normal functioning. Risk factors are behaviors or conditions that increase your chance of getting a disease. In this text, "heart disease" refers to coronary heart disease.

The five conditions listed below are metabolic risk factors for heart disease. A person can develop any one of these risk factors by itself, but they tend to occur together. Metabolic syndrome is diagnosed when a person has at least three of these heart disease risk factors:

- **A large waistline:** This is also called abdominal obesity or "having an apple shape." Excess fat in the abdominal area is a greater risk factor for heart disease than excess fat in other parts of the body, such as on the hips.

- **A higher than normal triglyceride level in the blood (or you're on medicine to treat high triglycerides):** Triglycerides are a type of fat found in the blood.

- **A lower than normal level of HDL cholesterol (high-density lipoprotein cholesterol) in the blood (or you're on medicine to treat low HDL):** HDL is considered "good" cholesterol because it lowers your chances of heart disease. Low levels of HDL increase your chances of heart disease.

- **Higher than normal blood pressure (or you're on medicine to treat high blood pressure):** Blood pressure is recorded as two numbers, usually written one on top of or before the other, such as 120/80. The top or first number, called the systolic blood pressure, measures the pressure in the bloodstream when your heart beats. The bottom or second number, called the diastolic blood pressure, measures the pressure in your bloodstream between heartbeats when the heart is relaxed.

- **Higher than normal fasting blood sugar (glucose) (or you're on medicine to treat high blood sugar):** Mildly high blood sugar can be an early warning sign of diabetes.

The more of these risk factors you have, the greater your chance of developing heart disease, diabetes, or a stroke. In general, a person with metabolic syndrome is twice as likely to develop heart disease and five times as likely to develop diabetes as someone without metabolic syndrome.

Other risk factors aside from those of the metabolic syndrome also increase your risk for heart disease. A high level of LDL cholesterol (low-density lipoprotein cholesterol; considered "bad" cholesterol) and smoking, for example, are key risk factors for heart disease, but they aren't components of metabolic syndrome. Even a single risk factor raises your risk for heart disease, and every risk factor should be lowered to reduce the risk.

The chance of developing metabolic syndrome is closely linked to being overweight or obese and to a lack of physical activity. Another cause is insulin resistance. Insulin resistance is a condition in which the body can't use its insulin properly. Insulin is a hormone the body uses to help change blood sugar into energy. Insulin resistance can lead to high blood sugar levels and is closely linked with being over-weight or obese.

Genetics (ethnicity and family history) and older age are other important underlying causes of metabolic syndrome.

Causes of Metabolic Syndrome

Metabolic syndrome has several causes that act together. Some can be controlled, while others can't.

Causes that can be controlled include overweight and obesity, lack of physical activity, and insulin resistance.

Some causes you can't control are growing older and genetics. Your chance of developing metabolic syndrome increases with age. Your genes can increase your chances of developing insulin resistance, for example, which can lead to metabolic syndrome, even if you have only a little extra weight around your waist.

Two other conditions are often found in people with metabolic syndrome, although it's not known if they cause it or worsen it. The two conditions are a tendency to form blood clots and a tendency to have a constant, low-grade inflammation throughout the body.

Additional conditions that are being studied to see whether they have links to metabolic syndrome include the following:

- Fatty liver (excess triglycerides and other fats in the liver)
- Polycystic ovarian syndrome (a tendency to develop cysts on the ovaries)
- Gallstones
- Breathing problems during sleep such as sleep apnea

Signs and Symptoms of Metabolic Syndrome

Metabolic syndrome is made up of a group of factors that can in-crease risk even if they are only moderately raised (borderline-high risk factors). Metabolic syndrome itself usually has no symptoms. Most of the risk factors linked to metabolic syndrome have no signs or symp-toms, although a large waistline is a visible sign.

Some people may have symptoms of high blood sugar (if diabetes is present) or, occasionally, high blood pressure. Symptoms of high blood sugar often include increased thirst; increased urination, especially at night; fatigue (tiredness); and blurred vision. High blood pressure is generally considered to have no signs or symptoms. However, a few people in the early stages of high blood pressure may have dull headaches, dizzy spells, or more nosebleeds than usual.

Section 6.4

Periodontal and Cardiovascular Disease

From "Study Finds Direct Association Between Cardiovascular Disease and Periodontal Bacteria," National Institutes of Health (NIH, www.nih.gov), February 7, 2005.

Researchers report this week that older adults who have higher proportions of four periodontal-disease-causing bacteria inhabiting their mouths also tend to have thicker carotid arteries, a strong predictor of stroke and heart attack. The study, published in a 2005 issue of the journal *Circulation,* was supported by four agencies of the National Institutes of Health.

According to the authors, these data mark the first report of a direct association between cardiovascular disease and bacteria involved in periodontal disease, inflammation of the gums that affects to varying degrees an estimated 200 million Americans. But the researchers say the findings are not proof that the bacteria cause cardiovascular disease, directly or indirectly.

"What was interesting to us was the specificity of the association," said Moïse Desvarieux, MD, PhD, the study's lead author and an infectious disease epidemiologist at Columbia University's Mailman School of Public Health and the University of Minnesota. "These same four bacteria were there, they were always there in the analysis, and the relationship seems to be pretty much, with one exception, limited to them."

Desvarieux stressed that although the new data further illuminate a long-standing scientific issue, they shed little light on the broader public health question related to cardiovascular disease. The 657 people in the study had their oral bacteria and carotid thickness evaluated at the same point in time. So Desvarieux said, "It's impossible to know which comes first, the periodontal disease or thickening of the carotid artery." The answer to that question is fundamental to establishing causality—in this case, whether chronic inflammation or infection could have led to the atherosclerosis of the carotid arteries.

He and his colleagues noted that the public health information could come soon. "We will re-examine the participants in less than 3 years, and, at that point, we can better evaluate the progression of the atherosclerosis and, hopefully, begin to establish a time frame underlying the diseases," said Ralph Sacco, MD, MS, associate chair of neurology, professor of neurology and epidemiology, and the director of the Stroke and Critical Care Division of Columbia University College of Physicians and Surgeons. He also is an author on the paper.

The idea that oral bacteria shed from chronic gum infections, enter the circulatory system, and possibly contribute to diseases of the heart and other body organs once was widely accepted in medicine. The concept, known as the "focal infection theory," fell out of fashion by the 1940s, then resurfaced four decades later with the publication of new data proposing a link.

Since then, a major sticking point in advancing the research has been simply how to pursue the hypothesis. Lacking the scientific tools to track oral bacteria in the body over several decades to determine if they directly trigger heart disease, most previous studies pursued indirect evidence. These included various measures of oral and cardiovascular health, which researchers then extrapolated to the influence of the oral pathogens. Conspicuously missing from the debate has been a large, well-designed study that in some way directly evaluates the role of the oral pathogens themselves.

To fill this void, the National Institute of Dental and Craniofacial Research launched the Oral Infections and Vascular Disease Epidemiology Study (INVEST), a multidisciplinary endeavor whose principal investigator is Dr. Desvarieux. The study, which is the source of the paper published in Circulation, will monitor the oral and cardiovascular health of a large, racially mixed group of people. All enrollees in the study live in a northern section of Manhattan in New York City and are age 55 or older. Participants are also members of the Northern Manhattan Study (NOMAS), a prospective cohort study supported by NIH's National Institute of Neurological Disorders and Stroke. Dr. Sacco is principal investigator of the companion NOMAS study.

"Although more than 600 bacteria have been shown to colonize the mouth, each person tends to carry different proportions of these microbes," said Panos N. Papapanou, DDS, PhD, an author on the paper and professor and chair of the Section of Oral and Diagnostics Sciences and director of the Division of Periodontics at Columbia University School of Dental and Oral Surgery. He noted that only a subset of bacteria tend to be dominant in dental plaque.

"We wanted to know during the baseline examination of the participants whether it was true that the greater the proportion of so-called 'bad' bacteria in the mouth, the higher the likelihood of a thickened carotid artery," added Papapanou, whose laboratory performed the periodontal microbiological analysis.

To get their answer, Desvarieux and colleagues collected on average seven dental plaque samples from a total of 657 older adults enrolled in INVEST who had not lost their teeth. The samples, taken from predetermined sites in the mouth, both diseased and healthy, were measured for 11 oral bacteria, including four bacteria widely regarded to be involved in causing periodontal disease: *Actinobacillus actinomycetemcomitans, Porphyromonas gingivalis, Tannerella forsythia,* and *Treponema denticola.* The other seven bacteria served as controls, as their role in periodontal disease was either neutral or has not yet been established.

Then, to evaluate their cardiovascular health, the participants received a carotid intima-media thickness (IMT) measurement and provided a blood sample to determine their C-reactive protein levels. C-reactive protein has been reported to be elevated in people with periodontal disease, and studies found that testing for this protein may be predictive of developing heart disease.

Controlling for several risk factors that might skew their data—such as smoking and diabetes, both of which are independently associated with these conditions—the scientists found the higher the levels of these periodontal-disease-causing bacteria, the more likely people were to have thicker carotid arteries. Interestingly, they noted no association between IMT, the periodontal pathogens, and C-reactive protein levels, suggesting the protein is involved in another cardiovascular disease pathway.

Next, the scientists wondered whether the broad association might be due to the four pathogens involved in causing periodontal disease, which combined accounted for only 23 percent of the bacteria in dental plaque. If so, the finding would provide added specificity to strengthen the case for the association.

"After reanalyzing the data, we found, with the exception of an oral bacterium called *Micromonas micros,* the relationship was limited to these four established oral pathogens," said David Jacobs, PhD, another author and a professor in the Division of Epidemiology at the University of Minnesota School of Public Health.

"In other words, it was exactly what we hypothesized," said Desvarieux.

However, he cautioned, "It now becomes crucial to follow the participants over time and see whether these baseline findings hold up and further translate into clinical disease."

Section 6.5

Sleep Apnea and Heart Disease

"Link between heart disease, sleep apnea should be probed,"
reprinted with permission. © 2009 American Heart Association, Inc.
(www.americanheart.org).

- Large-scale studies are needed to determine the exact relationship between heart disease and sleep apnea.

- Patients should ask their doctors about treatment and prevention for both their sleep apnea and their cardiovascular disease.

Medical researchers need to undertake large-scale studies to determine the exact relationship between heart disease and the different forms of sleep apnea, according to a joint statement from the American Heart Association and the American College of Cardiology, published online in *Circulation: Journal of the American Heart Association* and the *Journal of the American College of Cardiology*.

"There have been a number of studies on sleep apnea in the last decade, and those looking at cardiovascular diseases and their associations with sleep apnea are especially compelling," said Virend K. Somers, MD, DPhil, chair of the joint statement writing committee. "We feel it is important to alert the cardiovascular community to the implications of this emerging area of research. It is possible that diagnosing and treating sleep apnea may prove to be an important opportunity to advance our efforts at preventing and treating heart disease."

Though the link between sleep apnea and heart disease is not fully understood, the committee issued the statement because of the increasing evidence, the widespread prevalence of sleep apnea, and the rising levels of obesity, particularly in young people. Obesity is a major cause of sleep apnea, and "the epidemic of childhood obesity may be changing the epidemiology of obstructive sleep apnea in children," said Somers, who is professor of medicine and cardiovascular diseases at the Mayo Clinic in Rochester, Minnesota.

"We need to more clearly define the cause and effect relationship between sleep apnea and cardiovascular diseases and risk factors," Somers said. "There is evidence that sleep apnea may be a cause of some cases of high blood pressure, but for other cardiovascular conditions, the evidence is largely circumstantial."

The issues are more complex than the age-old "Which comes first?" debate, he said. People with sleep apnea often have other disorders, such as obesity, and people with heart disease often have additional medical issues, making it difficult to separate the role of sleep apnea in the cardiovascular disease process.

Sleep apnea has more effects than daytime tiredness. It can result in low oxygen levels, frequent arousals from sleep, and chronic sleep deprivation, with consequences that persist throughout the day. It can also affect the nervous system, lead to abnormal function of cells lining blood vessels, and promote abnormal chemical responses. In the longer term, it is possible that these changes may damage the heart and blood vessels.

"For now, until we have more clear information as to who should be treated and what the benefits of treatment would be, patients should be assessed on an individualized basis," Somers said. "Until we know the cause and effect relationship between sleep apnea and cardiovascular disease, it would be best to take a two-pronged approach and treat patients from both perspectives: In other words, treat both their sleep apnea and their cardiovascular disease."

The statement warns that sleep apnea cases are expected to increase due to the current epidemics of obesity, high blood pressure, atrial fibrillation, and heart failure in the United States.

Co-authors are: David P. White, MD (co-chair); Raouf Amin, MD (co-chair); William T. Abraham, MD; Fernando Costa, MD; Antonio Culebras, MD; Stephen Daniels, MD, PhD; John S. Floras, MD, DPhil; Carl E. Hunt, MD; Lyle J. Olson, MD; Thomas G. Pickering, MD, DPhil; Richard Russell, MD; Mary Woo, RN, PhD; and Terry Young, PhD.

Author disclosures are available on the manuscript.

The statement was written in collaboration with the National Heart, Lung, and Blood Institute's National Center on Sleep Disorders Research.

The American Heart Association/American Stroke Association receives funding primarily from individuals. In addition, foundations and corporations—including pharmaceutical, device manufacturers, and other companies—make donations and fund specific American Heart Association/American Stroke Association programs and events. Revenues from pharmaceutical and device corporations are disclosed at www.americanheart.org.

Section 6.6

Thyroid Disease Raises Risk of Heart Disease

Subclinical hypothyroidism, which is often the beginning of an underactive thyroid, appears to contribute more substantially toward the risk of heart disease in people up to the age of 65, according to a study that reviewed the medical literature. The study was presented Tuesday, June 5, 2007 at The Endocrine Society's 89th Annual Meeting in Toronto.

Subclinical hypothyroidism, which usually causes no symptoms of thyroid disease, is thought to be an early, mild form of hypothyroidism. As in hypothyroidism, the level of thyroid-stimulating hormone is too high in this early form, but unlike hypothyroidism, the level of the thyroid hormone thyroxine is within the normal range for the population, rather than low. Subclinical hypothyroidism affects 8 percent of all women and 3 percent of men, and becomes more prevalent with age, according to the study's lead author, Dr. Salman Razvi of the United Kingdom's Royal Victoria Infirmary.

It previously was unclear whether people with this thyroid condition have a higher risk of ischemic heart disease, because results from past studies have been inconsistent, Razvi said. Also called coronary artery disease or coronary heart disease, ischemic heart disease primarily results from narrowing of the arteries supplying the heart. It is the most common type of heart disease, according to the American Heart Association.

To better understand the risk of cardiovascular disease in this thyroid condition, Razvi and co-workers performed a systematic review of 32 studies of subclinical hypothyroidism that assessed ischemic heart disease and its risk factors. The studies were from the United States, Australia, and countries in Europe and Asia.

The occurrence of ischemic heart disease, as well as death due to it, was increased in people with subclinical hypothyroidism but only in studies that included people less than 65 years of age. This result is probably because people older than 65 increasingly have other risk factors for cardiovascular disease, so the risk due to thyroid abnormality becomes diluted, Razvi speculated.

The researchers also found that treatment of subclinical hypothyroidism reduced LDL ("bad") cholesterol and body mass index, a measure of obesity.

"Our analyses of large data sets suggest that there are age-related differences in the risk of cardiovascular disease attributable to subclinical hypothyroidism," Razvi said. "This has potentially important implications for therapy."

Patients with subclinical hypothyroidism may receive treatment with thyroid hormone medications if their doctors advise it, according to Razvi.

Chapter 7

Stress and Cardiovascular Disorders

Today scientists are looking at how stress makes people ill, and what can be done to help prevent illness caused by stress.

"This new science is forcing the medical community to take more seriously the popular notions of the mind-body connection," says Esther M. Sternberg, MD, director of the Integrative Neural Immune Program at the National Institute of Mental Health. In response to stressful events, our bodies pump out hormones. These hormones aren't necessarily harmful and can be very useful, says Dr. Sternberg, author of *The Balance Within: The Science Connecting Health and Emotions.* "The problem is when the stress response goes on for too long," she says. "That's when you get sick. Hormones weaken the immune system's ability to fight disease."

Dangers of Chronic Stress

Unhealthy levels of stress come in many guises. You may have to take care of a chronically ill person—and that's stressful. Or you may be stressed from being in constant pain. Work-related issues, marriage or family problems, and financial difficulties can generate chronic stress. Severe, chronic stress can damage our bodies in many ways.

From "How to Fight Stress and Ward Off Illness," by Celia Vimont, in *MedlinePlus: The Magazine,* by the National Library of Medicine (NLM, www.nlm.nih.gov), part of the National Institutes of Health, 2008.

"Chronic stress has been shown to prolong wound healing, decrease response to vaccines, and increase the frequency and severity of upper respiratory infections," Dr. Sternberg says.

Stress also can aggravate existing health problems. It can worsen angina, disturb heart rhythm, raise blood pressure, and lead to stroke. It can spark asthma and may affect the digestive system, making ulcers, acid reflux, or irritable bowel problems worse. Stress can play havoc with your nerves and muscles, causing backaches, tension headaches, or migraines.

Take Yourself Offline

"If you feel stressed all the time, you need to take yourself 'offline,'" Dr. Sternberg urges. "We reboot our computers when they are overworked, but we don't seem to do it with our bodies."

If you're exhausted from constantly working on deadline or caregiving, take a vacation—they're not luxuries, they're physical necessities. Find a place of peace where you can stop, look, and listen." If vacations are out of the question, Dr. Sternberg suggests meditation to rest body and mind. "Evidence shows that meditation bolsters immune function by reducing stress hormones that dampen immune cells' ability to fight infection," she says.

Exercise is a great way to improve your mood, and it changes the body's stress response, she says. If starting an exercise program seems too hard, then go slowly, she advises. "A few minutes are better than no minutes—you can gradually increase how much you exercise every day. You don't need to go jogging—walking has significant health benefits."

Yoga helps many people relax, while others find peace of mind through prayer, music, reading, or art. "We need to find our place of peace and try to go there every day," she says.

Getting enough sleep is very important for protection, Dr. Sternberg emphasizes. "Lack of sleep can change moods, cause irritability, weight gain, inability to perform, and poor memory."

When to Seek Professional Help

If the stress is bad enough that you can't fix it on your own, Dr. Sternberg recommends seeking professional help. In some people, what may seem like ongoing stress is actually depression.

Possible signs of depression include the following:

• Often waking up in the middle of the night with feelings of anxiety

- Suicidal thoughts
- Loss of weight and appetite
- Not wanting to be around other people
- Constant irritability

"Depression is an imbalance of hormones and nerve chemicals—it's a biological illness," Dr. Sternberg says. "And highly treatable."

Chapter 8

Genetics and Cardiovascular Disorders

International Effort Finds New Genetic Variants Associated with Lipid Levels, Risk for Coronary Artery Disease

Environmental and genetic factors influence a person's blood fat, or lipid levels, important risk factors for coronary artery disease (CAD). While there is some understanding of the environmental contribution, the role of genetics has been less defined. Now, in an international collaboration supported primarily by the National Institutes of Health (NIH), scientists have discovered more than 25 genetic variants in 18 genes connected to cholesterol and lipid levels. Seven of the 18 genes previously had not been connected to these levels, while the 11 others confirm previous discoveries. In the investigation, published online January 13 [2008] and in the February [2008] print issue of *Nature Genetics,* the associated genes were found through studies of more than 20,000 individuals and more than 2 million genetic variants, spanning the entire genome. These variants potentially open the door to strategies for the treatment and prevention of CAD.

This chapter includes text excerpted from "International Effort Finds New Genetic Variants Associated with Lipid Levels, Risk for Coronary Artery Disease," by the National Institute on Aging (NIA, www.nia.nih.gov), part of the National Institutes of Health, January 13, 2008, and from "Researchers Uncover Genetic Clues to Blood Pressure," by the National Human Genome Research Institute (NHGRI, www.genome.gov), May 10, 2009.

"Heart disease is a leading cause of illness, disability, and death in industrialized countries, particularly for older people," says National Institute on Aging (NIA) Director Richard J. Hodes, MD. "We know that certain lifestyle factors like smoking, diet, and physical activity greatly affect a person's lipid profiles. This study is an important, basic step in finding the genes that influence lipid levels and heart disease so that we can better understand the genetic contribution to cardiovascular risk."

The purpose of the study was to identify comprehensively genetic variants that influence lipid levels and to examine the relationships between these genetic variants and risk of CAD. High levels of low-density lipoprotein (LDL) ("bad" cholesterol) appear to increase the risk of CAD by narrowing or blocking arteries that carry blood to the heart. High levels of high-density lipoprotein (HDL) ("good" cholesterol) appear to lower the risk. High levels of triglycerides, which make up a large part of the body's fat and are also found in the bloodstream, are also associated with increased risk of CAD.

To identify genetic variants that play a role in lipid levels, researchers turned to a relatively new approach, known as a genome-wide association study (GWAS). The GWAS strategy enables researchers to survey the entire human genetic blueprint, or genome, not just the genetic variants in a few genes. The human genome contains approximately 3 billion base pairs, or letters, of DNA [deoxyribonucleic acid]. Small, single-letter variations naturally occur about once in every 1,000 letters of the DNA code. Most of these genetic variants have not yet been associated with particular traits or disease risks. However, in some instances, people with a certain trait, such as higher levels of LDL cholesterol, tend to have one version of the variant, while those with lower levels are more likely to have the other version. In such instances, researchers may infer that there is an association between the values of the trait and the variants in the gene.

Typically, GWAS studies have been carried out in samples where all individuals are examined with the same gene chip, an experimental device that allows investigators to measure more than 100,000 genetic variants in a single experiment. But in this study, investigators developed and employed new statistical methods that allowed them to combine data across different gene chips and thus examine much larger numbers of participants.

Researchers were able to identify variations in 18 genes that influence HDL, LDL, and/or triglyceride levels. This list of lipid-associated genes is substantially longer than what was generated by analyses of individual datasets, which had only pointed to one to three genes each.

Of the seven newly implicated genes, two were associated with HDL levels, one with LDL levels, three with triglyceride levels and one with both triglycerides and LDL levels.

"These results are yet another example of how genome-wide association studies are opening exciting new avenues for biomedical research," says NHGRI Director Francis S. Collins, MD, PhD, who is a coauthor of the study and an investigator in NHGRI's Genome Technology Branch. "While some of the genetic variants we identified are known to play a well-established role in lipid metabolism, others have no obvious connection. Further studies to identify the precise genes and biological pathways involved could shed new light on lipid metabolism."

Scientists estimate that the genetic contribution to lipid levels is about 30 to 40 percent; the genetic variants uncovered in the new study are responsible for about 5 to 8 percent of that contribution, the scientists note, which means there is more work to be done. "In this study we carried out a comprehensive search for common variants of large effect. The genetic factors still to be discovered might turn out to be common variants with smaller effects or rare variants with a large effect," says Karen L. Mohlke, PhD, of the University of North Carolina, Chapel Hill, who co-directed the study with Gonçalo R. Abecasis, PhD, of the University of Michigan's School of Public Health.

To determine if the genetic variants associated with lipid levels also influence risk of heart disease, the researchers compared their results with results from the Wellcome Trust Case Control Consortium's recent genome-wide association study of CAD involving 15,000 British individuals. They found that all gene variants associated with increased LDL levels also were more prevalent among people with CAD. People with the gene variant for high triglyceride levels also had an increased risk for CAD, although the relationship was not as strong. No relationship was found between HDL and CAD.

"It was surprising that while it was clear that genetic variants that increase your 'bad' cholesterol are also associated with increased risk of heart disease, we did not find that variants influencing your 'good' cholesterol were associated with decreased risk of coronary artery disease. Perhaps that result will lead us to re-examine the roles of good and bad cholesterol in susceptibility to heart disease," remarks Abecasis.

Identifying a correlation among genes influencing lipid levels and risk for coronary heart disease is a first step in a long path to potentially important clinical implications. "What we're looking for, ultimately, are novel therapeutics and/or lifestyle modifications that can be recommended to individuals to help manage blood lipid levels and reduce risk of heart disease," says David Schlessinger, PhD, chief of the NIA's Laboratory of Genetics and NIA Project Officer for SardiNIA.

This study also demonstrates the power of international collaboration in genetic analyses. None of the studies that cooperated to make this work possible were large enough to find all of these important associations alone. By working together, previously unsuspected genetic influences on lipid levels and heart disease were revealed.

Researchers Uncover Genetic Clues to Blood Pressure

An international research team has identified a number of unsuspected genetic variants associated with systolic blood pressure (SBP), diastolic blood pressure (DBP), and hypertension (high blood pressure), suggesting potential avenues of investigation for the prevention or treatment of hypertension. The research was funded in part by the National Heart, Lung, and Blood Institute (NHLBI) of the National Institutes of Health and by several other NIH institutes and centers.

The analysis of over 29,000 participants was published online in the journal *Nature Genetics* on May 10, 2009.

"This study provides important new insights into the biology of blood pressure regulation and, with continued research, may lead to the development of novel therapeutic approaches to combat hypertension and its complications," said NHLBI Director Elizabeth G. Nabel, MD.

About one in three adults (approximately 72 million people) in the United States has high blood pressure. Hypertension can lead to coronary heart disease, heart failure, stroke, kidney failure, and other health problems, and causes over 7 million deaths worldwide each year.

Blood pressure has a substantial genetic component and hypertension runs in families. Previous attempts to identify genes associated with blood pressure, however, have met with limited success.

In a genome-wide association study (GWAS), researchers scanned millions of common genetic variants of individuals from the Cohorts for Heart and Aging Research in Genomic Epidemiology (CHARGE) consortium to find variants associated with blood pressure and hypertension. This extensive resource includes white men and women from the Framingham Heart Study, Atherosclerosis Risk in Communities study, Cardiovascular Health Study, the Rotterdam Study, the

Rotterdam Extension Study, and the Age, Gene/Environment Susceptibility Reykjavik Study.

The investigators identified a number of genetic variants or single-
nucleotide polymorphisms (SNPs) associated with SBP, DBP, and
hypertension. When they jointly analyzed their findings with those
from the GWAS of over 34,000 participants in the Global BPgen Consortium (whose results are presented in an accompanying paper in
the same issue of *Nature Genetics*), they identified 11 genes showing
significant associations across the genome: four for SBP, six for DBP,
and one for hypertension.

"Large scale genome-wide association studies are providing a number of important insights into identifying genes that play a role in
diseases with major public health impact," said Dr. Daniel Levy, first
author of the study and director, the NHLBI's Framingham Heart
Study and Center for Population Studies. "We have identified eight
key genes, few of which would have been on anyone's short list of suspected blood pressure genes until now."

The international research team included Cornelia M. van Duijn,
PhD, Erasmus Medical Center, Rotterdam, the Netherlands; Aravinda
Chakravarti, PhD, Johns Hopkins University; Bruce Psaty, MD, PhD,
University of Washington; and Vilmundur Gudnason, MD, PhD, Ice-
landic Heart Association, Kopayogur, Iceland.

The blood pressure genes include ATP2B1, which encodes PMCA1,
a cell membrane enzyme that is involved in calcium transport;
CACNB2, which encodes part of a calcium channel protein; and
CYP17A1 which encodes an enzyme that is necessary for steroid production. One detected variant is within the gene SH2B3 and has been
associated with autoimmune diseases, hinting that pathways involved
with the immune response may influence blood pressure.

Blood pressure is measured in millimeters of mercury (mmHg), and
expressed with two numbers, for example, 120/80 mmHg. The first
number (systolic pressure) is the pressure when the heart beats while
pumping blood. The second number (diastolic pressure) is the pressure in large arteries when the heart is at rest between beats.

Researchers found that the top 10 gene variants, or SNPs, for systolic and diastolic blood pressure were each associated with around
a 1 and 0.5 mm Hg increase in systolic and diastolic blood pressure,
respectively. The prevalence of hypertension increased as the number of variants increased.

People who carry very few blood pressure genetic risk variants have
blood pressure levels that are several mmHg lower than those who carry
multiple risk variants. In practical terms this is enough to increase

the risk for cardiovascular disease. A prolonged increase in DBP of only 5 mmHg is associated with a 34 percent increase in risk for stroke and a 21 percent increase of coronary heart disease.

Chapter 9

How Aging Affects the Heart and Blood Vessels

The Effects of Normal Aging

The emerging methods of studying the heart have led to the growing realization that the many factors influencing the aging heart and blood vessels are interdependent. At least six major factors affect how the heart fills with blood and pumps it out. When scientists first discovered these factors, they thought they operated independently. But as investigators more closely examined these factors, they discovered that these six factors influence each other in various direct and indirect ways.

Structural Changes

The NIA's studies of normal aging have revealed a series of fine-tuned adjustments that allow the heart to meet the needs of the aging body. This picture is radically different from the one that prevailed several decades ago when marked declines in overall heart function were thought to be the norm. The revolution in perspective began in the 1970s when researchers came upon their first surprise: The walls of the left ventricle, as it ages, grow thicker.

Up until then, gerontologists thought that the heart shrank with age. One reason was that early researchers knew about the older heart

---

Excerpted from chapter 2 of "Aging Hearts and Arteries," a publication by the National Institute on Aging (NIA, www.nia.nih.gov), part of the National Institutes of Health, October 2008.

mainly through chest x-rays and autopsy studies of people who were institutionalized, often with chronic illnesses. These people's hearts, which were affected by disease or extremely sedentary lives, often were smaller than those of younger, healthier people.

Then, in the late 1950s, gerontologists began to study healthy volunteers, such as those who participate in the BLSA [Baltimore Longitudinal Study of Aging]. Soon afterward, scientists devised new technologies like echocardiography and radionuclide imaging. While x-rays provide a static, shadowy silhouette, echocardiography and other imaging techniques clearly show thickness, diameter, volume, and in some cases, shape of the heart and how these change with time during a given heart beat. Recently, gerontologists have begun using magnetic resonance imaging (MRI) to get a better look at the aging heart. MRI is a type of body scan that uses magnets and computers to provide high-quality images based on varying characteristics of the body's tissues. The technology allows physicians to noninvasively study the beating heart's overall structure and function continuously in three dimensions.

The thicker left ventricular walls supplied the first clue that the heart might be adjusting rather than simply declining with age. Scientists think that the increased thickness allows the walls to compensate for the extra stress they bear with age (stress imposed by pumping blood into stiffer blood vessels, for instance). When walls thicken, stress is spread out over a larger area of heart muscle.

Heart Filling

Other findings about the left side of the heart soon followed. While at the NIA, Gary Gerstenblith, MD, and his colleagues studied the left ventricle and the left atrium, the receiving chamber into which blood flows from the lungs before passing into the ventricle. Their echocardiograms with BLSA volunteers showed that in addition to the left ventricular wall growing thicker, the cavity of the left atrium increased.

This study also yielded one other finding, a curious one: The mitral valve—the gateway between the left atrium and ventricle—appeared to close more slowly in older people. As the ventricle fills, the two flaps of the mitral valve—like a trap door with two separate panels—float up on the rising pool of blood and come together to close the passage. If this valve were closing more slowly in older people, as the echocardiograms indicated, then perhaps the ventricle was filling more slowly.

To figure out why this occurs and if it makes any difference, investigators turned their attention to the fraction of a second between heart beats. During this momentary lull, called the diastole, the heart relaxes, fills with blood, and readies for the next contraction or systole.

Heart researchers divide the moments of diastole into even shorter periods. There is the early filling phase when blood from the left atrium pushes the mitral valve open, flows rapidly into the left ventricle, and floats the valve shut. This early diastolic filling is the phase that takes longer as people grow older, according to the Gerstenblith study. Then comes the late filling phase, when the left atrium contracts, forces open the mitral valve a second time, and delivers a last surge of blood to the ventricle, just before it too contracts.

Why should early diastolic filling slow down as people age? Could it be because the ventricle wall was not relaxing between heart beats as quickly as it once had?

This possibility intrigued NIA investigators because it fit neatly with another stray piece to the puzzle. In animal studies several years earlier, Dr. Edward Lakatta, chief of the Laboratory of Cardiovascular Science at NIA, had learned that rat hearts studied in the laboratory took longer to relax after a contraction when they were from older rats.

Later imaging studies in humans confirmed the animal studies: Between beats, the aging ventricle fills with blood more slowly because it is relaxing more slowly than it did when young.

But now another piece of the diastolic puzzle needed to be fit into place. If the older left ventricle fills more slowly with blood, does this mean it has less blood pooled at the end of diastole and thus less to send out to the body during the next contraction? The answer is no, and the reason was found in another of the adjustments that the heart makes with age. NIA investigators found that the heart compensates for the slower early filling rate by filling more quickly in the late diastolic period.

It happens like this: As the mitral valve slowly closes, incoming blood from the lungs pools in the left atrium, which is now larger and holds more blood than when young. In the last moments of the diastole, the SA [sinoatrial] node—the heart's pacemaker—triggers the first electrical impulse (the action potential), which will lead to contraction. The impulse spreads across the cells of the two atria.

The left atrium, stretched with a greater volume of blood in older hearts, contracts harder, pushing open the valves and propelling the blood into the ventricle. The late diastolic surge of blood into the left ventricle from the atrium's contraction occurs at all ages but is stronger in older hearts and delivers a greater volume of blood to the left

77

ventricle. As a result, at the end of diastole, the volume of blood in older hearts is about the same (in women) or slightly greater (in men) than in younger hearts. In younger people, about twice as much blood flows into the ventricle during the early filling period than during late filling. But as we age, this ratio changes so blood flow during early and late filling is about equal.

The next step in this chain of events is contraction or systole, and here the puzzle becomes more complex.

Picture the left ventricle at the end of diastole filled with a volume of blood that is equal to or slightly greater than the volume in younger hearts; this is called end diastolic volume. When the contraction occurs, it forces out a certain amount of blood—the stroke volume. However, not all of the blood in the heart is pumped out at once. A portion remains in the ventricle, and this is called the end systolic volume. The proportion of blood that is pumped out during each beat compared to the amount that remains in the heart at the beginning of the next beat is called the ejection fraction. Doctors frequently use the ejection fraction to estimate how well the heart is pumping.

These measurements are important because the links between end diastolic volume, stroke volume, end systolic volume, and ejection fraction make up a complex set of dynamics that researchers had to sort out as they attempted to understand what differences aging makes in the heart's pumping ability. The various cardiac volumes differ according to age, gender, body size and composition, and degree of physical activity. However, keep in mind that the various changes discussed in this text are what occur, on average, in older hearts. As we age, the differences in these measures between one individual and another will vary much more than in younger people. So, for instance, among 65- to 70-year-old women the range of end diastolic volumes and stroke volumes can be quite vast.

Pumping at Rest

When you are sitting in a chair reading a book or watching television, your heart—regardless of age—usually works well below its full capacity. Instead, the heart saves or reserves most of its capacity for times when it is really needed, such as playing tennis or shoveling snow.

In fact, at first glance, healthy young and old hearts don't seem very different—at least when resting. For instance, cardiac output—the amount of blood pumped through the heart each minute—averages 4 to 6 quarts per minute at rest depending on body size and doesn't change much with age. Similarly, while resting, both young and old hearts eject about two thirds of the blood in the left ventricle during each heart beat.

But on closer examination, there is at least one important difference between a healthy resting young heart and an older one: heart rate. When we're lying down, the rates of young and old hearts remain about the same. But when we're sitting, heart rate is less in older people compared to younger men and women, in part, because of age-associated changes in the sympathetic nervous system's signals to the heart's pacemaker. As we age, some of the pathways in this system may develop fibrous tissue and fat deposits. The SA node, the heart's natural pacemaker, loses some of its cells.

In men, the heart compensates partly for this decline in two ways. First, the increase in end diastolic volume that comes with age means there is more blood to pump; and second, the greater volume stretches the ventricular walls and brings into play a peculiar property of muscle cells—the more they are stretched, the more they contract. This phenomenon is called the Frank-Starling mechanism and together with the greater volume of blood to be pumped, it helps to make up for the lower heart rate.

In women, end diastolic volume while sitting does not increase with age, so stroke volume does not increase. The difference between the sexes probably reflects their different needs rather than a difference in their hearts' pumping abilities.

But while the resting older heart can keep pace with its younger counterpart, the older heart—even if in peak condition—is no match for a younger one during exercise or stress.

Pumping during Exercise

It's no secret that the ability to run, swim, and exert ourselves in other ways diminishes as we get older. In fact, the body's capacity to perform vigorous exercise declines by about 50 percent between the ages of 20 and 80. About half of this decline can be attributed to changes in the typical aging heart.

During any kind of activity—even moving from a sitting to a standing position—the heart must pump more blood to the working muscles. In younger people it does this by increasing the heart rate and squeezing harder during contractions, sending more blood with each beat. But age brings changes. Heart rate still rises, but it can no longer rise as high. In your 20s, for instance, your maximum heart rate is typically about 190 to 200 beats per minute; by age 80, this rate has diminished to about 145 beats per minute. A reduced response of heart cells to signals from the brain result in a substantial decline in the peak rate at which the older heart can beat. In addition, force of contraction during vigorous exercise increases, but not as much in older people as in younger ones.

As a result, the heart's cardiovascular reserve diminishes. Put another way, a typical 20-year-old can increase cardiac output during exercise to 3.5–4 times over resting levels. In comparison, by age 80, a person can only muster about two times as much cardiac output as at rest.

Yet the aging heart still must respond to many of the same demands as the younger heart. To do so, it takes advantage of its natural flexibility. The heart, which is composed of elastic-like material, can readily alter shape and size depending on the amount of blood within its chambers.

At rest, only a small portion of the body's blood supply is flowing into the heart at any given moment. But with exertion, your body sends out signals that increase blood flow from the veins back to the heart initially stretching and swelling it. This triggers the Frank-Starling mechanism. In response, the young heart pumps harder. Then the brain kicks in, releasing neurotransmitters that elevate heart rate, increase contraction strength, and boost ejection fraction. In addition, the young heart returns to its small, resting size at the start of each beat. All of these reactions help the young heart work more efficiently.

But the older heart doesn't respond in the same way. Although the brain still releases neurotransmitters that stimulate the heart to work harder during vigorous exercise, the older heart is less responsive to these signals than the younger heart. And unlike the young heart, it can't squeeze down to a small size at the end of a heart beat. So its ejection fraction increases only slightly from its resting level of about 65 percent during vigorous exercise. In addition, you might recall that the older heart can't increase its rate as much as the younger heart during exertion. So if it can't beat as fast or squeeze down as hard, then how does the older heart respond to the demands of exercise? The answer is: It adapts.

Because its pumping rate increases less during exercise, the older heart has more time than a younger heart to fill with blood between beats. This additional filling time, combined with a lower ejection fraction, causes the older heart to expand to a larger size during diastole than a young heart. As a result, during exercise the older, bigger heart has more blood in its chambers at the start of each beat than a younger heart. This extra blood volume allows the older heart to pump out just about as much blood with each beat as a younger, smaller heart, even though it has a lower ejection fraction. This represents the Frank-Starling mechanism working at its finest. However during vigorous exercise the older heart is still pumping less blood overall because it can't beat as fast as a young heart.

While this adaptation certainly helps the heart meet the immediate needs of the exercising older body, it does so at a cost. As the older heart dilates between beats, wall tension and pressure within its cavities rises. This increases load on the heart and forces it to work harder. In the long run, persistently elevated pressure promotes thickening and stiffening of the ventricular walls. As a result, the ventricles don't fully relax between beats, and this—combined with a greater filling volume—causes end diastolic left ventricular pressure to increase. When this happens the left atrial pressure increases and this pressure increase is transmitted to the lungs. As pressure rises, oxygenated blood has trouble getting from your lungs into the left side of your heart so it can be pumped out to the body. One outward sign of this scenario within the lungs is that you begin to feel short of breath while exerting yourself. How much exercise you can do before you experience this symptom depends, in part, on how much of the left ventricle's pumping capacity has been eroded. Regular aerobic exercise can help diminish the impact of many of these age-related changes.

Chapter 10

Warning Signs of Cardiovascular Disorders

Chapter Contents

Section 10.1

Heart Attack Warning Signs

From "Heart Attack Warning Signs," by the National Heart, Lung, and Blood Institute (NHLBI, www.nhlbi.nih.gov), part of the National Institutes of Health, 2002. Reviewed by David A. Cooke, MD, FACP, October 1, 2009.

A heart attack is a frightening event, and you probably don't want to think about it. But, if you learn the signs of a heart attack and what steps to take, you can save a life–maybe your own.

What are the signs of a heart attack? Many people think a heart attack is sudden and intense, like a movie heart attack, where a person clutches his or her chest and falls over.

The truth is that many heart attacks start slowly, as a mild pain or discomfort. If you feel such a symptom, you may not be sure what's wrong. Your symptoms may even come and go. Even those who have had a heart attack may not recognize their symptoms because the next attack can have entirely different ones.

Women may not think they're at risk of having a heart attack— but they are. Learn more about women and heart attack.

It's vital that everyone learn the warning signs of a heart attack, which include the following:

- **Chest discomfort:** Most heart attacks involve discomfort in the center of the chest that lasts for more than a few minutes or goes away and comes back. The discomfort can feel like uncomfortable pressure, squeezing, fullness, or pain.

- **Discomfort in other areas of the upper body:** This sign can include pain or discomfort in one or both arms, the back, neck, jaw, or stomach.

- **Shortness of breath:** This sign often comes along with chest discomfort, but it also can occur before chest discomfort.

- **Other symptoms:** This sign may include breaking out in a cold sweat, nausea, or light-headedness.

Learn the signs—but also remember: Even if you're not sure it's a heart attack, you should still have it checked out. Fast action can save lives—maybe your own.

Section 10.2

Orthostatic Hypotension: A Sign of a Heart Condition

Excerpted from "Orthostatic Hypotension Information Page," by the National Institute of Neurological Disorders and Stroke (NINDS, www .ninds.nih.gov), part of the National Institutes of Health, February 14, 2007.

What is orthostatic hypotension?

Orthostatic hypotension is a sudden fall in blood pressure that occurs when a person assumes a standing position. It may be caused by hypovolemia (a decreased amount of blood in the body), resulting from the excessive use of diuretics, vasodilators, or other types of drugs, dehydration, or prolonged bed rest. The disorder may be associated with Addison disease, atherosclerosis (build-up of fatty deposits in the arteries), diabetes, and certain neurological disorders including Shy-Drager syndrome and other dysautonomias. Symptoms, which generally occur after sudden standing, include dizziness, lightheadedness, blurred vision, and syncope (temporary loss of consciousness).

Is there any treatment?

When orthostatic hypotension is caused by hypovolemia due to medications, the disorder may be reversed by adjusting the dosage or by discontinuing the medication. When the condition is caused by prolonged bed rest, improvement may occur by sitting up with increasing frequency each day. In some cases, physical counterpressure such as elastic hose or whole-body inflatable suits may be required. Dehydration is treated with salt and fluids.

Section 10.3

Heart Palpitations

Excerpted from "Palpitations," by the National Heart, Lung, and Blood Institute (NHLBI, www.nhlbi.nih.gov), part of the National Institutes of Health, December 2007.

Palpitations are feelings that your heart is skipping a beat, fluttering, or beating too hard or fast. You may have these feelings in your chest, throat, or neck. They can occur during activity or even when you're sitting still or lying down.

Palpitations are very common. They usually aren't serious or harmful, but they can be bothersome. If you have them, your doctor can check to see whether you need treatment or ongoing care.

Causes of Palpitations

Many things can cause palpitations. You may feel palpitations even when your heart is beating normally or somewhat faster than normal. In these cases, nothing is wrong with your heart.

However, some palpitations are a sign of an actual heart problem. Sometimes, the cause of palpitations can't be found.

If you start having palpitations, you should see your doctor to have them checked out.

Causes Not Related to Heart Problems

Strong emotions: You may feel your heart pounding or racing during anxiety, fear, or stress. You also may have these feelings if you're having a panic attack.

Vigorous physical activity: Intense activity can make it feel as though your heart is beating too hard or fast, even though it's working normally. It also may cause an occasional premature (extra) heartbeat.

Medical conditions: Certain medical conditions can cause palpitations. This is because they can make the heart beat faster or stronger or cause premature (extra) heartbeats. These conditions include the following:

- An overactive thyroid
- A low blood sugar level
- Anemia
- Some types of low blood pressure
- Fever
- Dehydration (not enough fluid in the body)

Hormonal changes: The hormonal changes that happen during pregnancy, menstruation, and the perimenopausal period can sometimes cause palpitations. These palpitations will likely improve or go away as these conditions go away or change.

Some palpitations that occur during pregnancy may be due to anemia.

Medicines and stimulants: A number of medicines can trigger palpitations because they can make the heart beat faster or stronger or cause premature (extra) heartbeats. These include the following:

- Asthma inhalers may cause palpitations.
- Medicines to treat an underactive thyroid may cause palpitations. (Too much thyroid replacement hormone, used to treat an underactive thyroid, can cause palpitations by causing an overactive thyroid.)
- Medicines to prevent arrhythmias may cause palpitations. (Medicines used to treat these irregular heartbeats can sometimes cause other irregular heart rhythms.)
- Over-the-counter medicines that act as stimulants also may cause palpitations. (These include decongestants [found in cough and cold medicines] and some herbal or nutritional supplements.)
- Caffeine, nicotine (found in tobacco), alcohol, and illegal drugs (such as cocaine and amphetamines) also may cause palpitations.

Causes Related to Heart Problems

Sometimes, palpitations are the symptoms of arrhythmias. Arrhythmias are problems with the speed or rhythm of the heartbeat.

However, less than half of the people who have palpitations have arrhythmias.

During an arrhythmia, the heart can beat too fast, too slow, or with an irregular rhythm. An arrhythmia happens when some part of the heart's electrical system doesn't work as it should.

Palpitations are more likely to be related to an arrhythmia if you:

- have had a heart attack or are at risk for one;
- have heart disease or risk factors for heart disease;
- have other heart problems, such as heart failure, heart valve problems, or heart muscle problems;
- have abnormal electrolyte levels. Electrolytes are minerals, such as potassium and sodium, found in blood and body fluids. They're vital for normal health and functioning of the body.

Risk for Palpitations

Some people may be more likely to have palpitations, including people who:

- have anxiety, panic attacks, or are highly stressed;
- take certain medicines or stimulants;
- have certain medical conditions that aren't related to heart problems, such as an overactive thyroid;
- have certain heart problems, such as arrhythmias (irregular heartbeats), a previous heart attack, heart failure, heart valve problems, or heart muscle problems.

Women who are pregnant, menstruating, or perimenopausal also may be at higher risk, because hormonal changes can cause palpitations. Also, some palpitations that occur during pregnancy may be due to anemia.

Signs and Symptoms of Palpitations

Symptoms of palpitations include feelings that your heart is doing the following:

- Skipping a beat
- Fluttering
- Beating too hard or fast

You may have these feelings in your chest, throat, or neck. They can occur during activity or even when you're sitting still or lying down.

Often, palpitations are harmless and your heart is working normally. Palpitations can be a sign of a more serious problem if you also have the following problems:

- Feel dizzy or confused
- Are lightheaded, think you may faint, or do faint
- Have trouble breathing
- Have pain, pressure, or tightness in your chest, jaw, or arm
- Feel short of breath
- Have unusual sweating

If your doctor has already told you that your palpitations are harmless, talk to him or her again if they start to occur more often or are more noticeable or bothersome; or occur with other symptoms, such as those listed above.

Your doctor will want to check whether your palpitations are the symptom of a heart problem, such as an arrhythmia (irregular heartbeat).

Section 10.4

Signs of Stroke

Excerpted from "Know Stroke. Know the Signs. Act in Time," by the National Institute of Neurological Disorders and Stroke (NINDS, www .ninds.nih.gov), part of the National Institutes of Health, NIH Publication No. 08-4872, January 2008.

Stroke is the third leading cause of death in the United States and a leading cause of serious, long-term disability in adults. About 600,000 new strokes are reported in the United States each year. The good news is that treatments are available that can greatly reduce the damage caused by a stroke. However, you need to recognize the symptoms of a stroke and get to a hospital quickly. Getting treatment within 60 minutes can prevent disability.

What is a stroke?

A stroke, sometimes called a "brain attack," occurs when blood flow to the brain is interrupted. When a stroke occurs, brain cells in the immediate area begin to die because they stop getting the oxygen and nutrients they need to function.

What causes a stroke?

There are two major kinds of stroke. The first, called an ischemic stroke, is caused by a blood clot that blocks or plugs a blood vessel or artery in the brain. About 80 percent of all strokes are ischemic. The second, known as a hemorrhagic stroke, is caused by a blood vessel in the brain that breaks and bleeds into the brain. About 20 percent of strokes are hemorrhagic.

What disabilities can result from a stroke?

Although stroke is a disease of the brain, it can affect the entire body. The effects of a stroke range from mild to severe and can include paralysis, problems with thinking, problems with speaking, and emotional problems. Patients may also experience pain or numbness after a stroke.

What are the symptoms of a stroke?

Because stroke injures the brain, you may not realize that you are having a stroke. To a bystander, someone having a stroke may just look unaware or confused. Stroke victims have the best chance if someone around them recognizes the symptoms and acts quickly.

The symptoms of stroke are distinct because they happen quickly:

- Sudden numbness or weakness of the face, arm, or leg (especially on one side of the body)
- Sudden confusion, trouble speaking or understanding speech
- Sudden trouble seeing in one or both eyes
- Sudden trouble walking, dizziness, loss of balance or coordination
- Sudden severe headache with no known cause

What should a bystander do?

If you believe someone is having a stroke—if he or she suddenly loses the ability to speak, or move an arm or leg on one side, or experiences facial paralysis on one side—call 911 immediately.

Why is there a need to act fast?

Stroke is a medical emergency. Every minute counts when someone is having a stroke. The longer blood flow is cut off to the brain, the greater the damage.

Immediate treatment can save people's lives and enhance their chances for successful recovery.

Ischemic strokes, the most common type of strokes, can be treated with a drug called t-PA [tissue plasminogen activator], that dissolves blood clots obstructing blood flow to the brain. The window of opportunity to start treating stroke patients is 3 hours, but to be evaluated and receive treatment, patients need to get to the hospital within 60 minutes.

What is the benefit of treatment?

A 5-year study by the National Institute of Neurological Disorders and Stroke (NINDS) found that some stroke patients who received t-PA within 3 hours of the start of stroke symptoms were at least 30 percent more likely to recover with little or no disability after 3 months.

Chapter 11

Cardiovascular Emergencies: How to Help

Chapter Contents

Section 11.1

Cardiopulmonary Resuscitation (CPR)

CPR is a lifesaving procedure that is performed when someone's breathing or heartbeat has stopped, as in cases of electric shock, drowning, or heart attack. CPR is a combination of:

- rescue breathing, which provides oxygen to a person's lungs; and

- chest compressions, which keep the person's blood circulating.

Permanent brain damage or death can occur within minutes if a person's blood flow stops. Therefore, you must continue these procedures until the person's heartbeat and breathing return, or trained medical help arrives.

Considerations

CPR can be lifesaving, but it is best performed by those who have been trained in an accredited CPR course. The procedures described here are not a substitute for CPR training. (See www.americanheart.org for classes near you.)

Time is very important when dealing with an unconscious person who is not breathing. Permanent brain damage begins after only 4 minutes without oxygen, and death can occur as soon as 4–6 minutes later.

When a bystander starts CPR before emergency support arrives, the person has a much greater chance of surviving. Nevertheless, when most emergency workers arrive at a cardiac arrest, they usually find no one giving CPR.

Machines called automated external defibrillators (AEDs) can be found in many public places, and are available for home use. These machines have pads or paddles to place on the chest during a life-threatening emergency. They use computers to automatically check the heart rhythm and give a sudden shock if, and only if, that shock is needed to get the heart back into the right rhythm.

When using an AED, follow the instructions exactly.

Causes

In adults, major reasons that heartbeat and breathing stop include:

- drug overdose;
- excessive bleeding;
- heart disease (heart attack or abnormal heart rhythm);
- infection in the bloodstream (sepsis); and
- injuries and accidents.

Symptoms

- No breathing or difficulty breathing (gasping)
- No pulse
- Unconsciousness

First Aid

The following steps are based on instructions from the American Heart Association.

1. Check for responsiveness. Shake or tap the person gently. See if the person moves or makes a noise. Shout, "Are you OK?"

2. Call 911 if there is no response. Shout for help and send someone to call 911. If you are alone, call 911 and retrieve an AED (if available), even if you have to leave the person.

3. Carefully place the person on their back. If there is a chance the person has a spinal injury, two people should move the person to prevent the head and neck from twisting.

4. Open the airway. Lift up the chin with two fingers. At the same time, tilt the head by pushing down on the forehead with the other hand.

5. Look, listen, and feel for breathing. Place your ear close to the person's mouth and nose. Watch for chest movement. Feel for breath on your cheek.

6. If the person is not breathing or has trouble breathing:

   - cover their mouth tightly with your mouth;

   - pinch the nose closed;

   - keep the chin lifted and head tilted;

   - give two rescue breaths. Each breath should take about a second and make the chest rise.

7. Perform chest compressions:

   - Place the heel of one hand on the breastbone—right between the nipples.

   - Place the heel of your other hand on top of the first hand.

   - Position your body directly over your hands.

   - Give 30 chest compressions. These compressions should be **fast** and hard. Press down about 2 inches into the chest. Each time, let the chest rise completely. Count the 30 compressions quickly: "1,2,3,4,5,6,7,8,9,10,11,12,13,14,15,16, 17,18,19,20,21,22,23,24,25,26,27,28,29,30, off."

8. Give the person two more breaths. The chest should rise.

9. Continue CPR (30 chest compressions followed by 2 breaths, then repeat) until the person recovers or help arrives. If an AED for adults is available, use it as soon as possible.

   If the person starts breathing again, place them in the recovery position. Periodically recheck for breathing until help arrives.

Do Not

- If the person has normal breathing, coughing, or movement, **do not** begin chest compressions. Doing so may cause the heart to stop beating.

- Unless you are a health professional, **do not** check for a pulse. Only a health care professional is properly trained to check for a pulse.

When to Contact a Medical Professional

- If you have help, tell one person to call 911 while another person begins CPR.

- If you are alone, as soon as you determine that the person is unresponsive, call 911 immediately. Then begin CPR.

Prevention

To avoid injuries and heart problems that can lead to cardiac arrest:

- eliminate or reduce risk factors that contribute to heart disease, such as cigarette smoking, high cholesterol, high blood pressure, obesity, and stress;

- get plenty of exercise;

- see your doctor regularly;

- always use seat belts and drive safely; and

- avoid using illegal drugs.

Section 11.2

Automated External Defibrillators

"What is an Automated External Defibrillator?," reprinted with permission. © 2007 American Heart Association, Inc. (www.americanheart.org).

An automated external defibrillator (AED) is a lightweight, portable device that delivers an electric shock through the chest to the heart. The shock can stop an irregular rhythm and allow a normal rhythm to resume in a heart in sudden cardiac arrest. Sudden cardiac arrest is an abrupt loss of heart function. If it's not treated within minutes, it quickly leads to death. Most sudden cardiac arrests result from ventricular fibrillation. This is a rapid and unsynchronized heart rhythm originating in the heart's lower pumping chambers (the ventricles). The heart must be "defibrillated" quickly, because a victim's chance of surviving drops by 7 to 10 percent for every minute a normal heartbeat isn't restored.

Why are AEDs important?

AEDs make it possible for more people to respond to a medical emergency where defibrillation is required. Because AEDs are portable and can be used by nonmedical people, they can be made part of emergency response programs that also include rapid use of 911 and prompt delivery of CPR. All three of these activities are critical to improving survival from cardiac arrest.

How does an AED work?

A built-in computer checks a victim's heart rhythm through adhesive electrodes. The computer calculates whether defibrillation is needed. If it is, a recorded voice tells the rescuer to press the shock button on the AED. This shock momentarily stuns the heart and stops all activity and gives the heart an opportunity to resume beating effectively. Instructions guide the user through the process. AEDs advise a shock only for ventricular fibrillation or another life-threatening condition called pulseless ventricular tachycardia.

Who can use an AED?

Non-medical personnel such as police, fire service personnel, flight attendants, security guards, and other lay rescuers who have been properly trained can use AEDs.

Are AEDs safe to use?

AEDs are safe to use by anyone who's been trained to operate them. Studies have shown that 90 percent of the time AEDs are able to detect a rhythm that should be defibrillated.

And 95 percent of the time they are able to recommend **not** shocking when the computer shows defibrillation is not indicated.

Where should AEDs be placed?

All first-response vehicles, including ambulances, law-enforcement vehicles and many fire engines should have an AED. AEDs also should be placed in public areas such as sports arenas, gated communities, airports, office complexes, doctors' offices, and any other public or private place where large numbers of people gather or where people at high risk for heart attacks live.

Where can I get AED training?

The American Heart Association offers CPR and AED training through training centers.

To locate a training center, call your nearest American Heart Association office or 888-CPRLINE. You may also visit americanheart.org/cpr. Type in your ZIP code where requested on the home page to access contact information on training sites near you.

How can I learn more?

1. Talk to your doctor, nurse or other healthcare professionals. If you have heart disease or have had a stroke, members of your family also may be at higher risk. It's very important for them to make changes now to lower their risk.

2. Call 800-AHA-USA1 (800-242-8721) or visit americanheart.org to learn more about heart disease.

3. For information on stroke, call 888-4-STROKE (888-478-7653) or visit StrokeAssociation.org.

We have many other fact sheets and educational booklets to help you make healthier choices to reduce your risk, manage disease, or care for a loved one. Knowledge is power, so learn and live!

Part Two

Heart Disease

Chapter 12

Coronary Artery Disease

Coronary artery disease (CAD), also called coronary heart disease, is a condition in which plaque builds up inside the coronary arteries. These arteries supply your heart muscle with oxygen-rich blood.

Plaque is made up of fat, cholesterol, calcium, and other substances found in the blood. When plaque builds up in the arteries, the condition is called atherosclerosis.

Plaque narrows the arteries and reduces blood flow to your heart muscle. It also makes it more likely that blood clots will form in your arteries. Blood clots can partially or completely block blood flow.

Overview

When your coronary arteries are narrowed or blocked, oxygen-rich blood can't reach your heart muscle. This can cause angina or a heart attack.

Angina is chest pain or discomfort that occurs when not enough oxygen-rich blood is flowing to an area of your heart muscle. Angina may feel like pressure or squeezing in your chest. The pain also may occur in your shoulders, arms, neck, jaw, or back.

A heart attack occurs when blood flow to an area of your heart muscle is completely blocked. This prevents oxygen-rich blood from

Excerpted from text by the National Heart, Lung, and Blood Institute (NHLBI, www.nhlbi.nih.gov), part of the National Institutes of Health, February 2009.

reaching that area of heart muscle and causes it to die. Without quick treatment, a heart attack can lead to serious problems and even death.

Over time, CAD can weaken the heart muscle and lead to heart failure and arrhythmias. Heart failure is a condition in which your heart can't pump enough blood throughout your body. Arrhythmias are problems with the speed or rhythm of your heartbeat.

Outlook

CAD is the most common type of heart disease. It's the leading cause of death in the United States for both men and women. Lifestyle changes, medicines, and/or medical procedures can effectively prevent or treat CAD in most people.

Other Names for Coronary Artery Disease

- Atherosclerosis
- Coronary heart disease
- Hardening of the arteries
- Heart disease
- Ischemic heart disease
- Narrowing of the arteries

Causes of Coronary Artery Disease

Research suggests that coronary artery disease (CAD) starts when certain factors damage the inner layers of the coronary arteries. These factors include the following:

- Smoking
- High amounts of certain fats and cholesterol in the blood
- High blood pressure
- High amounts of sugar in the blood due to insulin resistance or diabetes

When damage occurs, your body starts a healing process. Excess fatty tissues release compounds that promote this process. This healing causes plaque to build up where the arteries are damaged.

The buildup of plaque in the coronary arteries may start in childhood. Over time, plaque can narrow or completely block some of your coronary arteries. This reduces the flow of oxygen-rich blood to your heart muscle.

Plaque also can crack, which causes blood cells called platelets to clump together and form blood clots at the site of the cracks. This narrows the arteries more and worsens angina or causes a heart attack.

Risk for Coronary Artery Disease

Coronary artery disease (CAD) is the leading cause of death in the United States for both men and women. Each year, more than half a million Americans die from CAD.

Certain traits, conditions, or habits may raise your chance of developing CAD. These conditions are known as risk factors.

You can control most risk factors and help prevent or delay CAD. Other risk factors can't be controlled.

Major Risk Factors

Many factors raise the risk of developing CAD. The more risk factors you have, the greater chance you have of developing CAD.

- **Unhealthy blood cholesterol levels:** This includes high LDL [low-density lipoprotein] cholesterol (sometimes called bad cholesterol) and low HDL [high-density lipoprotein] cholesterol (sometimes called good cholesterol).

- **High blood pressure:** Blood pressure is considered high if it stays at or above 140/90 mmHg [millimeters of mercury] over a period of time.

- **Smoking:** This can damage and tighten blood vessels, raise cholesterol levels, and raise blood pressure. Smoking also doesn't allow enough oxygen to reach the body's tissues.

- **Insulin resistance:** This condition occurs when the body can't use its own insulin properly. Insulin is a hormone that helps move blood sugar into cells where it's used.

- **Diabetes:** This is a disease in which the body's blood sugar level is high because the body doesn't make enough insulin or doesn't use its insulin properly.

- **Overweight or obesity:** Overweight is having extra body weight from muscle, bone, fat, and/or water. Obesity is having a high amount of extra body fat.

- **Metabolic syndrome:** Metabolic syndrome is the name for a group of risk factors linked to overweight and obesity that raise your chance for heart disease and other health problems, such as diabetes and stroke.

- **Lack of physical activity:** Lack of activity can worsen other risk factors for CAD.

- **Age:** As you get older, your risk for CAD increases. Genetic or lifestyle factors cause plaque to build in your arteries as you age. By the time you're middle-aged or older, enough plaque has built up to cause signs or symptoms. In men, the risk for CAD increases after age 45. In women, the risk for CAD risk increases after age 55.

- **Family history of early heart disease:** Your risk increases if your father or a brother was diagnosed with CAD before 55 years of age, or if your mother or a sister was diagnosed with CAD before 65 years of age.

Although age and a family history of early heart disease are risk factors, it doesn't mean that you will develop CAD if you have one or both.

Making lifestyle changes and/or taking medicines to treat other risk factors can often lessen genetic influences and prevent CAD from developing, even in older adults.

Emerging Risk Factors

Scientists continue to study other possible risk factors for CAD.

High levels of a protein called C-reactive protein (CRP) in the blood may raise the risk for CAD and heart attack. High levels of CRP are proof of inflammation in the body. Inflammation is the body's response to injury or infection. Damage to the arteries' inner walls seems to trigger inflammation and help plaque grow.

Research is under way to find out whether reducing inflammation and lowering CRP levels also can reduce the risk of developing CAD and having a heart attack.

High levels of fats called triglycerides in the blood also may raise the risk of CAD, particularly in women.

Other Factors That Affect Coronary Artery Disease

Other factors also may contribute to CAD. These include the following:

- **Sleep apnea:** Sleep apnea is a disorder in which your breathing stops or gets very shallow while you're sleeping. Untreated sleep apnea can raise your chances of having high blood pressure, diabetes, and even a heart attack or stroke.

- **Stress:** Research shows that the most commonly reported "trigger" for a heart attack is an emotionally upsetting event—particularly one involving anger.

- **Alcohol:** Heavy drinking can damage the heart muscle and worsen other risk factors for heart disease. Men should have no more than two drinks containing alcohol a day. Women should have no more than one drink containing alcohol a day.

Signs and Symptoms of Coronary Artery Disease

A common symptom of coronary artery disease (CAD) is angina. Angina is chest pain or discomfort that occurs when your heart muscle doesn't get enough oxygen-rich blood.

Angina may feel like pressure or a squeezing pain in your chest. You also may feel it in your shoulders, arms, neck, jaw, or back. This pain tends to get worse with activity and go away when you rest. Emotional stress also can trigger the pain.

Another common symptom of CAD is shortness of breath. This symptom happens if CAD causes heart failure. When you have heart failure, your heart can't pump enough blood throughout your body. Fluid builds up in your lungs, making it hard to breathe.

The severity of these symptoms varies. The symptoms may get more severe as the buildup of plaque continues to narrow the coronary arteries.

Signs and Symptoms of Heart Problems Linked to Coronary Artery Disease

Some people who have CAD have no signs or symptoms. This is called silent CAD. It may not be diagnosed until a person show signs and symptoms of a heart attack, heart failure, or an arrhythmia (an irregular heartbeat).

Heart attack: A heart attack happens when an area of plaque in a coronary artery breaks apart, causing a blood clot to form.

The blood clot cuts off most or all blood to the part of the heart muscle that's fed by that artery. Cells in the heart muscle die because they don't receive enough oxygen-rich blood. This can cause lasting damage to your heart.

The most common symptom of heart attack is chest pain or discomfort. Most heart attacks involve discomfort in the center of the chest that lasts for more than a few minutes or goes away and comes back. The discomfort can feel like pressure, squeezing, fullness, or pain. It can be mild or severe. Heart attack pain can sometimes feel like indigestion or heartburn.

Heart attacks also can cause upper body discomfort in one or both arms, the back, neck, jaw, or stomach. Shortness of breath or fatigue (tiredness) often may occur with or before chest discomfort. Other symptoms of heart attack are nausea (feeling sick to your stomach), vomiting, lightheadedness or fainting, and breaking out in a cold sweat.

Heart failure: Heart failure is a condition in which your heart can't pump enough blood to your body. Heart failure doesn't mean that your heart has stopped or is about to stop working. It means that your heart can't fill with enough blood or pump with enough force, or both.

This causes you to have shortness of breath and fatigue that tends to increase with activity. Heart failure also can cause swelling in your feet, ankles, legs, and abdomen.

Arrhythmia: An arrhythmia is a problem with the speed or rhythm of the heartbeat. When you have an arrhythmia, you may notice that your heart is skipping beats or beating too fast. Some people describe arrhythmias as a fluttering feeling in their chests. These feelings are called palpitations.

Some arrhythmias can cause your heart to suddenly stop beating. This condition is called sudden cardiac arrest (SCA). SCA can make you faint and it can cause death if it's not treated right away.

Diagnosing Coronary Artery Disease

Your doctor will diagnose coronary artery disease (CAD) based on the following:

- Your medical and family histories

- Your risk factors

- The results of a physical exam and diagnostic tests and procedures

Diagnostic Tests and Procedures

No single test can diagnose CAD. If your doctor thinks you have CAD, he or she will probably do one or more of the following tests.

EKG (electrocardiogram): An EKG is a simple test that detects and records the electrical activity of your heart. An EKG shows how fast your heart is beating and whether it has a regular rhythm. It also shows the strength and timing of electrical signals as they pass through each part of your heart.

Certain electrical patterns that the EKG detects can suggest whether CAD is likely. An EKG also can show signs of a previous or current heart attack.

Stress testing: During stress testing, you exercise to make your heart work hard and beat fast while heart tests are performed. If you can't exercise, you're given medicine to speed up your heart rate.

When your heart is beating fast and working hard, it needs more blood and oxygen. Arteries narrowed by plaque can't supply enough oxygen-rich blood to meet your heart's needs. A stress test can show possible signs of CAD, such as the following:

• Abnormal changes in your heart rate or blood pressure

• Symptoms such as shortness of breath or chest pain

• Abnormal changes in your heart rhythm or your heart's electrical activity

During the stress test, if you can't exercise for as long as what's considered normal for someone your age, it may be a sign that not enough blood is flowing to your heart. But other factors besides CAD can prevent you from exercising long enough (for example, lung diseases, anemia, or poor general fitness).

Some stress tests use a radioactive dye, sound waves, positron emission tomography (PET), or cardiac magnetic resonance imaging (MRI) to take pictures of your heart when it's working hard and when it's at rest.

These imaging stress tests can show how well blood is flowing in the different parts of your heart. They also can show how well your heart pumps blood when it beats.

Echocardiography: This test uses sound waves to create a moving picture of your heart. Echocardiography provides information about the size and shape of your heart and how well your heart chambers and valves are working.

The test also can identify areas of poor blood flow to the heart, areas of heart muscle that aren't contracting normally, and previous injury to the heart muscle caused by poor blood flow.

Chest x-ray: A chest x-ray takes a picture of the organs and structures inside the chest, including your heart, lungs, and blood vessels.

A chest x-ray can reveal signs of heart failure, as well as lung disorders and other causes of symptoms that aren't due to CAD.

Blood tests: Blood tests check the levels of certain fats, cholesterol, sugar, and proteins in your blood. Abnormal levels may show that you have risk factors for CAD.

Electron-beam computed tomography: Your doctor may recommend electron-beam computed tomography (EBCT). This test finds and measures calcium deposits (called calcifications) in and around the coronary arteries. The more calcium detected, the more likely you are to have CAD.

EBCT isn't used routinely to diagnose CAD, because its accuracy isn't yet known.

Coronary angiography and cardiac catheterization: Your doctor may ask you to have coronary angiography if other tests or factors show that you're likely to have CAD. This test uses dye and special x-rays to show the insides of your coronary arteries.

To get the dye into your coronary arteries, your doctor will use a procedure called cardiac catheterization. A long, thin, flexible tube called a catheter is put into a blood vessel in your arm, groin (upper thigh), or neck. The tube is then threaded into your coronary arteries, and the dye is released into your bloodstream. Special x-rays are taken while the dye is flowing through your coronary arteries.

Cardiac catheterization is usually done in a hospital. You're awake during the procedure. It usually causes little to no pain, although you may feel some soreness in the blood vessel where your doctor put the catheter.

Treating Coronary Artery Disease

Treatment for coronary artery disease (CAD) may include lifestyle changes, medicines, and medical procedures. The goals of treatments are to do the following:

- Relieve symptoms
- Reduce risk factors in an effort to slow, stop, or reverse the buildup of plaque
- Lower the risk of blood clots forming, which can cause a heart attack
- Widen or bypass clogged arteries
- Prevent complications of CAD

Lifestyle Changes

Making lifestyle changes can often help prevent or treat CAD. For some people, these changes may be the only treatment needed:

- Follow a heart-healthy eating plan to prevent or reduce high blood pressure and high blood cholesterol and to maintain a healthy weight
- Increase your physical activity. Check with your doctor first to find out how much and what kinds of activity are safe for you.
- Lose weight, if you're overweight or obese.
- Quit smoking, if you smoke. Avoid exposure to secondhand smoke.
- Learn to cope with and reduce stress.

Medicines

You may need medicines to treat CAD if lifestyle changes aren't enough. Medicines can do the following:

- Decrease the workload on your heart and relieve CAD symptoms
- Decrease your chance of having a heart attack or dying suddenly
- Lower your cholesterol and blood pressure
- Prevent blood clots
- Prevent or delay the need for a special procedure (for example, angioplasty or coronary artery bypass grafting [CABG])

Medicines used to treat CAD include anticoagulants, aspirin and other antiplatelet medicines, ACE [angiotensin-converting enzyme]

inhibitors, beta-blockers, calcium channel blockers, nitroglycerin, gly-
coprotein IIb-IIIa, statins, and fish oil and other supplements high
in omega-3 fatty acids.

Medical Procedures

You may need a medical procedure to treat CAD. Both angioplasty
and CABG are used as treatments.

Angioplasty opens blocked or narrowed coronary arteries. During
angioplasty, a thin tube with a balloon or other device on the end is
threaded through a blood vessel to the narrowed or blocked coronary
artery. Once in place, the balloon is inflated to push the plaque outward
against the wall of the artery. This widens the artery and restores the
flow of blood.

Angioplasty can improve blood flow to your heart, relieve chest pain,
and possibly prevent a heart attack. Sometimes a small mesh tube called
a stent is placed in the artery to keep it open after the procedure.

In CABG, arteries or veins from other areas in your body are used
to bypass (that is, go around) your narrowed coronary arteries. CABG
can improve blood flow to your heart, relieve chest pain, and possibly
prevent a heart attack.

You and your doctor can discuss which treatment is right for you.

Cardiac Rehabilitation

Your doctor may prescribe cardiac rehabilitation (rehab) for angina
or after CABG, angioplasty, or a heart attack. Cardiac rehab, when
combined with medicine and surgical treatments, can help you recover
faster, feel better, and develop a healthier lifestyle. Almost everyone
with CAD can benefit from cardiac rehab.

The cardiac rehab team may include doctors, nurses, exercise specialists, physical and occupational therapists, dietitians, and psychologists or other behavioral therapists.

Rehab has two parts:

- **Exercise training:** This part helps you learn how to exercise
  safely, strengthen your muscles, and improve your stamina. Your
  exercise plan will be based on your individual abilities, needs,
  and interests.

- **Education, counseling, and training:** This part of rehab
  helps you understand your heart condition and find ways to reduce your risk for future heart problems. The cardiac rehab

team will help you learn how to cope with the stress of adjusting to a new lifestyle and with your fears about the future.

Living with Coronary Artery Disease

Coronary artery disease (CAD) can cause serious complications. However, if you follow your doctor's advice and change your habits, you can prevent or reduce the chances of the following:

- Dying suddenly from heart problems
- Having a heart attack and permanently damaging your heart muscle
- Damaging your heart because of reduced oxygen supply
- Having arrhythmias (irregular heartbeats)

Ongoing Health Care Needs

Doing physical activity regularly, taking prescribed medicines, following a heart-healthy eating plan, and watching your weight can help control CAD.

See your doctor regularly to keep track of your blood pressure and blood cholesterol and blood sugar levels. A cholesterol blood test will show your levels of LDL ("bad") cholesterol, HDL ("good") cholesterol, and triglycerides. A fasting blood glucose test will check your blood sugar level and show if you're at risk for or have diabetes. These tests will show whether you need more treatments for your CAD.

Talk to your doctor about how often you should schedule office visits or blood tests. Between those visits, call your doctor if you develop any new symptoms or if your symptoms worsen.

CAD raises your risk for heart attack. Learn the symptoms of heart attack and arrhythmia. Call 911 if you have any of these symptoms for more than 5 minutes:

- Chest discomfort or pain, such as uncomfortable pressure, squeezing, fullness, or pain in the center of the chest that can be mild or strong (This discomfort or pain lasts more than a few minutes or goes away and comes back.)
- Upper body discomfort in one or both arms, the back, neck, jaw, or stomach
- Shortness of breath, which may occur with or before chest discomfort

113

It's important to know the difference between angina and a heart attack. During a heart attack, the pain is usually more severe than angina, and it doesn't go away when you rest or take medicine. If you don't know whether your chest pain is angina or a heart attack, call 911.

Let the people you see regularly know you're at risk for a heart attack. They can seek emergency care if you suddenly faint, collapse, or develop other severe symptoms.

You may feel depressed or anxious if you've been diagnosed with CAD and/or had a heart attack. You may worry about heart problems or making lifestyle changes that are necessary for your health. Your doctor may recommend medicine, professional counseling, or relaxation therapy if you have depression or anxiety.

Physical activity can improve mental well-being, but you should talk to your doctor before starting any fitness activities. It's important to treat any anxiety or depression that develops because it raises your risk of having a heart attack.

Chapter 13

Angina

Angina is chest pain or discomfort that occurs when an area of your heart muscle doesn't get enough oxygen-rich blood. Angina may feel like pressure or squeezing in your chest. The pain also may occur in your shoulders, arms, neck, jaw, or back. It can feel like indigestion.

Angina itself isn't a disease. Rather, it's a symptom of an underlying heart problem. Angina is usually a symptom of coronary artery disease (CAD), the most common type of heart disease.

CAD occurs when a fatty material called plaque builds up on the inner walls of the coronary arteries. These arteries carry oxygen-rich blood to your heart. When plaque builds up in the arteries, the condition is called atherosclerosis.

Plaque causes the coronary arteries to become narrow and stiff. The flow of oxygen-rich blood to the heart muscle is reduced. This causes pain and can lead to a heart attack.

Types of Angina

The three types of angina are stable, unstable, and variant (Prinzmetal). Knowing how the types are different is important. This is because they have different symptoms and require different treatment.

Excerpted from text by the National Heart, Lung, and Blood Institute (NHLBI, www.nhlbi.nih.gov), part of the National Institutes of Health, November 2007.

115

Stable Angina

Stable angina is the most common type. It occurs when the heart is working harder than usual. Stable angina has a regular pattern. If you know you have stable angina, you can learn to recognize the pattern and predict when the pain will occur.

The pain usually goes away in a few minutes after you rest or take your angina medicine.

Stable angina isn't a heart attack, but it makes a heart attack more likely in the future.

Unstable Angina

Unstable angina doesn't follow a pattern. It can occur with or without physical exertion and isn't relieved by rest or medicine.

Unstable angina is very dangerous and needs emergency treatment. It's a sign that a heart attack may happen soon.

Variant (Prinzmetal) Angina

Variant angina is rare. It usually occurs while you're at rest. The pain can be severe. It usually happens between midnight and early morning. This type of angina is relieved by medicine.

Overview

It's thought that nearly 7 million people in the United States suffer from angina. About 400,000 patients go to their doctors with new cases of angina every year.

Angina occurs equally in men and women. It can be a sign of heart disease, even when initial tests don't show evidence of CAD.

Not all chest pain or discomfort is angina. A heart attack, lung problems (such as an infection or a blood clot), heartburn, or a panic attack also can cause chest pain or discomfort. All chest pain should be checked by a doctor.

Other Names for Angina

- Angina pectoris
- Acute coronary syndrome
- Chest pain
- Coronary artery spasms

- Prinzmetal angina
- Stable or common angina
- Unstable angina
- Variant angina

Causes of Angina

Underlying Causes

Angina is a symptom of an underlying heart condition. Angina pain is the result of reduced blood flow to an area of heart muscle. Coronary artery disease (CAD) usually causes the reduced blood flow.

This means that the underlying causes of angina are generally the same as the underlying causes of CAD.

Research suggests that damage to the inner layers of the coronary arteries causes CAD. Smoking, high levels of fat and cholesterol in the blood, high blood pressure, and a high level of sugar in the blood (due to insulin resistance or diabetes) can damage the coronary arteries.

When damage occurs, your body starts a healing process. Excess fatty tissues release compounds that promote this process. This healing causes plaque to build up where the arteries are damaged. Plaque narrows or blocks the arteries, reducing blood flow to the heart muscle.

Some plaque is hard and stable and leads to narrowed and hardened arteries. Other plaque is soft and is more likely to break open and cause blood clots.

The buildup of plaque on the arteries' inner walls can cause angina in two ways. It can 1) narrow the arteries and greatly reduce blood flow to the heart and 2) form blood clots that partially or totally block the arteries.

Immediate Causes

There are different triggers for angina pain, depending on the type of angina you have.

Stable angina: Physical exertion is the most common trigger of stable angina. Severely narrowed arteries may allow enough blood to reach the heart when the demand for oxygen is low (such as when you're sitting). But with exertion, like walking up a hill or climbing stairs, the heart works harder and needs more oxygen.

Other triggers of stable angina include the following:

- Emotional stress
- Exposure to very hot or cold temperatures
- Heavy meals
- Smoking

Unstable angina: Blood clots that partially or totally block an artery cause unstable angina. If plaque in an artery ruptures or breaks open, blood clots may form. This creates a larger blockage. A clot may grow large enough to completely block the artery and cause a heart attack.

Blood clots may form, partly dissolve, and later form again. Angina can occur each time a clot blocks an artery.

Variant angina: A spasm in a coronary artery causes variant angina. The spasm causes the walls of the artery to tighten and narrow. Blood flow to the heart slows or stops. Variant angina may occur in people with or without CAD.

Other causes of spasms in the coronary arteries include the following:

- Exposure to cold
- Emotional stress
- Medicines that tighten or narrow blood vessels
- Smoking
- Cocaine use

Risk for Angina

Angina is a symptom of an underlying heart condition, usually coronary artery disease (CAD). So if you're at risk for CAD, you're also at risk for angina.

Risk factors for CAD include the following:

- Unhealthy cholesterol levels
- High blood pressure
- Cigarette smoking
- Insulin resistance or diabetes
- Overweight or obesity
- Metabolic syndrome

- Lack of physical activity
- Age (The risk increases for men after 45 years of age and for women after 55 years of age.)
- Family history of early heart disease

Populations Affected

People sometimes think that because men have more heart attacks than women, men also suffer from angina more often. In fact, angina occurs equally among women and men. It can be a sign of heart disease, even when initial tests don't show evidence of CAD.

Unstable angina occurs more often in older adults.

Variant angina is rare. It accounts for only about two out of 100 cases of angina. People who have variant angina are often younger than those who have other forms of angina.

Signs and Symptoms of Angina

Pain and discomfort are the main symptoms of angina. Angina is often described as pressure, squeezing, burning, or tightness in the chest. It usually starts in the chest behind the breastbone.

Pain from angina also can occur in the arms, shoulders, neck, jaw, throat, or back. It may feel like indigestion.

Some people say that angina discomfort is hard to describe or that they can't tell exactly where the pain is coming from.

Symptoms such as nausea (feeling sick to your stomach), fatigue (tiredness), shortness of breath, sweating, lightheadedness, or weakness also may occur. Women are more likely to feel discomfort in their back, shoulders, and abdomen.

Symptoms vary based on the type of angina.

Stable Angina

The pain or discomfort has the following characteristics:

- Occurs when the heart must work harder, usually during physical exertion
- Doesn't come as a surprise, and episodes of pain tend to be alike
- Usually lasts a short time (5 minutes or less)
- Is relieved by rest or medicine

- May feel like gas or indigestion
- May feel like chest pain that spreads to the arms, back, or other areas

Unstable Angina

The pain or discomfort has the following characteristics:

- Often occurs at rest, while sleeping at night, or with little physical exertion
- Comes as a surprise
- Is more severe and lasts longer (as long as 30 minutes) than episodes of stable angina
- Is usually not relieved with rest or medicine
- May get continually worse
- May mean that a heart attack will happen soon

Variant Angina

The pain or discomfort has the following characteristics:

- Usually occurs at rest and during the night or early morning hours
- Tends to be severe
- Is relieved by medicine

Lasting Chest Pain

Chest pain that lasts longer than a few minutes and isn't relieved by rest or angina medicine may mean you're having (or are about to have) a heart attack. Call 911 right away.

Diagnosing Angina

The most important issues to address when you go to the doctor with chest pain are what's causing the chest pain and whether you're having or are about to have a heart attack.

Angina is a symptom of an underlying heart problem, usually coronary artery disease (CAD). The type of angina pain you have can be a sign of how severe the CAD is and whether it's likely to cause a heart attack.

If you have chest pain, your doctor will want to find out whether it's angina. He or she also will want to know whether the angina is stable or unstable. If it's unstable, you may need emergency medical attention to try to prevent a heart attack.

To diagnose chest pain as stable or unstable angina, your doctor will do a physical exam, ask about your symptoms, and ask about your risk factors and your family history of CAD or other heart disease.

He or she may also ask questions about your symptoms, such as the following:

- What brings on the pain or discomfort and what relieves it?
- What does the pain or discomfort feel like (for example, heaviness or tightness)?
- How often does the pain occur?
- Where do you feel the pain or discomfort?
- How severe is the pain or discomfort?
- How long does the pain or discomfort last?

Diagnostic Tests and Procedures

If your doctor suspects that you have unstable angina or that your angina is related to a serious heart condition, he or she may order one or more tests.

EKG (electrocardiogram): An EKG is a simple test that detects and records the electrical activity of your heart. An EKG shows how fast your heart is beating and whether it has a regular rhythm. It also shows the strength and timing of electrical signals as they pass through each part of your heart.

Certain electrical patterns that the EKG detects can suggest whether CAD is likely. An EKG also can show signs of a previous or current heart attack.

However, some people with angina have a normal EKG.

Stress testing: During stress testing, you exercise to make your heart work hard and beat fast while heart tests are performed. If you can't exercise, you're given medicine to speed up your heart rate.

During exercise stress testing, your blood pressure and EKG readings are checked while you walk or run on a treadmill or pedal a bicycle. Other heart tests, such as nuclear heart scanning or echocardiography, also can be done at the same time.

121

If you're unable to exercise, a medicine can be injected into your bloodstream to make your heart work hard and beat fast. Nuclear heart scanning or echocardiography is then usually done.

When your heart is beating fast and working hard, it needs more blood and oxygen. Arteries narrowed by plaque can't supply enough oxygen-rich blood to meet your heart's needs.

A stress test can show possible signs of CAD, such as the following:

• Abnormal changes in your heart rate or blood pressure

• Symptoms such as shortness of breath or chest pain

• Abnormal changes in your heart rhythm or your heart's electrical activity

Chest x-ray: A chest x-ray takes a picture of the organs and structures inside the chest, including your heart, lungs, and blood vessels. A chest x-ray can reveal signs of heart failure, as well as lung disorders and other causes of symptoms that aren't due to CAD.

Coronary angiography and cardiac catheterization: Your doctor may ask you to have coronary angiography if other tests or factors show that you're likely to have CAD. This test uses dye and special x-rays to show the insides of your coronary arteries.

To get the dye into your coronary arteries, your doctor will use a procedure called cardiac catheterization. A long, thin, flexible tube called a catheter is put into a blood vessel in your arm, groin (upper thigh), or neck. The tube is then threaded into your coronary arteries, and the dye is released into your bloodstream. Special x-rays are taken while the dye is flowing through the coronary arteries.

Cardiac catheterization is usually done in a hospital. You're awake during the procedure. It usually causes little to no pain, although you may feel some soreness in the blood vessel where your doctor put the catheter.

Blood tests: Blood tests check the levels of certain fats, cholesterol, sugar, and proteins in your blood. Abnormal levels may show that you have risk factors for CAD.

Your doctor may order a blood test to check the level of C-reactive protein (CRP) in your blood. Some studies suggest that high levels of CRP in the blood may increase the risk for CAD and heart attack.

Your doctor also may order a blood test to check for low hemoglobin in your blood. Hemoglobin is an iron-rich protein in the red blood cells that carries oxygen from the lungs to all parts of your body. If you have low hemoglobin, you may have a condition called anemia.

Treating Angina

Treatments for angina include lifestyle changes, medicines, medical procedures, and cardiac rehabilitation (rehab). The main goals of treatment are to reduce pain and discomfort and how often it occurs and prevent or lower the risk of heart attack and death by treating the underlying heart condition.

Lifestyle changes and medicines may be the only treatments needed if your symptoms are mild and aren't getting worse. When lifestyle changes and medicines don't control angina, you may need medical procedures or cardiac rehab.

Unstable angina is an emergency condition that requires treatment in the hospital.

Chapter 14

Heart Attack (Myocardial Infarction)

A heart attack occurs when blood flow to a section of heart muscle becomes blocked. If the flow of blood isn't restored quickly, the section of heart muscle becomes damaged from lack of oxygen and begins to die.

Heart attack is a leading killer of both men and women in the United States. But fortunately, today there are excellent treatments for heart attack that can save lives and prevent disabilities. Treatment is most effective when started within 1 hour of the beginning of symptoms. If you think you or someone you're with is having a heart attack, call 911 right away.

Overview

Heart attacks occur most often as a result of a condition called coronary artery disease (CAD). In CAD, a fatty material called plaque builds up over many years on the inside walls of the coronary arteries (the arteries that supply blood and oxygen to your heart). Eventually, an area of plaque can rupture, causing a blood clot to form on the surface of the plaque. If the clot becomes large enough, it can mostly or completely block the flow of oxygen-rich blood to the part of the heart muscle fed by the artery.

Excerpted from "Heart Attack," by the National Heart, Lung, and Blood Institute (NHLBI, www.nhlbi.nih.gov), part of the National Institutes of Health, March 2008.

During a heart attack, if the blockage in the coronary artery isn't treated quickly, the heart muscle will begin to die and be replaced by scar tissue. This heart damage may not be obvious, or it may cause severe or long-lasting problems.

Severe problems linked to heart attack can include heart failure and life-threatening arrhythmias (irregular heartbeats). Heart failure is a condition in which the heart can't pump enough blood throughout the body. Ventricular fibrillation is a serious arrhythmia that can cause death if not treated quickly.

Get Help Quickly

Acting fast at the first sign of heart attack symptoms can save your life and limit damage to your heart. Treatment is most effective when started within 1 hour of the beginning of symptoms.

The most common heart attack signs and symptoms are the following:

- Chest discomfort or pain, such as uncomfortable pressure, squeezing, fullness, or pain in the center of the chest that can be mild or strong (This discomfort or pain lasts more than a few minutes or goes away and comes back.)

- Upper body discomfort in one or both arms, the back, neck, jaw, or stomach

- Shortness of breath may occur with or before chest discomfort

- Other signs include nausea (feeling sick to your stomach), vomiting, lightheadedness or fainting, or breaking out in a cold sweat

If you think you or someone you know may be having a heart attack, take the following steps:

- Call 911 within a few minutes—5 at the most—of the start of symptoms.

- If your symptoms stop completely in less than 5 minutes, still call your doctor.

- Only take an ambulance to the hospital. Going in a private car can delay treatment.

- Take a nitroglycerin pill if your doctor has prescribed this type of medicine.

Outlook

Each year, about 1.1 million people in the United States have heart attacks, and almost half of them die. CAD, which often results in a heart attack, is the leading killer of both men and women in the United States.

Many more people could recover from heart attacks if they got help faster. Of the people who die from heart attacks, about half die within an hour of the first symptoms and before they reach the hospital.

Other Names for a Heart Attack

- Myocardial infarction or MI
- Acute myocardial infarction or AMI
- Acute coronary syndrome
- Coronary thrombosis
- Coronary occlusion

Causes of Heart Attack

Most heart attacks occur as a result of coronary artery disease (CAD). CAD is the buildup over time of a material called plaque on the inner walls of the coronary arteries. Eventually, a section of plaque can break open, causing a blood clot to form at the site. A heart attack occurs if the clot becomes large enough to cut off most or all of the blood flow through the artery.

The blocked blood flow prevents oxygen-rich blood from reaching the part of the heart muscle fed by the artery. The lack of oxygen damages the heart muscle. If the blockage isn't treated quickly, the damaged heart muscle begins to die.

Heart attack also can occur due to problems with the very small, microscopic blood vessels of the heart. This condition is called microvascular disease. It's believed to be more common in women than in men.

Another less common cause of heart attack is a severe spasm (tightening) of a coronary artery that cuts off blood flow through the artery. These spasms can occur in coronary arteries that don't have CAD. It's not always clear what causes a coronary artery spasm, but sometimes it can be related to the following:

- Taking certain drugs, such as cocaine

- Emotional stress or pain
- Exposure to extreme cold
- Cigarette smoking

Risk for Heart Attack

Certain risk factors make it more likely that you will develop coronary artery disease (CAD) and have a heart attack. Some risk factors for heart attack can be controlled, while others can't.

Major risk factors for heart attack that you can control include the following:

- Smoking
- High blood pressure
- High blood cholesterol
- Overweight and obesity
- Physical inactivity
- Diabetes (high blood sugar)

Risk factors that you can't change include the following:

- **Age:** Risk increases for men older than 45 years and for women older than 55 years (or after menopause).
- **Family history of early CAD:** Your risk increases if your father or a brother was diagnosed with CAD before 55 years of age, or if your mother or a sister was diagnosed with CAD before 65 years of age.

Certain CAD risk factors tend to occur together. When they do, it's called metabolic syndrome. In general, a person with metabolic syndrome is twice as likely to develop heart disease and five times as likely to develop diabetes as someone without metabolic syndrome.

Signs and Symptoms of a Heart Attack

Not all heart attacks begin with a sudden, crushing pain that is often shown on TV or in the movies. The warning signs and symptoms of a heart attack aren't the same for everyone. Many heart attacks start slowly as mild pain or discomfort. Some people don't have symptoms at all (this is called a silent heart attack).

Chest Pain or Discomfort

The most common symptom of heart attack is chest pain or discomfort. Most heart attacks involve discomfort in the center of the chest that lasts for more than a few minutes or goes away and comes back. The discomfort can feel like uncomfortable pressure, squeezing, fullness, or pain. It can be mild or severe. Heart attack pain can sometimes feel like indigestion or heartburn.

The symptoms of angina can be similar to the symptoms of a heart attack. Angina is pain in the chest that occurs in people with coronary artery disease, usually when they're active. Angina pain usually lasts for only a few minutes and goes away with rest. Angina that doesn't go away or that changes from its usual pattern (occurs more frequently or occurs at rest) can be a sign of the beginning of a heart attack and should be checked by a doctor right away.

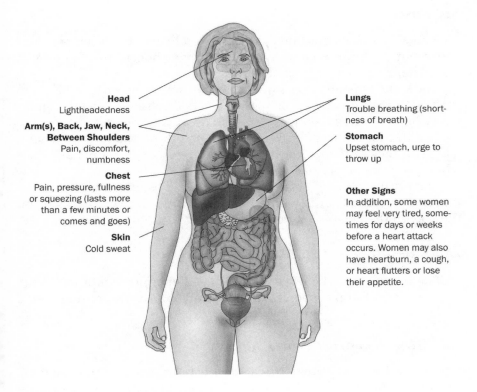

Head
Lightheadedness

Arm(s), Back, Jaw, Neck, Between Shoulders
Pain, discomfort, numbness

Chest
Pain, pressure, fullness or squeezing (lasts more than a few minutes or comes and goes)

Skin
Cold sweat

Lungs
Trouble breathing (shortness of breath)

Stomach
Upset stomach, urge to throw up

Other Signs
In addition, some women may feel very tired, sometimes for days or weeks before a heart attack occurs. Women may also have heartburn, a cough, or heart flutters or lose their appetite.

Figure 14.1. Heart attack warning signs.

Other Common Signs and Symptoms

Other common signs and symptoms that a person can have during a heart attack include the following:

- Upper body discomfort in one or both arms, the back, neck, jaw, or stomach
- Shortness of breath may often occur with or before chest discomfort
- Nausea (feeling sick to your stomach), vomiting, lightheadedness or fainting, or breaking out in a cold sweat

Not everyone having a heart attack experiences the typical symptoms. If you've already had a heart attack, your symptoms may not be the same for another one. The more signs and symptoms you have, the more likely it is that you're having a heart attack.

Act Fast

Sometimes the signs and symptoms of a heart attack happen suddenly, but they can also develop slowly, over hours, days, and even weeks before a heart attack occurs.

Know the warning signs of a heart attack so you can act fast to get treatment for yourself or someone else. The sooner you get emergency help, the less damage there will be to your heart.

Call 911 for help within 5 minutes if you think you may be having a heart attack or if your chest pain doesn't go away as it usually does when you take prescribed medicine.

Don't drive yourself or anyone else to the hospital. Call an ambulance so that medical personnel can begin life-saving treatment on the way to the emergency room.

Diagnosing Heart Attack

The diagnosis of heart attack is based on your symptoms, your personal and family medical history, and the results of diagnostic tests.

EKG (Electrocardiogram)

This test detects and records the electrical activity of the heart. Certain changes in the appearance of the electrical waves on an EKG are strong evidence of a heart attack. An EKG also can show if you're having arrhythmias (abnormal heartbeats), which a heart attack (and other conditions) can cause.

Blood Tests

During a heart attack, heart muscle cells die and burst open, letting certain proteins out in the bloodstream. Blood tests can measure the amount of these proteins in the bloodstream. Higher than normal levels of these proteins in the bloodstream is evidence of a heart attack.

Commonly used blood tests include troponin tests, CK or CK–MB tests, and serum myoglobin tests. Blood tests are often repeated to check for changes over time.

Coronary Angiography

Coronary angiography is a special x-ray exam of the heart and blood vessels. It's often done during a heart attack to help pinpoint blockages in the coronary arteries.

The doctor passes a catheter (a thin, flexible tube) through an artery in your arm or groin (upper thigh) and threads it to your heart. This procedure—called cardiac catheterization—is part of coronary angiography.

A dye that can be seen on x-ray is injected into the bloodstream through the tip of the catheter. The dye lets the doctor study the flow of blood through the heart and blood vessels. If a blockage is found, another procedure, called angioplasty, may be used to restore blood flow through the artery.

Sometimes during angioplasty, the doctor will place a stent (a small mesh tube) in the artery to help keep the artery open.

Treating Heart Attack

Early treatment can prevent or limit damage to the heart muscle. Acting fast, at the first symptoms of heart attack, can save your life. Medical personnel can begin diagnosis and treatment even before you get to the hospital.

Certain treatments are usually started right away if a heart attack is suspected, even before the diagnosis is confirmed. These include the following:

- Oxygen
- Aspirin to prevent further blood clotting

- Nitroglycerin, to reduce the workload on the heart and improve blood flow through the coronary arteries
- Treatment for chest pain

Once the diagnosis of heart attack is confirmed or strongly suspected, treatments to try to restore blood flow to the heart are started as soon as possible. Treatments include medicines and medical procedures.

Medicines

A number of different kinds of medicines may be used to treat heart attack. They include the following.

Thrombolytic medicines: These medicines (also called clot busters) are used to dissolve blood clots that are blocking the coronary arteries. To be most effective, these medicines must be given within 1 hour after the start of heart attack symptoms.

Beta-blockers: These medicines decrease the workload on your heart. Beta-blockers also are used to relieve chest pain or discomfort and to help prevent additional heart attacks. Beta-blockers also are used to correct arrhythmias (irregular heartbeats).

Angiotensin-converting enzyme (ACE) inhibitors: These medicines lower blood pressure and reduce the strain on your heart. They also help slow down further weakening of the heart muscle.

Anticoagulants: These medicines thin the blood and prevent clots from forming in your arteries.

Antiplatelet medicines: These medicines (such as aspirin and clopidogrel) stop platelets (a type of blood cell) from clumping together and forming unwanted clots.

Other medicines: Medicines may also be given to relieve pain and anxiety, and to treat arrhythmias, which often occur during a heart attack.

Medical Procedures

If medicines can't stop a heart attack, medical procedures—surgical or nonsurgical—may be used. These procedures include the following.

Angioplasty: This nonsurgical procedure can be used to open coronary arteries that are blocked by a blood clot. During angioplasty, a catheter (a thin, flexible tube) with a balloon on the end is threaded through a blood vessel to the blocked coronary artery. Then, the balloon is inflated to push the plaque against the wall of the artery. This widens the inside of the artery, restoring blood flow.

During angioplasty, a small mesh tube called a stent may be put in the artery to help keep it open. Some stents are coated with medicines that help prevent the artery from becoming blocked again.

Coronary artery bypass grafting: Coronary artery bypass grafting is a surgery in which arteries or veins are taken from other areas of your body and sewn in place to bypass (that is, go around) blocked coronary arteries. This provides a new route for blood flow to the heart muscle.

Treatment after You Leave the Hospital

Most people spend several days in the hospital after a heart attack. When you leave the hospital, treatment doesn't stop. At home, your treatment may include daily medicines and cardiac rehabilitation (rehab). Your doctor may recommend lifestyle changes, including quitting smoking, losing weight, changing your diet, and increasing your physical activity, to lower your chances of having another heart attack.

Cardiac rehabilitation: Your doctor may prescribe cardiac rehab to help you recover from a heart attack and to help prevent another heart attack. Almost everyone who has had a heart attack can benefit from rehab. The heart is a muscle, and the right exercise will strengthen it.

But cardiac rehab isn't only about exercise. It also includes education, counseling, and learning about reducing your risk factors. Rehab will help you learn the best way to take care of yourself after having a heart attack and how to prevent having another one.

The cardiac rehab team may include doctors (your family doctor, a cardiologist, and/or a surgeon), nurses, exercise specialists, physical and occupational therapists, dietitians, and psychologists or other behavioral therapists.

Preventing Heart Attack

Lowering your risk factors for coronary artery disease (CAD) can help you prevent a heart attack. Even if you already have CAD, you can still take steps to lower your risk of heart attack.

Reducing the risk of heart attack usually means making healthy lifestyle choices. You also may need treatment for medical conditions that raise your risk.

To help prevent heart attack, do the following:

• Follow a low-fat diet rich in fruits and vegetables. Pay careful attention to the amounts and types of fat in your diet. Lower your salt intake. These changes can help lower high blood pressure and high blood cholesterol.

• Lose weight if you're overweight or obese.

• Quit smoking.

• Do physical activity to improve heart fitness. Ask your doctor how much and what kinds of physical activity are safe for you.

Treat Related Conditions

In addition to making lifestyle changes, you can help prevent heart attacks by treating conditions you have that make a heart attack more likely:

• **High blood cholesterol:** You may need medicine to lower your cholesterol if diet and exercise aren't enough.

• **High blood pressure:** You may need medicine to keep your blood pressure under control.

• **Diabetes (high blood sugar):** If you have diabetes, control your blood sugar levels through diet and physical activity as your doctor recommends). If needed, take medicine as prescribed.

Have an Emergency Action Plan

Make sure that you have an emergency action plan in case you or someone else in your family has a heart attack. This is especially important if you're at high risk or have already had a heart attack.

Talk with your doctor about the signs and symptoms of heart attack, when you should call 911, and steps you can take while waiting for medical help to arrive.

Life after a Heart Attack

Many people survive heart attacks and live active and full lives. If you get help quickly, treatment can limit the damage to your heart muscle. Less heart damage improves your chances for a better quality of life after a heart attack.

Medical Followup

After a heart attack, you will need treatment for coronary artery disease to prevent another heart attack. Your doctor may recommend the following:

- Lifestyle changes, such as quitting smoking, following a healthy diet, increasing your physical activity, and losing weight, if needed
- Medicines to control chest pain or discomfort, blood pressure, blood cholesterol, and your heart's workload
- Participation in a cardiac rehabilitation program

Returning to Normal Activities

After a heart attack, most people without chest pain or discomfort or other complications can safely return to most of their normal activities within a few weeks. Most can begin walking immediately. Sexual activity also can begin within a few weeks for most patients. Discuss with your doctor a safe schedule for returning to your normal activities.

If allowed by state law, driving can usually begin within a week for most patients who don't have chest pain or discomfort or other complications. Each state has rules about driving a motor vehicle following a serious illness. People with complications shouldn't drive until their symptoms have been stable for a few weeks.

Anxiety and Depression after a Heart Attack

After a heart attack, many people worry about having another heart attack. Sometimes they feel depressed and have trouble adjusting to the new lifestyle that's needed to limit further heart trouble. Your doctor may recommend medicine or professional counseling if you have depression or anxiety. Physical activity can improve mental well-being, but you should consult with your doctor before starting any fitness activities.

Risk of a Repeat Heart Attack

Once you've had a heart attack, you're at higher risk for another one. It's important to know the difference between angina and a heart attack. The pain of angina usually occurs after exertion and goes away in a few minutes when you rest or take medicine as directed. During a heart attack, the pain is usually more severe than angina, and it doesn't go away when you rest or take medicine. If you don't know whether your chest pain is angina or a heart attack, call 911.

Remember, the symptoms of a second heart attack may not be the same as those of a first heart attack. Don't take a chance if you're in doubt. Always call 911 within 5 minutes if you or someone you're with has symptoms of a heart attack.

Unfortunately, most heart attack victims wait 2 hours or more after their symptoms begin before they seek medical help. This delay can result in lasting heart damage or death.

Chapter 15

Sudden Cardiac Arrest

Sudden cardiac arrest (SCA) is a condition in which the heart suddenly and unexpectedly stops beating. When this happens, blood stops flowing to the brain and other vital organs.

SCA usually causes death if it's not treated within minutes.

To understand SCA, it helps to understand how the heart works. The heart has an internal electrical system that controls the rate and rhythm of the heartbeat. Problems with the electrical system can cause abnormal heart rhythms called arrhythmias.

There are many types of arrhythmias. During an arrhythmia, the heart can beat too fast, too slow, or with an irregular rhythm. Some arrhythmias can cause the heart to stop pumping blood to the body. These are the type of arrhythmias that cause SCA.

SCA is not the same as a heart attack. A heart attack occurs when blood flow to part of the heart muscle is blocked. During a heart attack, the heart usually doesn't suddenly stop beating. SCA, however, may happen after or during recovery from a heart attack.

People who have heart disease are at increased risk for SCA. However, most SCAs happen in people who appear healthy and have no known heart disease or other risk factors for SCA.

Ninety-five percent of people who have SCA die from it—most within minutes. Rapid treatment of SCA with a defibrillator can be

Excerpted from text by the National Heart, Lung, and Blood Institute (NHLBI, www.nhlbi.nih.gov), part of the National Institutes of Health, February 2009.

lifesaving. A defibrillator is a device that sends an electric shock to the heart to try to restore its normal rhythm.

Automated external defibrillators (AEDs), which often are found in public places like airports and office buildings, can be used by bystanders to save the lives of people who are having SCA.

Causes of Sudden Cardiac Arrest

Most cases of sudden cardiac arrest (SCA) are due to ventricular fibrillation (v-fib). V-fib is a type of arrhythmia. In v-fib, the ventricles (the heart's lower chambers) don't beat normally. Instead, they quiver very rapidly and irregularly.

When this happens, the heart pumps little or no blood to the body. V-fib is fatal if not treated within a few minutes.

Other electrical problems in the heart also can cause SCA. For example, SCA can occur if the rate of the heart's electrical signals becomes very slow and stops. SCA also can occur if the heart muscle doesn't respond to the heart's electrical signals.

Several factors can cause the electrical problems that lead to SCA. These factors include the following:

- Coronary artery disease (CAD), which reduces blood flow to the heart muscle

- Severe physical stress, which raises the risk for abnormal electrical activity in the heart

- Inherited disorders that disrupt the heart's electrical activity

- Structural changes in the heart that cause electrical signals to spread abnormally

Several research studies are under way to try to find the exact causes of SCA and how to prevent them.

Risk for Sudden Cardiac Arrest

Each year, between 250,000 and 450,000 Americans have sudden cardiac arrest (SCA). SCA occurs most often in people in their midthirties to mid-forties. It appears to affect men twice as often as women.

SCA rarely occurs in children unless they have inherited problems that make them likely to have SCA. Only a very small number of children have SCA each year.

Signs and Symptoms of Sudden Cardiac Arrest

Usually, the first sign of sudden cardiac arrest (SCA) is loss of consciousness (fainting). At the same time, no heartbeat (or pulse) can be felt.

Some people may have a racing heartbeat or feel dizzy or lightheaded just before they faint. Within an hour before SCA, some people have chest pain, shortness of breath, nausea (feeling sick to the stomach), or vomiting.

Diagnosing Sudden Cardiac Arrest

Sudden cardiac arrest (SCA) happens without warning. It requires immediate emergency treatment. Doctors rarely can diagnose SCA with medical tests as it's happening.

Instead, SCA often is diagnosed after it happens. Doctors do this by ruling out other causes of a person's sudden collapse.

Treating Sudden Cardiac Arrest

Emergency Treatment

Sudden cardiac arrest (SCA) requires immediate treatment with a defibrillator. This device sends an electric shock to the heart. The electric shock may restore a normal rhythm to a heart that's stopped beating.

To work well, defibrillation must be done within minutes of SCA. With every minute that passes, the chances of surviving SCA drop rapidly.

Police, emergency medical technicians, and other first responders usually are trained and equipped to use a defibrillator. Call 911 right away if someone has signs or symptoms of SCA. The sooner help is called, the sooner potentially lifesaving treatment can be done.

Automated External Defibrillators

Automated external defibrillators (AEDs) are special defibrillators that untrained bystanders can use. These devices are becoming more available in public places like airports, office buildings, and shopping centers.

AEDs are programmed to give an electric shock if they detect a dangerous arrhythmia, such as ventricular fibrillation. This prevents giving a shock to someone who may have fainted but isn't having SCA.

Cardiopulmonary resuscitation (CPR) should be given to a person having SCA until defibrillation can be done.

People who are at risk for SCA may want to consider having an AED at home. Currently, one AED, the Phillips HeartStart Home Defibrillator, is sold over-the-counter for home use.

A 2008 study by the National Heart, Lung, and Blood Institute and the National Institutes of Health found that AEDs in the home are safe and effective. However, the benefits of home-use AEDs are still debated.

Some people feel that placing these devices in homes will save many lives, because many SCAs occur at home.

Others note that no evidence supports the idea that home-use AEDs save more lives. These people fear that people who have AEDs in their homes will delay calling for help during an emergency. They're also concerned that people who have home-use AEDs will not properly maintain the devices or forget where they are.

When considering a home-use AED, talk to your doctor. He or she can help you decide whether having an AED in your home will benefit you.

Treatment in a Hospital

If you survive SCA, you usually will be admitted to a hospital for observation and treatment. In the hospital, your medical team will closely watch your heart. They may give you medicines to try to reduce the chance of another SCA.

While in the hospital, your medical team will try to find out what caused your SCA. If you're diagnosed with coronary artery disease, you may have angioplasty or coronary artery bypass grafting. These procedures help restore blood flow through narrowed or blocked coronary arteries.

Often, people who have SCA get a device called an implantable cardioverter defibrillator (ICD). This small device is surgically placed under the skin in your chest or abdomen. An ICD uses electric pulses or shocks to help control dangerous arrhythmias.

Chapter 16

Cardiogenic Shock

Cardiogenic shock is a state in which a weakened heart isn't able to pump enough blood to meet the body's needs. It is a medical emergency and is fatal if not treated right away. The most common cause of cardiogenic shock is damage to the heart muscle from a severe heart attack.

Not everyone who has a heart attack develops cardiogenic shock. In fact, less than 10 percent of people who have a heart attack develop it. But when cardiogenic shock does occur, it's very dangerous. For people who die from a heart attack in a hospital, cardiogenic shock is the most common cause.

What Is Shock?

The medical term "shock" refers to a state in which not enough blood and oxygen reach important organs in the body, such as the brain and kidneys. In a state of shock, a person's blood pressure is very low.

Shock can have a number of different causes. Cardiogenic shock is only one cause of shock. Other causes of shock include the following:

- **Hypovolemic shock:** This is shock due to not enough blood in the body. The most common cause is severe bleeding.

Excerpted from text by the National Heart, Lung, and Blood Institute (NHLBI, www.nhlbi.nih.gov), part of the National Institutes of Health, June 2007.

- **Vasodilatory shock:** In this type of shock, the blood vessels relax too much and cause very low blood pressure. When the blood vessels are too relaxed, there isn't enough pressure to push the blood through them. Without enough pressure, blood doesn't reach the organs. A bacterial infection in the bloodstream, a severe allergic reaction, or damage to the nervous system (brain and nerves) may cause vasodilatory shock.

When a person is in shock (from any cause), not enough blood or oxygen is reaching the body's organs. If shock lasts more than several minutes, the lack of oxygen to the organs starts to damage them. If shock isn't treated quickly, the organ damage can become permanent, and the person can die.

Some of the signs and symptoms of shock include the following:

- Confusion or lack of alertness
- Loss of consciousness
- A sudden, rapid heartbeat
- Sweating
- Pale skin
- Weak pulse
- Rapid breathing
- Decreased or no urine output
- Cool hands and feet

If you suspect that you or someone with you is in shock, call 911 and get emergency treatment right away. Prompt treatment can help prevent or limit lasting damage to the brain and other organs and can prevent death.

Outlook

In the past, almost no one survived cardiogenic shock. Now, thanks to improved treatments, around 50 percent of people who go into cardiogenic shock survive.

The reason more people are able to survive cardiogenic shock is because of treatments (medicines and devices) that restore blood flow to the heart and help the heart pump better. In some cases, devices that take over the pumping function of the heart are used. Implanting these devices requires major surgery.

Causes of Cardiogenic Shock

Immediate Causes

Cardiogenic shock happens when the heart can't pump enough blood to the body. This mostly occurs when the left ventricle isn't working because the muscle isn't getting enough blood or oxygen due to an ongoing heart attack. The weakened heart muscle can't pump enough oxygen-rich blood to the rest of the body.

In about 3 percent of the cases of cardiogenic shock, the right ventricle isn't working. This means the heart can't effectively pump blood to the lungs, where the blood picks up oxygen to bring back to the heart and the rest of the body.

When the heart isn't pumping enough blood to the rest of the body, organs (such as the brain and kidneys) don't get enough oxygen and can be damaged. Some of the things that might happen include the following.

- Cardiogenic shock may result in death if the flow of blood and oxygen to the organs isn't restored quickly. This is why emergency medical treatment is essential.

- When organs don't get enough blood or oxygen and stop working, cells in the organs die, and the organs may never go back to working normally.

- As some organs stop working, they may cause problems with other bodily functions. This, in turn, can make the shock worse. Here are some examples:

    - When the kidneys aren't working right, the levels of important chemicals in the body change. This may cause the heart and other muscles to become even weaker, limiting blood flow even more.

    - When the liver isn't working right, the body stops making proteins that cause the blood to clot. This can lead to more bleeding if the shock is due to blood loss.

    - How well the brain, kidneys, and other organs recover depends on how long a person is in shock. The shorter the time in shock, the less damage to the organs. This is another reason why it's so important to get emergency treatment right away.

143

Underlying Causes

The underlying causes of cardiogenic shock are conditions that weaken the heart and make it unable to pump enough blood and oxygen to the body.

These conditions include the following:

- Heart attack: Coronary artery disease (CAD) usually causes heart attack. CAD is a condition in which a material called plaque narrows or blocks the coronary arteries.

- Serious heart conditions that may cause a heart attack and lead to cardiogenic shock, such as:

  - Ventricular septal rupture. This is when the wall between the two ventricles breaks down because cells in part of the wall have died due to a heart attack. If the ventricles aren't separated, they can't pump properly.

  - Papillary muscle infarction or rupture. This is when the muscles that help anchor the heart valves stop working or break because their blood supply is cut off due to a heart attack. When this happens, blood doesn't flow in the right way between the different chambers of the heart, and they can't pump properly.

- Serious heart conditions that may happen with or without a heart attack, including the following:

  - Myocarditis, or inflammation of the heart muscle

  - Endocarditis, or infection of the heart valves

  - Arrhythmias, or problems with the speed or rhythm of the heartbeat

  - Pericardial tamponade, or too much fluid or blood around the heart (The fluid squeezes the heart muscle so it can't pump properly.)

  - Pulmonary embolism (This is a sudden blockage in a lung artery, usually due to a blood clot that traveled to the lung from a vein in the leg.)

Risk for Cardiogenic Shock

The most common risk factor for cardiogenic shock is having a heart attack.

If you've had a heart attack, the following factors can further increase your risk for cardiogenic shock:

- Older age
- Having a history of heart attacks or heart failure
- Having coronary artery disease in all the major heart blood vessels

Signs and Symptoms of Cardiogenic Shock

A lack of blood and oxygen reaching the brain, kidneys, skin, and other parts of the body causes the symptoms of cardiogenic shock.

The signs and symptoms of cardiogenic shock include the following:

- Confusion or lack of alertness
- Loss of consciousness
- A sudden, rapid heartbeat
- Sweating
- Pale skin
- Weak pulse
- Rapid breathing
- Decreased or no urine output
- Cool hands and feet

If you or someone with you is having these signs and symptoms, call 911 right away for emergency treatment. Prompt treatment can help prevent or limit lasting damage to the heart and other organs and can prevent sudden death.

Treating Cardiogenic Shock

Cardiogenic shock is life threatening and requires emergency medical treatment. In most cases, cardiogenic shock is diagnosed after a person has been admitted to the hospital for a heart attack. If the person isn't already in the hospital, emergency treatment can start as soon as medical personnel arrive.

The goals of emergency treatment for cardiogenic shock are first to treat the shock and then to treat the underlying cause or causes of the shock.

Sometimes both the shock and its cause are treated at the same time. For example, doctors may quickly open a blocked blood vessel that's causing damage to the heart. Often, opening the blood vessel can get the patient out of shock with little or no additional treatment.

Emergency Life Support

Emergency life support treatment is required for any type of shock. This treatment helps get blood and oxygen flowing to the brain, kidneys, and other organs. Restoring blood flow to the organs is essential to keep the patient alive and to try to prevent long-term damage to the organs. Emergency life support treatment includes giving the patient extra oxygen to breathe so that more oxygen reaches the lungs, the heart, and the rest of the body; and giving the patient fluids, including blood and blood products, through a needle inserted in a vein (when the shock is due to blood loss). Putting more blood into the bloodstream can help get more blood to important organs and to the rest of the body. This is usually not done for cardiogenic shock because the heart can't pump the blood that's already in the body and too much fluid is in the lungs, making it difficult to breathe.

Medicines

During and after emergency life support treatment, doctors try to find out what is causing the shock. If the reason for the shock is that the heart isn't pumping strongly enough, then the diagnosis is cardiogenic shock.

Depending on what is causing the cardiogenic shock, treatment may include medicines to do the following:

- Increase the force with which the heart muscle contracts

- Treat the heart attack that may have caused the shock

Medical Devices and Procedures

In addition to medicines, there are medical devices that can help the heart pump and improve blood flow. The devices most commonly used to treat cardiogenic shock include the following:

- **Intra-aortic balloon pump:** This device is placed in the aorta (the main blood vessel that carries blood from the heart to the body). A large balloon at the tip of the device is inflated and deflated in a rhythm that exactly matches the rhythm of the heart's pumping action. This helps the weakened heart muscle pump as much blood as it can, and gets more blood to vital organs such as the brain and kidneys.

- **Angioplasty and stents:** Angioplasty is a procedure used to restore blood flow through blocked coronary arteries and to treat an ongoing heart attack. A stent is a small device that's placed in a coronary artery during angioplasty to help keep it open.

Surgery

Sometimes medicine and medical devices aren't enough to treat cardiogenic shock. Surgery can restore blood flow to the heart and the rest of the body and repair damage to the heart. Surgery can help keep a patient alive while recovering from shock and improve the chances for long-term survival.

The types of surgery used to treat underlying causes of cardiogenic shock include the following:

- Coronary artery bypass grafting: In this surgery, arteries or veins from other parts of the body are used to bypass (that is, go around) narrowed coronary arteries.

- Surgery to repair damaged heart valves

- Surgery to repair a break in the wall between two chambers of the heart: This break is called a septal rupture.

- Surgery to implant a device to help the heart pump blood to the body: This device is called a left ventricular assist device (LVAD) or mechanical circulatory assist. This surgery may be done if damage to the left ventricle is causing the shock. The implanted device is a battery-operated pump that takes over part of the pumping action of the heart.

- Heart transplant: This is rarely done during an emergency situation like cardiogenic shock due to the other available devices and surgery options. Also, doctors need to do very careful tests to make sure a patient will benefit from a heart transplant and to find a matching heart from a donor.

Still, in some cases, doctors may recommend a transplant if they feel it's the best way to improve the patient's chances of long-term survival.

Chapter 17

Heart Failure

Heart failure is a condition in which the heart can't pump blood the way it should. In some cases, the heart can't fill with enough blood. In other cases, the heart can't send blood to the rest of the body with enough force. Some people have both problems.

Heart failure doesn't mean that your heart has stopped or is about to stop working. However, it's a serious condition that requires medical care.

Heart failure develops over time as the pumping of the heart grows weaker. It can affect the right side of the heart only or both the left and right sides of the heart. Most cases involve both sides of the heart.

Right-side heart failure occurs when the heart can't pump blood to the lungs, where it picks up oxygen. Left-side heart failure occurs when the heart can't pump enough oxygen-rich blood to the rest of the body.

Right-side heart failure may cause fluid to build up in the feet, ankles, legs, liver, abdomen, and, rarely, the veins in the neck. Right-side and left-side heart failure also cause shortness of breath and fatigue (tiredness).

The leading causes of heart failure are diseases that damage the heart. These include coronary artery disease (CAD), high blood pressure, and diabetes.

Excerpted from text by the National Heart, Lung, and Blood Institute (NHLBI, www.nhlbi.nih.gov), part of the National Institutes of Health, December 2007.

Heart failure is a very common condition. About 5 million people in the United States have heart failure, and it results in about 300,000 deaths each year.

Both children and adults can have heart failure, although the symptoms and treatments differ. This text focuses on heart failure in adults.

Taking steps to prevent CAD can help prevent heart failure. These steps include following a heart healthy diet, not smoking, doing physical activity, and losing weight if you're overweight or obese. Working with your doctor to control high blood pressure and diabetes also can help prevent heart failure.

People who have heart failure can live longer and more active lives if it's diagnosed early and they follow their treatment plans. For most, treatment includes medicines and lifestyle measures.

Currently, there's no cure for heart failure. However, researchers are finding and testing new treatments. These treatments offer hope for better ways to delay heart failure and its complications.

Other Names for Heart Failure

- Dropsy

- Left-side, or systolic, heart failure (This is when the heart can't pump enough oxygen-rich blood to the body.)

- Right-side, or diastolic, heart failure (This is when the heart can't fill with enough blood.)

Some people have only right-side heart failure. But all people who have left-side heart failure also have right-side heart failure. Treatments for right-side heart failure alone differ from treatments for both right-side and left-side heart failure. Your doctor will plan your treatment based on your type of heart failure and your unique needs.

Causes of Heart Failure

Conditions that damage the heart muscle or make it work too hard can cause heart failure. Over time, the heart weakens. It isn't able to fill with and/or pump blood as well as it should.

As the heart weakens, certain proteins and other substances may be released into the blood. They have a toxic effect on the heart and blood flow, and they cause heart failure to worsen.

150

Major Causes

The most common causes of heart failure are coronary artery disease (CAD), high blood pressure, and diabetes. Treating these problems can prevent or improve heart failure.

Coronary artery disease: CAD occurs when a fatty material called plaque builds up in your coronary arteries. These arteries supply oxygen-rich blood to your heart. Plaque narrows the arteries, causing less blood to flow to your heart muscle. This can lead to chest pain, heart attack, and heart damage.

High blood pressure: Blood pressure is the force of blood pushing against the walls of the arteries. Blood pressure is "high" if it stays at or above 140/90 mmHg over a period of time. High blood pressure stiffens blood vessels and makes the heart work harder. Without treatment, the heart may be damaged.

Diabetes: This disease occurs when the level of sugar in the blood is high. The body doesn't make enough insulin or doesn't use its insulin properly. Insulin is a hormone that helps convert food to energy. High sugar levels can damage blood vessels around the heart.

Other Causes

Other diseases and conditions that can lead to heart failure include the following:

- **Heart muscle diseases:** These diseases may be present at birth or due to injury or infection.

- **Heart valve disorders:** These problems may be present at birth or due to infections, heart attacks, or damage from heart disease.

- **Arrhythmias, or irregular heartbeats:** These heart problems may be present at birth or due to heart disease or heart defects.

- **Congenital heart defects:** These heart problems are present at birth.

Other factors also can injure the heart muscle and lead to heart failure. These include the following:

- Treatments for cancer, such as radiation and chemotherapy

- Thyroid disorders (having either too much or too little thyroid hormone in the body)

- Alcohol abuse

- HIV/AIDS [human immunodeficiency virus/acquired immuno-deficiency syndrome]

- Cocaine and other illegal drug use

- Too much vitamin E

Heart damage from obstructive sleep apnea may cause heart failure to worsen. In obstructive sleep apnea, your breathing stops or gets very shallow while you're sleeping. This can deprive the heart of oxygen and increase its workload. Treating this sleep problem may improve heart failure.

Risk Factors for Heart Failure

About 5 million people in the United States have heart failure, and it results in about 300,000 deaths each year. The number of people who have heart failure is growing. Each year, another 550,000 people are diagnosed for the first time. Heart failure is more common in the following people:

- **People who are 65 or older:** Aging can weaken the heart muscle. Older people also may have had a disease for many years that causes heart failure. Heart failure is the number-one reason for hospital visits in this age group.

- **African Americans:** African Americans are more likely than people of other races to have heart failure and to suffer from more severe forms of it. They're also more likely than other groups to have symptoms at a younger age, get worse faster, have more hospital visits due to heart failure, and die from heart failure.

- **People who are overweight or obese:** Excess weight puts a greater strain on the heart. It also can lead to type 2 diabetes, which adds to the risk of heart failure.

Men have a higher rate of heart failure than women. But in actual numbers, more women have the condition. This is because many more women than men live into their seventies and eighties when it's common.

Children with congenital heart defects also can develop heart failure. Children are born with these defects when the heart, heart valves, and/or blood vessels near the heart don't form correctly. This can weaken the heart muscle and lead to heart failure.

Children don't have the same symptoms or get the same treatment for heart failure as adults. This text focuses on heart failure in adults.

Signs and Symptoms of Heart Failure

The most common signs and symptoms of heart failure include the following:

- Shortness of breath or trouble breathing
- Fatigue (tiredness)
- Swelling in the ankles, feet, legs, abdomen, and, rarely, the veins in your neck

All of these symptoms are due to the buildup of fluid in your body. When symptoms start, you may feel tired and short of breath after routine physical effort—like climbing stairs.

As the heart grows weaker, symptoms get worse. You may begin to feel tired and short of breath after getting dressed or walking across the room. Some people have shortness of breath while lying flat.

Fluid buildup from heart failure also causes weight gain, frequent urination, and a cough that's worse at night and when you're lying down. This cough may be a sign of a condition called acute pulmonary edema. This is when too much fluid is in your lungs. This severe condition requires emergency treatment.

Treating Heart Failure

Early diagnosis and treatment can help people with heart failure live longer, more active lives. How heart failure is treated will depend on your type and stage of heart failure (how severe it is).

The goals of treatment for all stages of heart failure are to do the following:

- Treat the underlying cause of your heart failure, such as coronary artery disease (CAD), high blood pressure, or diabetes
- Reduce your symptoms

- Stop your heart failure from getting worse
- Increase your lifespan and improve your quality of life

For people with any stage of heart failure, treatment will include lifestyle measures, medicines, and ongoing care. People who have more severe heart failure also may need medical procedures and surgery.

Chapter 18

Cardiomyopathy

Chapter Contents

Section 18.1

Overview of Cardiomyopathy

Excerpted from "Cardiomyopathy," by the National Heart, Lung, and Blood Institute (NHLBI, www.nhlbi.nih.gov), part of the National Institutes of Health, December 2008.

Cardiomyopathy refers to diseases of the heart muscle. These diseases have a variety of causes, symptoms, and treatments.

In cardiomyopathy, the heart muscle becomes enlarged, thick, or rigid. In rare cases, the muscle tissue in the heart is replaced with scar tissue.

As cardiomyopathy worsens, the heart becomes weaker. It's less able to pump blood through the body and maintain a normal electrical rhythm. This can lead to heart failure or arrhythmia. In turn, heart failure can cause fluid to build up in the lungs, ankles, feet, legs, or abdomen.

The weakening of the heart also can cause other severe complications, such as heart valve problems.

Overview

The four main types of cardiomyopathy include the following:

- Dilated cardiomyopathy
- Hypertrophic cardiomyopathy
- Restrictive cardiomyopathy
- Arrhythmogenic right ventricular dysplasia (ARVD)

The different types of the disease have different causes, signs and symptoms, and outcomes.

Cardiomyopathy can be acquired or inherited. Acquired means you aren't born with the disease but you develop it due to another disease, condition, or factor. Inherited means your parents passed the gene for the disease on to you. In many cases, the cause of cardiomyopathy isn't known.

Cardiomyopathy can affect people of all ages. However, certain age groups are more likely to have certain types of cardiomyopathy. This text focuses on cardiomyopathy in adults.

Outlook

Some people who have cardiomyopathy have no signs or symptoms and need no treatment. For other people, the disease develops rapidly, symptoms are severe, and serious complications occur.

Treatments for cardiomyopathy include lifestyle changes, medicines, surgery, implanted devices to correct arrhythmias, and a nonsurgical procedure. These treatments can control symptoms, reduce complications, and stop the disease from getting worse.

Types of Cardiomyopathy

Dilated Cardiomyopathy

Dilated cardiomyopathy is the most common type of the disease. It mostly occurs in adults aged 20 to 60. Men are more likely than women to have this type of cardiomyopathy.

Dilated cardiomyopathy affects the heart's ventricles and atria. These are the lower and upper chambers of the heart, respectively.

The disease often starts in the left ventricle, the heart's main pumping chamber. The heart muscle begins to dilate (stretch and become thinner). This causes the inside of the chamber to enlarge. The problem often spreads to the right ventricle and then to the atria as the disease gets worse.

When the chambers dilate, the heart muscle doesn't contract normally. Also, the heart can't pump blood very well. Over time, the heart becomes weaker and heart failure can occur. Symptoms of heart failure include fatigue (tiredness); swelling of the ankles, feet, legs, and abdomen; and shortness of breath.

Dilated cardiomyopathy also can lead to heart valve problems, arrhythmias, and blood clots in the heart.

Hypertrophic Cardiomyopathy

Hypertrophic cardiomyopathy is very common and can affect people of any age. About one out of every 500 people has this type of cardiomyopathy. It affects men and women equally. Hypertrophic cardiomyopathy is the most common cause of sudden cardiac arrest (SCA) in young people, including young athletes.

This type of cardiomyopathy occurs when the walls of the ventricles (usually the left ventricle) thicken. Despite this thickening, the ventricle size often remains normal.

Hypertrophic cardiomyopathy may block blood flow out of the ventricle. When this happens, the condition is called obstructive hypertrophic cardiomyopathy. In some cases, the septum thickens and bulges into the left ventricle. (The septum is the wall that divides the left and right sides of the heart.) In both cases, blood flow out of the left ventricle is blocked.

As a result of the blockage, the ventricle must work much harder to pump blood out to the body. Symptoms can include chest pain, dizziness, shortness of breath, or fainting.

Hypertrophic cardiomyopathy also can affect the heart's mitral valve, causing blood to leak backward through the valve.

Sometimes the thickened heart muscle doesn't block blood flow out of the left ventricle. This is called nonobstructive hypertrophic cardiomyopathy. The entire ventricle may become thicker, or the thickening may happen only at the bottom of the heart. The right ventricle also may be affected.

In both types (obstructive and nonobstructive), the thickened muscle makes the inside of the left ventricle smaller, so it holds less blood. The walls of the ventricle also may stiffen. As a result, the ventricle is less able to relax and fill with blood.

These changes cause increased blood pressure in the ventricles and the blood vessels of the lungs. Changes also occur to the cells in the damaged heart muscle. This may disrupt the heart's electrical signals and lead to arrhythmias.

Rarely, people who have hypertrophic cardiomyopathy have no signs or symptoms, and the condition doesn't affect their lives. Others have severe symptoms and complications, such as serious arrhythmias, an inability to exercise, or extreme fatigue with little physical activity.

Rarely, people who have this type of cardiomyopathy can have SCA during very vigorous physical activity. The physical activity can trigger dangerous arrhythmias. If you have this type of cardiomyopathy, talk to your doctor about what types and amounts of physical activity are safe for you.

Restrictive Cardiomyopathy

Restrictive cardiomyopathy tends to mostly affect older adults. In this type of the disease, the ventricles become stiff and rigid. This is due to abnormal tissue, such as scar tissue, replacing the normal heart muscle.

As a result, the ventricles can't relax normally and fill with blood, and the atria become enlarged. Over time, blood flow in the heart is reduced. This can lead to problems such as heart failure or arrhythmias.

Arrhythmogenic Right Ventricular Dysplasia

Arrhythmogenic right ventricular dysplasia (ARVD) is a rare type of cardiomyopathy. ARVD occurs when the muscle tissue in the right ventricle dies and is replaced with scar tissue.

This process disrupts the heart's electrical signals and causes arrhythmias. Symptoms include palpitations and fainting after physical activity.

ARVD usually affects teens or young adults. It can cause SCA in young athletes. Fortunately, such deaths are rare.

Causes of Cardiomyopathy

Cardiomyopathy can be acquired or inherited. Acquired means you aren't born with the disease, but you develop it due to another disease, condition, or factor.

Inherited means your parents passed the gene for the disease on to you. Researchers continue to look for the genetic links to cardiomyopathy. They also continue to explore how these links cause or contribute to the various types of cardiomyopathy.

Many times, the cause of cardiomyopathy isn't known. This is often the case when the disease occurs in children.

Risk for Cardiomyopathy

People of all ages can have cardiomyopathy. However, certain types of the disease are more common in certain groups.

Dilated cardiomyopathy is more common in African Americans than in Whites. This type of the disease also is more common in men than women.

Teens and young adults are more likely than older people to have arrhythmogenic right ventricular dysplasia, although it's rare in both groups.

Major Risk Factors

Certain diseases, conditions, or factors can raise your risk for cardiomyopathy. Major risk factors include the following:

- A family history of cardiomyopathy, heart failure, or sudden cardiac arrest (SCA)

- A disease or condition that can lead to cardiomyopathy, such as coronary artery disease, heart attack, or a viral infection that inflames the heart muscle

- Diabetes, other metabolic diseases, or severe obesity

- Diseases that can damage the heart, such as hemochromatosis, sarcoidosis, or amyloidosis

- Long-term alcoholism

- Long-term high blood pressure

Some people who have cardiomyopathy never have signs or symptoms. That's why it's important to identify people who may be at high risk for the disease. This can help prevent future problems, such as serious arrhythmias or SCA.

Signs and Symptoms of Cardiomyopathy

Some people who have cardiomyopathy never have signs or symptoms. Others don't have signs or symptoms in the early stages of the disease.

As cardiomyopathy worsens and the heart weakens, signs and symptoms of heart failure usually occur. These signs and symptoms include the following:

- Shortness of breath or trouble breathing

- Fatigue (tiredness)

- Swelling in the ankles, feet, legs, and abdomen (Rarely, swelling may occur in the veins of your neck.)

Other signs and symptoms can include dizziness, lightheadedness, fainting during physical activity, chest pain, arrhythmias, and heart murmur (an extra or unusual sound heard during a heartbeat).

Section 18.2

Cardiomyopathy Often Cause of Sudden Death in Athletes

"Proper Heart Screening and Awareness Is Vital for Athletes," American College of Sports Medicine, News Release, April 16, 2004. Reprinted with permission. Reviewed by David A. Cooke, MD, FACP, October 1, 2009.

Sudden death is often the first and last sign of underlying heart ailment. Athletes and active people at every stage of life should focus more on heart health and be aware of potentially fatal dangers associated with undiagnosed heart ailments. That message was delivered in a keynote address by cardiologist and team physician John D. Cantwell, MD, at the eighth annual ACSM [American College of Sports Medicine] Health & Fitness Summit & Exposition.

Cantwell, who has served as team physician for the Atlanta Braves and Georgia Tech University, as well as holding the position of Chief Medical Officer for the 1996 Atlanta Olympic Games, warns against beginning or continuing strenuous activity without proper screening for heart problems from birth defects to problems developing over time.

"For most athletes, there is no warning sign or symptom," said Cantwell. "We become aware of these silent but deadly heart conditions only after it's too late. You have to know yourself and don't just get up and go without first being screened for trouble, and if someone is already active, he or she must be screened routinely for a variety of heart ailments."

Speaking before an audience of health and fitness professionals, Cantwell detailed several occurrences of sudden death in high-profile athletes such as basketball players Len Bias and Reggie Lewis and baseball player Daryl Kile. He recommends a standard questionnaire, cardiac examination, and an electrocardiogram for all athletes and additional screening tools such as CT [computed tomography] scans for older athletes and a limited echocardiogram in selected others.

"Through advances in technology, we can and do discover these conditions with routine and advanced screening and tests," said Cantwell.

"Because of our ability to do so, awareness is the key, particularly for people who are just taking up an exercise program or increasing the intensity of their regimen."

Cantwell explained how technology can reveal birth defects such as hypertrophic cardiomyopathy, a dangerously enlarged heart muscle, which is present in one in 500 humans. This is one example of a potentially fatal condition that disqualifies athletes from strenuous activity. He adds as athletes and active people reach and exceed the age of 30, care and consideration should be given to additional dangers to the heart such as high cholesterol and calcium in the coronary arteries.

Cantwell also advocated the widespread availability of automated external defibrillators (AEDs) at athletic events, which can be quickly utilized to stimulate the heart in cases of cardiac arrest. He said spectators, coaches, and referees could also be aided by AEDs if necessary, and that this form of immediate care tends to be more effective than emergency response.

The American College of Sports Medicine is the largest sports medicine and exercise science organization in the world. More than 20,000 International, National and Regional members are dedicated to promoting and integrating scientific research, education, and practical applications of sports medicine and exercise science to maintain and enhance physical performance, fitness, health and quality of life.

The American College of Sports Medicine gratefully acknowledges the following Health & Fitness Summit & Exposition sponsors: LifeFitness (Premier Sponsor), Gatorade Sports Science Institute, Gatorade, Reebok (Educational Partner), Amino Vital, Centers for Disease Control and Prevention, EAS, Lippincott Williams & Wilkins, BSDI, and SPRI Products, Inc.

Chapter 19

Arrhythmias

Chapter Contents

Section 19.1

Overview of Arrhythmias

Excerpted from "Arrhythmia," by the National Heart, Lung,
and Blood Institute (NHLBI, www.nhlbi.nih.gov), part of the
National Institutes of Health, May 2007.

An arrhythmia, sometimes called dysrhythmia, is a problem with
the rate or rhythm of the heartbeat. During an arrhythmia, the heart
can beat too fast, too slow, or with an irregular rhythm.

A heartbeat that is too fast is called tachycardia. A heartbeat that
is too slow is called bradycardia.

Most arrhythmias are harmless, but some can be serious or even
life threatening. When the heart rate is too fast, too slow, or irregular, the heart may not be able to pump enough blood to the body. Lack
of blood flow can damage the brain, heart, and other organs.

Understanding the Heart's Electrical System

To understand arrhythmias, it helps to understand the heart's internal electrical system. The heart's electrical system controls the rate
and rhythm of the heartbeat.

With each heartbeat, an electrical signal spreads from the top of
the heart to the bottom. As the signal travels, it causes the heart to
contract and pump blood. The process repeats with each new heartbeat.

Each electrical signal begins in a group of cells called the sinus
node or sinoatrial (SA) node. The SA node is located in the right
atrium, which is the upper right chamber of the heart. In a healthy
adult heart at rest, the SA node fires off an electrical signal to begin
a new heartbeat 60 to 100 times a minute.

From the SA node, the electrical signal travels through special
pathways in the right and left atria. This causes the atria to contract and pump blood into the heart's two lower chambers, the ventricles.

The electrical signal then moves down to a group of cells called
the atrioventricular (AV) node, located between the atria and the

ventricles. Here, the signal slows down just a little, allowing the ventricles time to finish filling with blood.

The electrical signal then leaves the AV node and travels along a pathway called the bundle of His. This pathway divides into a right bundle branch and a left bundle branch. The signal goes down these branches to the ventricles, causing them to contract and pump blood out to the lungs and the rest of the body.

The ventricles then relax, and the heartbeat process starts all over again in the SA node.

A problem with any part of this process can cause an arrhythmia. For example, in atrial fibrillation, a common type of arrhythmia, electrical signals travel through the atria in a fast and disorganized way. This causes the atria to quiver instead of contract.

Outlook

There are many types of arrhythmia. Most arrhythmias are harmless, but some are not. The outlook for a person who has an arrhythmia depends on the type and severity of the arrhythmia.

Even serious arrhythmias often can be successfully treated. Most people who have arrhythmias are able to live normal, healthy lives.

Types of Arrhythmia

The four main types of arrhythmia are premature (extra) beats, supraventricular arrhythmias, ventricular arrhythmias, and brady-arrhythmias.

Premature (Extra) Beats

Premature beats are the most common type of arrhythmia. They're harmless most of the time and often don't cause any symptoms.

When symptoms do occur, they usually feel like fluttering in the chest or a feeling of a skipped beat. Most of the time, premature beats need no treatment, especially in healthy people.

Premature beats that occur in the atria are called premature atrial contractions, or PACs. Premature beats that occur in the ventricles are called premature ventricular contractions, or PVCs.

In most cases, premature beats occur naturally, not due to any heart disease. But certain heart diseases can cause premature beats. They also can happen because of stress, too much exercise, or too much caffeine or nicotine.

Supraventricular Arrhythmias

Supraventricular arrhythmias are tachycardias (fast heart rates) that start in the atria or the atrioventricular (AV) node. The AV node is a group of cells located between the atria and the ventricles.

Types of supraventricular arrhythmias include atrial fibrillation (AF), atrial flutter, paroxysmal supraventricular tachycardia (PSVT), and Wolff-Parkinson-White (WPW) syndrome.

Atrial fibrillation: AF is the most common type of serious arrhythmia. It's a very fast and irregular contraction of the atria.

In AF, the heart's electrical signal doesn't begin in the SA node. Instead, the signal begins in another part of the atria or in the nearby pulmonary veins and is conducted abnormally.

When this happens, the electrical signal doesn't travel through the normal pathways in the atria. Instead, it spreads throughout the atria in a fast and disorganized manner.

This causes the walls of the atria to quiver very fast (fibrillate) instead of beating normally. As a result, the atria aren't able to pump blood into the ventricles the way they should.

In AF, electrical signals can travel through the atria at a rate of more than 300 per minute. Some of these abnormal electrical signals can travel to the ventricles, causing them to beat too fast and with an irregular rhythm. AF usually isn't life threatening, but it can be dangerous when it causes the ventricles to beat very fast.

The two most serious complications of chronic (long-term) AF are stroke and heart failure. Stroke can happen if a blood clot travels to an artery in the brain, blocking off blood flow.

In AF, blood clots can form because some of the blood "pools" in the fibrillating atria instead of flowing into the ventricles. If a piece of a blood clot in the left atrium breaks off, it can travel to the brain, causing a stroke. People who have AF often are treated with blood-thinning medicines to lower their risk for blood clots.

Heart failure is when the heart can't pump enough blood to meet the body's needs. AF can cause heart failure if the ventricles beat too fast and don't have enough time to fill with blood to pump out to the body. Heart failure causes fatigue (tiredness), leg swelling, and shortness of breath.

AF and other supraventricular arrhythmias can occur for no apparent reason. But most of the time, an underlying condition that damages the heart muscle and its ability to conduct electrical impulses causes AF. These conditions include high blood pressure, coronary heart disease (also called coronary artery disease), heart failure, and rheumatic heart disease.

Other conditions also can lead to AF, including an overactive thyroid gland (too much thyroid hormone produced) and heavy alcohol use. AF also becomes more common as people get older.

Atrial flutter: Atrial flutter is similar to AF, but instead of the electrical signals spreading through the atria in a fast and irregular rhythm, they travel in a fast and regular rhythm.

Atrial flutter is much less common than AF, but it has similar symptoms and complications.

Paroxysmal supraventricular tachycardia: PSVT is a very fast heart rate that begins and ends suddenly. PSVT occurs due to problems with the electrical connection between the atria and the ventricles.

In PSVT, electrical signals that begin in the atria and travel to the ventricles can reenter the atria, causing extra heartbeats. This type of arrhythmia usually isn't dangerous and tends to occur in young people. It can happen during vigorous exercise.

A special type of PSVT is called Wolff-Parkinson-White syndrome. WPW syndrome is a condition in which the heart's electrical signals travel along an extra pathway from the atria to the ventricles.

This extra pathway disrupts the timing of the heart's electrical signals and can cause the ventricles to beat very fast. This type of arrhythmia can be life threatening.

Ventricular Arrhythmias

These arrhythmias start in the ventricles. They can be very dangerous and usually need medical attention right away.

Ventricular arrhythmias include ventricular tachycardia and ventricular fibrillation (v-fib). Coronary heart disease, heart attack, weakened heart muscle, and other problems can cause ventricular arrhythmias.

Ventricular tachycardia: Ventricular tachycardia is a fast, regular beating of the ventricles that may last for only a few seconds or for much longer.

A few beats of ventricular tachycardia often don't cause problems. However, episodes that last for more than a few seconds can be dangerous. Ventricular tachycardia can turn into other, more dangerous arrhythmias, such as v-fib.

Ventricular fibrillation: V-fib occurs when disorganized electrical signals make the ventricles quiver instead of pump normally. Without the ventricles pumping blood out to the body, you'll lose consciousness within seconds and die within minutes if not treated.

To prevent death, the condition must be treated right away with an electric shock to the heart called defibrillation.

V-fib may happen during or after a heart attack or in someone whose heart is already weak because of another condition. Health experts think that most of the sudden cardiac deaths that occur every year (about 335,000) are due to v-fib.

Torsades de pointes (torsades) is a type of v-fib that causes a unique pattern on an EKG (electrocardiogram). Certain medicines or imbalanced amounts of potassium, calcium, or magnesium in the bloodstream can cause this condition.

People who have long QT syndrome are at higher risk for torsades. People who have this condition need to be careful about taking certain antibiotics, heart medicines, and over-the-counter medicines.

Bradyarrhythmias

Bradyarrhythmias are arrhythmias in which the heart rate is slower than normal. If the heart rate is too slow, not enough blood reaches the brain. This can cause you to lose consciousness.

In adults, a heart rate slower than 60 beats per minute is considered a bradyarrhythmia. Some people normally have slow heart rates, especially people who are very physically fit. For them, a heartbeat slower than 60 beats per minute isn't dangerous and doesn't cause symptoms. But in other people, bradyarrhythmia can be due to a serious disease or other condition.

Bradyarrhythmias can be caused by the following:

• Heart attack

• Conditions that harm or change the heart's electrical activity, such as an underactive thyroid gland or aging

• An imbalance of chemicals or other substances, such as potassium, in the blood

• Some medicines, such as beta-blockers

Bradyarrhythmias also can happen as a result of severe bundle branch block. Bundle branch block is a condition in which an electrical signal traveling down either or both of the bundle branches is delayed or blocked.

When this happens, the ventricles don't contract at exactly the same time, as they should. As a result, the heart has to work harder to pump blood to the body. The cause of bundle branch block often is an existing heart condition.

Arrhythmias in Children

A child's heart rate normally decreases as he or she gets older. A newborn's heart beats between 95 to 160 times a minute. A 1-year-old's heart beats between 90 to 150 times a minute, and a 6- to 8-year-old's heart beats between 60 to 110 times a minute.

A baby or child's heart can beat faster or slower than normal for many reasons. Like adults, when children are active, their hearts will beat faster. When they're sleeping, their hearts will beat slower. Their heart rates can speed up and slow down as they breathe in and out. All of these changes are normal.

Some children are born with heart defects that cause arrhythmias. In other children, arrhythmias can develop later in childhood. Doctors use the same tests to diagnose arrhythmias in children and adults.

Treatments for children who have arrhythmias include medicines, defibrillation (electric shock), surgically implanted devices that control the heartbeat, and other procedures that fix abnormal electrical signals in the heart.

Causes of Arrhythmia

An arrhythmia can occur if the electrical signals that control the heartbeat are delayed or blocked. This can happen if the special nerve cells that produce electrical signals don't work properly, or if electrical signals don't travel normally through the heart.

An arrhythmia also can occur if another part of the heart starts to produce electrical signals. This adds to the signals from the special nerve cells and disrupts the normal heartbeat.

Smoking, heavy alcohol use, use of certain drugs (such as cocaine or amphetamines), use of certain prescription or over-the-counter medicines, or too much caffeine or nicotine can lead to arrhythmias in some people.

Strong emotional stress or anger can make the heart work harder, raise blood pressure, and release stress hormones. In some people, these reactions can lead to arrhythmias.

A heart attack or an underlying condition that damages the heart's electrical system also can cause arrhythmias. Examples of such conditions include high blood pressure, coronary heart disease, heart failure, overactive or underactive thyroid gland (too much or too little thyroid hormone produced), and rheumatic heart disease.

In some arrhythmias, such as Wolff-Parkinson-White syndrome, the underlying heart defect that causes the arrhythmia is congenital (present at birth). Sometimes, the cause of an arrhythmia can't be found.

Risk for Arrhythmia

Millions of Americans have arrhythmias. They're very common in older adults. About 2.2 million Americans have atrial fibrillation (a common type of arrhythmia that can cause problems).

Most serious arrhythmias affect people older than 60. This is because older adults are more likely to have heart disease and other health problems that can lead to arrhythmias.

Older adults also tend to be more sensitive to the side effects of medicines, some of which can cause arrhythmias. Some medicines used to treat arrhythmias can even cause arrhythmias as a side effect.

Some types of arrhythmia happen more often in children and young adults. Paroxysmal supraventricular tachycardias (PSVTs), including Wolff-Parkinson-White syndrome, are more common in young people. PSVT is a fast heart rate that begins and ends suddenly.

Major Risk Factors

Arrhythmias are more common in people who have diseases or conditions that weaken the heart, such as the following:

- Heart attack
- Heart failure or cardiomyopathy, which weakens the heart and changes the way electrical signals move around the heart
- Heart tissue that's too thick or stiff or that hasn't formed normally
- Leaking or narrowed heart valves, which make the heart work too hard and can lead to heart failure
- Congenital heart defects (problems that are present at birth) that affect the heart's structure or function

Other conditions also can increase the risk for arrhythmias, such as the following:

- High blood pressure

- Infections that damage the heart muscle or the sac around the heart

- Diabetes, which increases the risk of high blood pressure and coronary heart disease

- Sleep apnea (when breathing becomes shallow or stops during sleep), which can stress the heart because the heart doesn't get enough oxygen

- An overactive or underactive thyroid gland (too much or too little thyroid hormone in the body)

Also, several other risk factors can increase risk for arrhythmias. Examples include heart surgery, certain drugs (such as cocaine or amphetamines), or an imbalance of chemicals or other substances (such as potassium) in the bloodstream.

Signs and Symptoms of an Arrhythmia

Many arrhythmias cause no signs or symptoms. When signs or symptoms are present, the most common ones include the following:

- Palpitations (feelings that your heart is skipping a beat, fluttering, or beating too hard or fast)

- A slow heartbeat

- An irregular heartbeat

- Feeling pauses between heartbeats

More serious signs and symptoms include the following:

- Anxiety

- Weakness, dizziness, and lightheadedness

- Fainting or nearly fainting

- Sweating

- Shortness of breath

- Chest pain

Treating Arrhythmias

Common arrhythmia treatments include medicines, medical procedures, and surgery. Treatment is needed when an arrhythmia causes serious symptoms, such as dizziness, chest pain, or fainting.

Treatment also is needed if an arrhythmia increases your risk for complications, such as heart failure, stroke, or sudden cardiac arrest.

Medicines

Medicines can be used to speed up a heart that's beating too slow or slow down a heart that's beating too fast. They also can be used to convert an abnormal heart rhythm to a normal, steady rhythm. Medicines that do this are called antiarrhythmics.

Some of the medicines used to slow a fast heart rate are beta-blockers (such as metoprolol and atenolol), calcium channel blockers (such as diltiazem and verapamil), and digoxin (digitalis). These medicines often are used to slow the heart rate in people who have atrial fibrillation.

Some of the medicines used to restore an abnormal heartbeat to a normal rhythm are amiodarone, sotalol, flecainide, propafenone, dofetilide, ibutilide, quinidine, procainamide, and disopyramide. These medicines often have side effects. Some of the side effects can make an arrhythmia worse or even cause a different kind of arrhythmia.

People who have atrial fibrillation and some other arrhythmias often are treated with anticoagulants, or blood thinners, to reduce the risk of blood clots forming. Aspirin, warfarin (Coumadin®), and heparin are commonly used blood thinners.

Medicines also can control an underlying medical condition, such as heart disease or a thyroid condition, that might be causing an arrhythmia.

Medical Procedures

Some arrhythmias are treated with a pacemaker. A pacemaker is a small device that's placed under the skin of your chest or abdomen to help control abnormal heart rhythms.

This device uses electrical pulses to prompt the heart to beat at a normal rate. Most pacemakers contain a sensor that activates the device only when the heartbeat is abnormal.

Some arrhythmias are treated with a jolt of electricity delivered to the heart. This type of treatment is called cardioversion or defibrillation, depending on which type of arrhythmia is being treated.

Some people who are at risk for ventricular fibrillation are treated with a device called an implantable cardioverter defibrillator (ICD). Like a pacemaker, an ICD is a small device that's placed under the skin in the chest. This device uses electrical pulses or shocks to help control life-threatening arrhythmias.

An ICD continuously monitors the heartbeat. If it senses a dangerous ventricular arrhythmia, it sends an electric shock to the heart to restore a normal heartbeat.

A procedure called catheter ablation is sometimes used to treat certain types of arrhythmia when medicines don't work.

During this procedure, a long, thin, flexible tube is put into a blood vessel in your arm, groin (upper thigh), or neck. The tube is guided to your heart through the blood vessel. A special machine sends energy through the tube to your heart.

This energy finds and destroys small areas of heart tissue where abnormal heartbeats may cause an arrhythmia to start. Catheter ablation usually is done in a hospital as part of an electrophysiology study.

Surgery

Sometimes, an arrhythmia is treated with surgery. This often occurs when surgery is already being done for another reason, such as repair of a heart valve.

One type of surgery for atrial fibrillation is called "maze" surgery. In this operation, the surgeon makes small cuts or burns in the atria that prevent the spread of disorganized electrical signals.

If coronary heart disease is causing arrhythmias, coronary artery bypass grafting may be recommended. This surgery improves blood supply to the heart muscle.

Other Treatments

Vagal maneuvers are another arrhythmia treatment. These simple exercises sometimes can stop or slow down certain types of supraventricular arrhythmias. They do this by affecting the vagus nerve, which helps control the heart rate.

Some vagal maneuvers include the following:

- Gagging
- Holding your breath and bearing down (Valsalva maneuver)
- Immersing your face in ice-cold water
- Coughing
- Putting your fingers on your eyelids and pressing down gently

Vagal maneuvers aren't an appropriate treatment for everyone. Discuss with your doctor whether vagal maneuvers are an option for you.

Section 19.2

Atrial Fibrillation

Excerpted from text by the National Heart, Lung, and Blood Institute
(NHLBI, www.nhlbi.nih.gov), part of the National Institutes of Health,
June 2007.

Atrial fibrillation, or AF, is the most common type of arrhythmia. An arrhythmia is a problem with the rate or rhythm of the heartbeat. During an arrhythmia, the heart can beat too fast, too slow, or with an irregular rhythm.

AF occurs when rapid, disorganized electrical signals cause the atria, the two upper chambers of the heart, to fibrillate. The term "fibrillate" means to contract very fast and irregularly.

In AF, blood pools in the atria and isn't pumped completely into the ventricles, the heart's two lower chambers. As a result, the heart's upper and lower chambers don't work together as they should.

Often, people who have AF may not feel symptoms. However, even when not noticed, AF can increase the risk of stroke. In some people, AF can cause chest pain or heart failure, particularly when the heart rhythm is very rapid.

AF may occur rarely or every now and then, or it may become a persistent or permanent heart rhythm lasting for years.

Outlook

People who have AF can live normal, active lives. For some people, treatment can cure AF and restore normal heart rhythms.

For people who have permanent AF, treatment can successfully control symptoms and prevent complications. Treatments include medicines, medical procedures, and lifestyle changes.

Types of Atrial Fibrillation

Paroxysmal Atrial Fibrillation

In paroxysmal atrial fibrillation (AF), the abnormal electrical signals and rapid heart rate begin suddenly and then stop on their own.

Symptoms can be mild or severe and last for seconds, minutes, hours, or days.

Persistent Atrial Fibrillation

Persistent AF is a condition in which the abnormal heart rhythm continues until it's stopped with treatment.

Permanent Atrial Fibrillation

Permanent AF is a condition in which a normal heart rhythm can't be restored with the usual treatments. Both paroxysmal and persistent AF may become more frequent and, over time, result in permanent AF.

Other Names for Atrial Fibrillation

- A fib
- Auricular fibrillation

Causes of Atrial Fibrillation

Atrial fibrillation (AF) occurs when the electrical signals traveling through the heart are conducted abnormally and become very rapid and disorganized.

This is the result of damage to the heart's electrical system. The damage most often is the result of other conditions, such as coronary heart disease (also called coronary artery disease) or high blood pressure, that affect the health of the heart.

Sometimes, the cause of AF is unknown.

Risk for Atrial Fibrillation

More than 2 million people in the United States have atrial fibrillation (AF). It affects both men and women.

The risk of AF increases as you age. This is mostly because as you get older, your risk for heart disease and other conditions that can cause AF also increases. However, about half of the people who have AF are younger than 75.

AF is uncommon in children.

Major Risk Factors

AF is more common in people who have heart diseases or conditions, such as the following:

- Coronary heart disease

- Heart failure

- Rheumatic heart disease

- Structural heart defects, such as mitral valve disorders

- Pericarditis (a condition in which the membrane, or sac, around your heart is inflamed)

- Congenital heart defects

- Sick sinus syndrome (a condition in which the heart's electrical signals don't fire properly and the heart rate slows down; sometimes the heart will switch back and forth between a slow rate and a fast rate)

AF also is more common in people who are having heart attacks or who have just had surgery.

Other Risk Factors

Other conditions that increase AF risk include hyperthyroidism (too much thyroid hormone), obesity, high blood pressure, diabetes, and lung disease.

Other factors also can increase your risk of AF. For example, drinking large amounts of alcohol, especially binge drinking, increases your risk. Even modest amounts of alcohol can trigger AF in some people. Caffeine or psychological stress also may trigger AF in some people.

Some evidence suggests that people who have sleep apnea are at greater risk for AF. Sleep apnea is a common disorder in which you have one or more pauses in breathing or shallow breaths while you sleep.

Metabolic syndrome also increases your risk of AF. People who have this condition have a group of risk factors that increase their risk of heart disease and other health problems.

Recent research suggests that people who receive high-dose steroid therapy are at increased risk of AF. This therapy, which is commonly used for asthma and certain inflammatory conditions, may act as a trigger in people who already have other AF risk factors.

Signs and Symptoms of Atrial Fibrillation

Atrial fibrillation (AF) usually causes the ventricles to contract faster than normal. When this happens, the ventricles don't have enough time to fill completely with blood to pump to the lungs and body.

This inefficient pumping can cause signs and symptoms, such as the following:

- Palpitations (feelings that your heart is skipping a beat, fluttering, or beating too hard or fast)
- Shortness of breath
- Weakness or difficulty exercising
- Chest pain
- Dizziness or fainting
- Fatigue (tiredness)
- Confusion

Atrial Fibrillation Complications

AF has two major complications—stroke and heart failure.

Stroke: During AF, the atria don't pump all of their blood to the ventricles. Some blood pools in the atria. When this happens, a blood clot (also called a thrombus) can form.

If the clot breaks off and travels to the brain, it can cause a stroke. (A clot that forms in one part of the body and travels in the bloodstream to another part of the body is called an embolus.)

Blood-thinning medicines to reduce the risk of stroke are a very important part of treatment for people who have AF.

Heart failure: Heart failure occurs when the heart can't pump enough blood to meet the body's needs. AF can lead to heart failure because the ventricles are beating very fast and aren't able to properly fill with blood to pump out to the body.

Fatigue and shortness of breath are common symptoms of heart failure. A buildup of fluid in the lungs causes these symptoms. Fluid also can build up in the feet, ankles, and legs, causing weight gain.

Lifestyle changes, medicines, and sometimes special care (rarely, a mechanical heart pump or heart transplant) are the main treatments for heart failure.

Treating Atrial Fibrillation

Treatment for atrial fibrillation (AF) depends on how severe or frequent the symptoms are and whether you already have heart disease. General treatment options include medicines, medical procedures, and lifestyle changes.

Section 19.3

Heart Block

Excerpted from text by the National Heart, Lung, and Blood Institute
(NHLBI, www.nhlbi.nih.gov), part of the National Institutes of Health,
April 2008.

Heart block is a problem that occurs with the heart's electrical system. This system controls the rate and rhythm of heartbeats. ("Rate" refers to the number of times your heart beats in a minute.)

With each heartbeat, an electrical signal spreads across the heart from the upper to the lower chambers. As it travels, the signal causes the heart to contract and pump blood. This process repeats with each new heartbeat.

Heart block occurs when the electrical signal is slowed or disrupted as it moves through the heart.

Outlook

The symptoms and severity of heart block depend on which type you have. First-degree heart block rarely causes severe symptoms.

Second-degree heart block may result in the heart skipping a beat or beats. This type of heart block also can make you feel dizzy or faint.

Third-degree heart block limits the heart's ability to pump blood to the rest of the body. This type of heart block may cause fatigue (tiredness), dizziness, and fainting. Third-degree heart block requires prompt treatment, because it can be fatal.

A medical device called a pacemaker is used to treat third-degree heart block and some cases of second-degree heart block. This device uses electrical pulses to make the heart beat at a normal rate.

Understanding the Heart's Electrical System and EKG Results

Doctors use a test called an EKG (electrocardiogram) to help diagnose heart block. This test detects and records the heart's electrical activity. An EKG records the strength and timing of electrical signals as they pass through each part of the heart.

The data is recorded on a graph so your doctor can study your heart's electrical activity. Different parts of the graph show each step of an electrical signal's journey through the heart.

Each electrical signal begins in a group of cells called the sinus node or sinoatrial (SA) node. The SA node is located in the right atrium, which is the upper right chamber of the heart. In a healthy adult heart at rest, the SA node fires off an electrical signal to begin a new heartbeat 60 to 100 times a minute.

From the SA node, the signal travels to the right and left atria. This causes the atria to contract and pump blood into the heart's two lower chambers, the ventricles. This is recorded as the P wave on the EKG.

The signal passes between the atria and ventricles through a group of cells called the atrioventricular (AV) node. The signal slows down as it passes through the AV node. This slowing allows the ventricles time to finish filling with blood. On the EKG, this is the flat line between the end of the P wave and beginning of the Q wave.

The electrical signal then leaves the AV node and travels along a pathway called the bundle of His. From there the signal travels into the right and left bundle branches. On the EKG, this is the Q wave.

As the signal spreads across the right and left ventricles, they contract and pump blood out to the lungs and the rest of the body. On the EKG, R marks the contraction of the left ventricle and S marks the contraction of the right ventricle.

The ventricles then relax (shown as the T wave on the EKG). This entire process continues over and over with each new heartbeat.

Causes of Heart Block

Heart block has a number of causes. You can be born with this disorder (congenital) or acquire it.

Congenital Heart Block

One form of congenital heart block occurs in the babies of women who have autoimmune diseases, such as lupus. People who have these diseases make proteins called antibodies.

In pregnant women, these antibodies can cross the placenta. (The placenta is the organ that attaches the umbilical cord to the mother's womb.) They can damage the baby's heart and lead to congenital heart block.

Congenital heart defects (problems with heart's structure) also may cause congenital heart block. Often, doctors don't know what causes these defects.

Acquired Heart Block

A number of factors, such as diseases, surgery, medicines, and other conditions, can cause acquired heart block.

The most common cause of acquired heart block is damage to the heart from a heart attack. Other diseases that can cause heart block include coronary artery disease, myocarditis (inflammation of the heart muscle), heart failure, rheumatic fever, and cardiomyopathy.

Other diseases may increase the risk for heart block. These include sarcoidosis and the degenerative muscle disorders Lev disease and Lenègre disease.

Certain types of surgery also may damage the heart's electrical system and lead to heart block.

Exposure to toxic substances and taking certain medicines, including digitalis and beta-blockers, also may cause heart block. Doctors closely watch people who are taking these medicines for signs of problems.

In some cases, atrioventricular (AV) heart block has been linked to genetic mutations (changes in the genes).

An overly active vagus nerve can cause first-degree heart block. Activity in this nerve slows the heart rate.

Well-trained athletes and young people are at higher risk for first-degree heart block due to this cause.

In some cases, acquired heart block may go away if the factor causing it is treated or resolved. For example, heart block that occurs after a heart attack or surgery may go away after recovery.

Also, if a medicine is causing heart block, the condition may go away if the medicine is stopped or the dosage is lowered. However, you shouldn't change the way you take your medicines unless your doctor tells you to.

Signs and Symptoms of Heart Block

Signs and symptoms depend on the type of heart block you have. First-degree heart block rarely causes symptoms.

Symptoms of second- and third-degree heart block include the following:

• Fainting

• Feeling dizzy or lightheaded

• Fatigue (tiredness)

- Shortness of breath
- Chest pain

These symptoms may point to other health problems as well. If these symptoms are new or severe, call 911 or go to the hospital emergency room. If you have milder symptoms, talk to your doctor right away to find out whether you need prompt treatment.

Treating Heart Block

Treatment depends on the type of heart block you have. First-degree heart block usually needs no treatment.

If you have second-degree heart block, you may need a pacemaker. A pacemaker is a small device that's placed under the skin of your chest or abdomen. This device uses electrical pulses to stimulate the heart to beat at a normal rate.

If you have third-degree heart block, you will need a pacemaker. In an emergency, a temporary pacemaker may be used until you can get a permanent one. Most people who have third-degree heart block need pacemakers for the rest of their lives.

Some people with third-degree congenital heart block don't need a pacemaker for many years. Others may need a pacemaker at a young age or during infancy.

In some cases, acquired heart block may go away if the factor causing it is treated or resolved. For example, heart block that occurs after a heart attack or surgery may go away.

Also, if a medicine is causing heart block, the condition may go away if the medicine is stopped or the dosage is lowered. However, you shouldn't change the way you take your medicines unless your doctor tells you to.

Section 19.4

Long QT Syndrome

Excerpted from text by the National Heart, Lung, and Blood Institute (NHLBI, www.nhlbi.nih.gov), part of the National Institutes of Health, July 2007.

Long QT syndrome (LQTS) is a disorder of the heart's electrical activity. It may cause you to develop a sudden, uncontrollable, and dangerous heart rhythm called an arrhythmia in response to exercise or stress.

Arrhythmias also can develop for no known reason in people who have LQTS. Not everyone who has LQTS develops dangerous heart rhythms. However, if one does occur, it may be fatal.

The term "long QT" refers to an abnormal pattern seen on an EKG (electrocardiogram). An EKG is a test that detects and records the heart's electrical activity. The QT interval, recorded on the EKG, corresponds to the time during which the lower chambers of your heart are triggered to contract and then build the potential to contract again. These chambers are called ventricles.

The timing of the heartbeat's electrical activity is complex, and the body carefully controls it. Normally the QT interval of the heartbeat lasts about a third of each heartbeat cycle on the EKG.

However, in people who have LQTS, the QT interval usually lasts longer than normal. This can upset the careful timing of the heartbeat and trigger a dangerous, abnormal rhythm.

Overview

On the surface of each muscle cell in the heart are tiny pores called ion channels. Ion channels open and close to let electrically charged sodium, calcium, and potassium atoms (ions) flow into and out of the cell. This generates the heart's electrical activity.

This activity causes each heart cell to contract. Normally, the electrical activity spreads from one heart cell to the next in an orderly and coordinated way. This allows the heart to pump blood.

During each normal heartbeat, the muscle cells in the upper chambers of the heart, the atria, contract. The contraction pumps blood from the atria to the ventricles. Then the muscle cells in the ventricles contract, pumping blood from the ventricles to the lungs and the rest of the body.

This coordinated contraction of the atria and ventricles represents one normal heartbeat.

In people who have LQTS, problems with the ion channels in the heart cells may disrupt the timing of the electrical activity in the ventricles. The ion channels may not work properly, or there may be too few of them. In this situation, the heart may suddenly develop a fast and abnormal heart rhythm that can be life threatening.

Many cases of LQTS are inherited, which means you're born with the condition and have it your whole life. There are seven known types of inherited LQTS. The most common ones are called LQTS 1, LQTS 2, and LQTS 3.

Emotional stress or exercise (especially swimming) that makes the heart beat fast tends to trigger abnormal heart rhythms if you have LQTS 1. In LQTS 2, abnormal rhythms may be triggered by surprise or other extreme emotions. In LQTS 3, a slow heart rate during sleep may trigger an abnormal heart rhythm.

Acquired, or noninherited, LQTS may be brought on by certain medicines or other medical conditions.

Outlook

More than half of the people who have an untreated, inherited form of LQTS die within 10 years. But for many people who have LQTS, lifestyle changes and medical treatments can help prevent dangerous complications and lengthen life expectancy.

Some of these lifestyle changes and treatments include the following:

- Avoiding strenuous physical activity or startling noises

- Adding more potassium to your diet

- Taking heart medicines called beta-blockers, which are very effective at preventing sudden cardiac arrest

- Having an implanted medical device, such as a pacemaker or implantable cardioverter defibrillator, that helps control abnormal heart rhythms

Discuss with your doctor which lifestyle changes and treatments are appropriate for you and the type of LQTS you have.

Signs and Symptoms of Long QT Syndrome

Major Signs and Symptoms

If you have long QT syndrome (LQTS), you're prone to developing a sudden and dangerous arrhythmia (abnormal heartbeat). Signs and symptoms of LQTS-related arrhythmias often first appear during childhood and include the following:

- **Unexplained fainting:** This happens because your heart isn't pumping enough blood to your brain. Fainting may occur when you're under physical or emotional stress. Some people will have fluttering feelings in their chests before they faint.

- **Unexplained seizures:** Those around you may mistake your fainting from LQTS as a seizure due to epilepsy. In children, fainting may be seen as a hysterical reaction to a stressful situation.

- **Unexplained drowning or near drowning:** This may be due to fainting while swimming.

- **Unexplained sudden cardiac arrest (SCA) or death:** This means that your heart suddenly stops beating for no obvious reason. People who have SCA will die within minutes unless they receive treatment. Most people who have SCA die. In about one out of 10 patients, SCA or sudden death is the first sign of LQTS.

Other Signs and Symptoms

Often, people who have LQTS 3 will develop an abnormal heartbeat during sleep. This may cause them to have noisy gasping while sleeping.

Long QT Syndrome without Symptoms

People who have LQTS may not have any signs or symptoms (silent LQTS). Doctors often advise family members of people who have the condition to be tested for it, even if they have no symptoms.

Medical and genetic tests may reveal whether they have LQTS and what type of the condition they have.

Chapter 20

Heart Valve Disease

Chapter Contents

Section 20.1

*Overview of
Heart Valve Disease*

Excerpted from "Heart Valve Disease," by the National Heart,
Lung, and Blood Institute (NHLBI, www.nhlbi.nih.gov), part of the
National Institutes of Health, December 2007.

Heart valve disease is a condition in which one or more of your
heart valves don't work properly. The heart has four valves: the tricuspid, pulmonary, mitral, and aortic valves.

These valves have tissue flaps that open and close with each heartbeat. The flaps make sure blood flows in the right direction through
your heart's four chambers and to the rest of your body.

Birth defects, age-related changes, infections, or other conditions
can cause one or more of your heart valves to not open fully or to let
blood leak back into the heart chambers. This can make your heart
work harder and affect its ability to pump blood.

Heart Valve Problems

Heart valves can have three basic kinds of problems:

- Regurgitation, or backflow, occurs when a valve doesn't close
  tightly. Blood leaks back into the chamber rather than flowing
  forward through the heart or into an artery. In the United States,
  backflow is most often due to prolapse. "Prolapse" is when the
  flaps of the valve flop or bulge back into an upper heart chamber
  during a heartbeat. Prolapse mainly affects the mitral valve,
  but it can affect the other valves as well.

- Stenosis occurs when the flaps of a valve thicken, stiffen, or fuse
  together. This prevents the heart valve from fully opening, and not
  enough blood flows through the valve. Some valves can have both
  stenosis and backflow problems.

- Atresia occurs when a heart valve lacks an opening for blood to
  pass through.

You can be born with heart valve disease or you can acquire it later in life. Heart valve disease that develops before birth is called a congenital valve disease. Congenital heart valve disease can occur alone or with other congenital heart defects.

Congenital heart valve disease usually involves pulmonary or aortic valves that don't form properly. These valves may not have enough tissue flaps, they may be the wrong size or shape, or they may lack an opening through which blood can flow properly.

Acquired heart valve disease usually involves the aortic or mitral valves. Although the valve is normal at first, disease can cause problems to develop over time.

Both congenital and acquired heart valve disease can cause stenosis or backflow.

Outlook

Many people have heart valve defects or disease but don't have symptoms. For some people, the condition will stay largely the same over their lifetime and not cause any problems.

For other people, the condition will worsen slowly over time until symptoms develop. If not treated, advanced heart valve disease can cause heart failure, stroke, blood clots, or sudden death due to sudden cardiac arrest.

Currently, no medicines can cure heart valve disease. However, lifestyle changes and medicines can relieve many of the symptoms and problems linked to heart valve disease. They also can lower your risk of developing a life-threatening condition, such as stroke or sudden cardiac arrest. Eventually, you may need to have your faulty heart valve repaired or replaced.

Some types of congenital heart valve disease are so severe that the valve is repaired or replaced during infancy or childhood or even before birth. Other types may not cause problems until you're middle-aged or older, if at all.

Other Names for Heart Valve Disease

- Aortic regurgitation
- Aortic stenosis
- Aortic sclerosis
- Aortic valve disease
- Bicuspid aortic valve

- Congenital heart defect
- Congenital valve disease
- Mitral regurgitation
- Mitral stenosis
- Mitral valve disease
- Mitral valve prolapse
- Pulmonic regurgitation
- Pulmonic stenosis
- Pulmonic valve disease
- Tricuspid regurgitation
- Tricuspid stenosis
- Tricuspid valve disease

Causes of Heart Valve Disease

Heart conditions and other disorders, age-related changes, rheumatic fever, and infections can cause acquired heart valve disease. These factors change the shape or flexibility of once-normal valves.

The cause of congenital heart valve defects isn't known. These defects occur before birth as the heart is forming. Congenital heart valve defects can occur alone or with other types of congenital heart defects.

Heart Conditions and Other Disorders

Heart valves can be stretched and distorted by the following:

- Damage and scar tissue due to a heart attack or injury to the heart can stretch and distort the heart valves.
- Advanced high blood pressure and heart failure can stretch and distort the heart valves. These conditions can enlarge the heart or the main arteries.
- Narrowing of the aorta due to the buildup of a fatty material called plaque inside the artery can cause damage. The aorta is the main artery that carries oxygen-rich blood to the body. The buildup of plaque inside an artery is called atherosclerosis.

Age-Related Changes

Men older than 65 and women older than 75 are prone to developing calcium and other deposits on their heart valves. These deposits stiffen and thicken the valve flaps and limit blood flow (stenosis).

The aortic valve is especially prone to this problem. The deposits resemble those seen in the narrowed and hardened blood vessels of people who have atherosclerosis. Some of the same processes may cause both atherosclerosis and heart valve disease.

Rheumatic Fever

Some people have heart valve disease due to untreated strep throat or other infections with strep bacteria, which progress to rheumatic fever.

When the body tries to fight the strep infection, one or more heart valves may be damaged or scarred in the process. The aortic and mitral valves are most often affected. Symptoms due to heart valve damage often don't appear until many years after recovery from rheumatic fever.

Today, most people with strep infections are treated with antibiotics before rheumatic fever develops. It's very important to take the entire amount of antibiotics your doctor prescribes for strep throat, even if you feel better.

Heart valve disease due to rheumatic fever mainly affects older people who had strep infections before antibiotics were available. It also affects people from developing countries, where rheumatic fever is more common.

Infections

Common germs that enter through the bloodstream and get carried to the heart can sometimes infect the inner surface of the heart, including the heart valves. This rare, but sometimes life-threatening, infection is called endocarditis.

The germs can enter the bloodstream through needles, syringes, or other medical devices and through breaks in the skin or gums. Usually the body's defenses fight off the germs and no infection occurs. Sometimes these defenses fail, which leads to endocarditis.

Endocarditis can develop in people who already have abnormal blood flow through a heart valve due to congenital or acquired heart valve disease. The abnormal blood flow causes blood clots to form on the surface of the valve. The blood clots make it easier for germs to attach to and infect the valve.

Endocarditis can worsen existing heart valve disease.

189

Other Conditions and Factors Linked to Heart Valve Disease

A number of other conditions and factors are sometimes linked to heart valve disease. However, it's often unknown how these conditions actually cause heart valve disease.

- **Systemic lupus erythematosus (SLE):** SLE and other immune diseases can affect the aortic and mitral valves.

- **Carcinoid syndrome:** Tumors in the digestive tract that spread to the liver or lymph nodes can affect the tricuspid and pulmonary valves.

- **Metabolic disorders:** Relatively uncommon diseases, such as Fabry disease and hyperlipidemia, can affect the heart valves.

- **Diet medicines:** The use of fenfluramine and phentermine ("Fen-Phen") has sometimes been linked to heart valve problems. These problems typically stabilize or improve after the medicine is stopped.

- **Radiation therapy:** Radiation therapy to the chest area can cause heart valve disease. This therapy is used to treat cancer. Heart valve disease due to radiation therapy may not cause symptoms for as many as 20 years after the therapy ends.

- **Marfan syndrome:** Congenital disorders, such as Marfan syndrome, and other connective tissue disorders mainly affect the structure of the body's main arteries. However, these conditions also can also affect the heart valves.

Risk for Heart Valve Disease

Populations Affected

Older people are more likely to develop heart valve disease. It's estimated that one in eight people age 75 or older have at least moderate heart valve disease.

People who have a history of endocarditis, rheumatic fever, heart attack, or heart failure—or previous heart valve disease—are more likely to develop heart valve disease.

About 1 to 2 percent of people are born with an aortic valve that has two flaps instead of three. Sometimes an aortic valve may have three flaps, but two flaps are fused together and act as one flap. This is called a bicuspid or bicommissural aortic valve. People who have this congenital condition are more likely to develop aortic heart valve disease.

Major Risk Factors

The major risk factors for acquired heart valve disease are the following:

- Age

- Heart disease risk factors, such as unhealthy blood cholesterol levels, high blood pressure, smoking, insulin resistance, diabetes, overweight or obesity, lack of physical activity, and a family history of early heart disease

- Risk factors for endocarditis, such as intravenous drug use

Signs and Symptoms of Heart Valve Disease

Major Signs and Symptoms

The main sign of heart valve disease is an unusual heart sound called a heart murmur. Your doctor can hear a heart murmur with a stethoscope.

However, many people have heart murmurs without having heart valve disease or any other heart problems. Others may have heart murmurs due to heart valve disease, but have no other signs or symptoms.

Heart valve disease often worsens over time, so signs and symptoms may develop years after a heart murmur is first heard. Many people who have heart valve disease don't have any symptoms until they're middle-aged or older.

Other common signs and symptoms of heart valve disease relate to heart failure, which heart valve disease can eventually cause. These symptoms include the following:

- Unusual fatigue (tiredness)

- Shortness of breath, especially when you exert yourself or when you're lying down

- Swelling of your ankles, feet, or sometimes the abdomen

Other Signs and Symptoms

Heart valve disease can cause chest pain that may only happen when you exert yourself. You also may notice a fluttering, racing, or irregular heartbeat. Some types of heart valve disease, such as aortic or mitral valve stenosis, can cause dizziness or fainting.

Treating Heart Valve Disease

The goals of heart valve disease treatment are to do the following:

- Prevent, treat, or relieve the symptoms of other related heart conditions

- Protect your valve from further damage

- Repair or replace faulty valves when they cause severe symptoms or become life threatening (Man-made or biological valves are used as replacements.)

Currently, no medicines can cure heart valve disease. However, lifestyle changes and medicines often can successfully treat symptoms and delay complications for many years. Eventually, though, you may need surgery to repair or replace a faulty heart valve.

Section 20.2

Mitral Valve Prolapse

Excerpted from text by the National Heart, Lung, and
Blood Institute (NHLBI, www.nhlbi.nih.gov), part of the
National Institutes of Health, May 2008.

Mitral valve prolapse (MVP) is a condition in which one of the heart's valves, the mitral valve, doesn't work properly. The flaps of the valve are "floppy" and don't close tightly.

Much of the time, MVP doesn't cause any problems. Rarely, blood can leak the wrong way through the floppy valve, which may cause shortness of breath, palpitations (strong or rapid heartbeats), chest pain, and other symptoms.

Normal Mitral Valve

The mitral valve controls the flow of blood between the two chambers on the left side of the heart. The two chambers are the left atrium and the left ventricle.

The mitral valve allows blood to flow from the left atrium to the left ventricle, but not back the other way. (The heart also has a right atrium and ventricle, separated by the tricuspid valve.)

At the beginning of a heartbeat, the atria contract and push blood through to the ventricles. The flaps of the mitral and tricuspid valves swing open to let the blood through. Then, the ventricles contract to pump the blood out of the heart.

When the ventricles contract, the flaps of the mitral and tricuspid valves swing shut. They form a tight seal that prevents blood from flowing back into the atria.

Mitral Valve Prolapse

In MVP, when the left ventricle contracts, one or both flaps of the mitral valve flop or bulge back (prolapse) into the left atrium. This can prevent the valve from forming a tight seal.

As a result, blood may flow backward from the ventricle into the atrium. The backflow of blood is called regurgitation.

Backflow doesn't occur in all cases of MVP. In fact, most people who have MVP don't have backflow and never have any symptoms or complications. In these people, even though the valve flaps prolapse, the valve still can form a tight seal.

When backflow does occur, it can cause symptoms and complications such as shortness of breath, arrhythmias, or chest pain. Arrhythmias are problems with the rate or rhythm of the heartbeat.

Backflow can get worse over time. It can lead to changes in the heart's size and higher pressures in the left atrium and lungs. Backflow also increases the risk for heart valve infections.

Medicines can treat troublesome MVP symptoms and prevent complications. Some people will need surgery to repair or replace their mitral valves.

MVP was once thought to affect as much as 5 to 15 percent of the population. It's now believed that many people who were diagnosed with MVP in the past didn't actually have an abnormal mitral valve.

They may have had a slight bulging of the valve flaps due to other conditions, such as dehydration or a small heart. However, their valves were normal, and there was little or no backflow of blood through their valves.

Now, diagnosing MVP is more precise because of a test called echocardiography. This test allows doctors to easily identify true MVP and detect troublesome backflow.

As a result, it's now believed that less than 3 percent of the population actually has true MVP, and an even smaller percentage has serious complications from it.

Outlook

Most people who have MVP have no symptoms or medical problems and don't need treatment. These people are able to lead normal, active lives; they may not even know they have the condition.

A small number of people who have MVP may need medicines to relieve their symptoms. Very few people who have MVP need heart valve surgery to repair their mitral valves.

Rarely, MVP can cause complications such as arrhythmias (irregular heartbeats) or infective endocarditis. Endocarditis is an infection of the inner lining of the heart chambers and valves. Bacteria that enter the bloodstream can cause the infection.

Other Names for Mitral Valve Prolapse

- Balloon mitral valve
- Barlow syndrome
- Billowing mitral valve
- Click-murmur syndrome
- Floppy valve syndrome
- Myxomatous mitral valve
- Prolapsing mitral valve syndrome

Causes of Mitral Valve Prolapse

The exact cause of mitral valve prolapse (MVP) isn't known. Most people who have the condition are born with it. MVP tends to run in families and is more common in people who were born with connective tissue disorders, such as Marfan syndrome.

The mitral valve can be abnormal in two ways. First, the valve flaps may be oversized and thickened. Second, the valve flaps may be "floppy." The tissue of the flaps and their supporting "strings" are too stretchy, and parts of the valve flop or bulge back into the atrium.

Some people's valves are abnormal in both ways. Either way can keep the valve from making a tight seal.

Risk for Mitral Valve Prolapse

Mitral valve prolapse (MVP) occurs in all age groups and in men and women. MVP with complications or severe symptoms most often occurs in men older than 50.

Certain conditions increase the risk for MVP, including the following:

- Connective tissue disorders, such as Marfan syndrome
- Scoliosis and other skeletal problems
- Some types of muscular dystrophy
- Graves disease

Signs and Symptoms of Mitral Valve Prolapse

Most people who have mitral valve prolapse (MVP) aren't affected by the condition. This is because they don't have any symptoms or major mitral valve backflow.

Among those who do have symptoms, palpitations (strong or rapid heartbeats) are reported most often. Other symptoms include shortness of breath, cough, dizziness, fatigue (tiredness), anxiety, migraine headaches, and chest discomfort.

MVP symptoms can vary from one person to another. They tend to be mild but can worsen over time, mainly when complications occur.

Mitral Valve Prolapse Complications

Complications of MVP are rare. When present, they're most often due to the backflow of blood through the mitral valve.

Mitral valve backflow is most common among men and people who have high blood pressure. People who have severe cases of backflow may need valve surgery to prevent complications.

Mitral valve backflow causes blood to flow backward from the left ventricle into the left atrium. Blood can even back up from the atrium into the lungs, causing shortness of breath.

The backflow of blood puts a strain on the muscles of both the atrium and the ventricle. Over time, the strain can lead to arrhythmias. Backflow also increases the risk of infective endocarditis (IE), an infection of the inner lining of your heart chambers and valves.

Arrhythmias: Mitral valve backflow can cause arrhythmias. Arrhythmias are problems with the rate or rhythm of the heartbeat.

There are many types of arrhythmia. The most common arrhythmias are harmless. Others can be serious or even life threatening.

When the heart rate is too slow, too fast, or irregular, the heart may not be able to pump enough blood to the body. Lack of blood flow can damage the brain, heart, and other organs.

One troublesome arrhythmia that MVP can cause is atrial fibrillation (AF). In AF, the walls of the atria quiver instead of beating normally. As a result, the atria aren't able to pump blood into the ventricles the way they should.

AF is bothersome but rarely life threatening, unless the atria contract very fast or blood clots form in the atria. Blood clots can occur because some of the blood "pools" in the atria instead of flowing into the ventricles. If a blood clot breaks off and goes into the bloodstream, it can reach the brain and cause a stroke.

Infection of the mitral valve: A deformed mitral valve flap attracts bacteria that may be in the bloodstream. The bacteria attach to the valve and can cause a serious infection called infective endocarditis (IE). Signs and symptoms of a bacterial infection include fever, chills, body aches, or headaches.

IE doesn't happen often, but when it does, it's serious. MVP is the most common heart condition that puts people at risk for this infection.

You can take steps to prevent this infection. Floss and brush your teeth regularly. Gum infections and tooth decay can cause IE.

Treating Mitral Valve Prolapse

Most people who have mitral valve prolapse (MVP) don't need treatment because they don't have complications and have few or no symptoms. Even people who do have symptoms may not need treatment.

The presence of symptoms doesn't always mean that the backflow of blood through the valve is significant.

People who have MVP and troublesome mitral valve backflow usually need treatment. MVP is treated with medicines, surgery, or both.

The goals of treating MVP include the following:

- Preventing infective endocarditis (IE), arrhythmias, and other complications

- Relieving symptoms

- Correcting the underlying mitral valve problem, when necessary

Medicines

Medicines called beta-blockers have been used to treat symptoms such as palpitations (strong or rapid heartbeats) and chest discomfort in people who have MVP and little or no mitral valve backflow.

If you have MVP and significant backflow and symptoms, your doctor may prescribe the following:

- Vasodilators widen your blood vessels and reduce the workload of your heart. Examples of vasodilators are isosorbide dinitrate and hydralazine.

- Digoxin strengthens your heartbeat.

- Diuretics (water pills) remove excess fluid in your lungs.

- Medicines such as flecainide and procainamide regulate your heart rhythms.

- Blood-thinning medicines reduce the risk of blood clots forming if you have atrial fibrillation. Examples of blood-thinning medicines include aspirin and warfarin.

Surgery

Surgery on the mitral valve is done only when the valve is very abnormal and blood is flowing back into the atrium. The main goal of surgery is to improve symptoms and reduce the risk of heart failure.

The timing of the surgery is very important. If it's done too early and your leaking valve is working fairly well, you may be put at needless risk from surgery. If it's done too late, heart damage may have already occurred that can't be fixed.

Surgical approaches: Traditionally, mitral valve repair and replacement are done by making an incision (cut) in the breastbone and exposing the heart.

A small but growing number of heart surgeons are using another approach that uses one or more smaller cuts through the side of the chest wall. This results in less cutting, reduced blood loss, and a shorter hospital stay. However, this approach isn't yet available in all hospitals.

Valve repair and valve replacement: In mitral valve surgery, the valve is repaired or replaced completely. Valve repair is preferred when possible. Repair is less likely to weaken the heart. It also lowers the risk of infection and decreases the need for lifelong use of blood-thinning medicines.

If repair isn't an option, then the valve can be replaced. Mechanical valves and biological valves are available as replacement valves.

Mechanical valves are man-made and can last a lifetime. People who have mechanical valves must take blood-thinning medicines for the rest of their lives.

Biological valves are taken from cows or pigs or made from human tissue. Many people who have biological valves don't need to take blood-thinning medicines for the rest of their lives. The major drawback of biological valves is that they weaken and often only last about 10 years.

After surgery, a patient usually stays in the intensive care unit in the hospital for 2 to 3 days. Overall, most people spend about 1 to 2 weeks in the hospital. Complete recovery takes a few weeks to several months, depending on your health before surgery.

If you've had valve repair or replacement, you may need antibiotics before dental work and surgery that can allow bacteria into the bloodstream. These medicines can help prevent IE, a serious heart valve infection. Discuss with your doctor whether you need to take antibiotics before such procedures.

Experimental approaches: Some researchers are testing the repair of leaky valves using a catheter (tube) inserted through a large blood vessel.

Although this approach is less invasive and can prevent a patient from having open-heart surgery, it's only being done at a few medical centers. Large studies haven't yet shown that this new approach is better than traditional approaches.

Section 20.3

Rheumatic Heart Disease

What are rheumatic heart disease and rheumatic fever?

Rheumatic (roo-MAT'ik) heart disease is a condition in which the heart valves are damaged by rheumatic fever.

Rheumatic fever begins with a strep throat (also called strep pharyngitis). Strep throat is caused by Group A *Streptococcus* bacteria. It is the most common bacterial infection of the throat.

Rheumatic fever is an inflammatory disease. It can affect many of the body's connective tissues—especially those of the heart, joints, brain, or skin. Anyone can get acute rheumatic fever, but it usually occurs in children 5 to 15 years old. The rheumatic heart disease that results can last for life.

The incidence of rheumatic fever/rheumatic heart disease is low in the United States and most other developed countries. However, it continues to be the leading cause of cardiovascular death during the first 5 decades of life in the developing world.

What are the symptoms of strep throat?

Symptoms include (but are not limited to):

- sudden onset of sore throat;
- pain on swallowing;
- fever, usually 101–104 degrees Fahrenheit;
- headache;
- red throat/tonsils;
- abdominal pain, nausea, and vomiting may also occur, especially in children.

In some people, strep throat is very mild with just a few symptoms. Also, sore throats are caused more often by viruses than by a strep infection. Viral throat infections don't raise the risk of rheumatic fever and are not treatable with antibiotics.

What are the symptoms of rheumatic fever?

Symptoms may include:

- fever;
- painful, tender, red swollen joints;
- pain in one joint that migrates to another one;
- heart palpitations;
- chest pain;
- shortness of breath;
- skin rashes;
- fatigue;
- small, painless nodules under the skin.

The symptoms of rheumatic fever usually appear about 3 weeks after the strep throat.

How can I prevent rheumatic heart disease?

The best defense against rheumatic heart disease is to prevent rheumatic fever from ever occurring. By treating strep throat with penicillin or other antibiotics, doctors can usually stop acute rheumatic fever from developing.

People who've already had rheumatic fever are more susceptible to recurrent attacks and heart damage. That's why they're given continuous monthly or daily antibiotic treatment, maybe for life. If their heart has been damaged by rheumatic fever, they're also at increased risk for developing infective endocarditis (also known as bacterial endocarditis), an infection of the heart's lining or valves.

In 2007, the American Heart Association updated its guidelines for prevention of endocarditis and concluded that there is no convincing evidence linking dental, gastrointestinal, or genitourinary tract procedures with the development of endocarditis. The prophylactic use of antibiotics prior to a dental procedure is now recommended **only** for those patients with the highest risk of adverse outcome resulting from endocarditis, such as patients with a prosthetic cardiac valve, previous endocarditis, or those with specific forms of congenital heart disease. The guidelines no longer recommend prophylaxis prior to a dental procedure for patients with rheumatic heart disease unless they also have one of the underlying cardiac conditions listed above.

Antibiotic prophylaxis solely to prevent endocarditis is no longer recommended for patients who undergo a gastrointestinal or genitourinary tract procedure.

Chapter 21

Endocarditis

Endocarditis is an infection of the inner lining of your heart chambers and valves. This lining is called the endocardium. The condition also is called infective endocarditis (IE).

The term "endocarditis" also is used to describe an inflammation of the endocardium due to other conditions. This text only discusses endocarditis related to infection.

IE occurs if bacteria, fungi, or other germs invade your bloodstream and attach to abnormal areas of your heart. The infection can damage the heart and cause serious and sometimes fatal complications.

IE can develop quickly or slowly. How the infection develops depends on what type of germ is causing it and whether you have an underlying heart problem. When IE develops quickly, it's called acute infective endocarditis. When it develops slowly, it's called subacute infective endocarditis.

Overview

IE mainly affects people who have the following conditions:

- Damaged or artificial heart valves
- Congenital heart defects (defects present at birth)
- Implanted medical devices in the heart or blood vessels

Excerpted from text by the National Heart, Lung, and Blood Institute (NHLBI, www.nhlbi.nih.gov), part of the National Institutes of Health, November 2008.

People who have normal heart valves also can get IE. However, the condition is much more common in people who have abnormal hearts.

Certain factors make it easier for bacteria to enter your bloodstream. These factors also put you at higher risk for the infection. For example, if you've had IE before, you're at higher risk for the infection.

Other risk factors include having poor dental hygiene and unhealthy teeth and gums, using intravenous (IV) drugs, and having catheters or other medical devices in your body for long periods.

Common symptoms of IE are fever and other flu-like symptoms. Because the infection can affect people in different ways, the signs and symptoms vary. IE also can cause complications in many other parts of the body besides the heart.

If you're at high risk for IE, seek medical care if you have signs or symptoms of the infection, especially a fever that persists or unexplained fatigue (tiredness).

Outlook

IE is treated with antibiotics for several weeks. You also may need heart surgery to repair or replace heart valves or remove infected heart tissue.

Most people who are treated with the proper antibiotics recover. But if the infection isn't treated, or if it persists despite treatment (for example, if the bacteria are resistant to antibiotics), it's usually fatal.

If you have signs or symptoms of IE, you should see your doctor as soon as you can, especially if you have abnormal heart valves.

Causes of Endocarditis

Infective endocarditis (IE) occurs when bacteria, fungi, or other germs invade your bloodstream and attach to abnormal areas of your heart. Certain factors increase the risk of germs attaching to a heart valve or chamber and causing an infection.

A common underlying factor in IE is a structural heart defect, especially faulty heart valves. Usually your immune system will kill germs in your bloodstream. However, if your heart has a rough lining or abnormal valves, the invading germs can attach and multiply in the heart.

Other factors, such as those that allow germs to build up in your bloodstream, also can play a role in causing IE. Common activities, such as brushing your teeth or having certain dental procedures, can allow bacteria to enter your bloodstream. This is even more likely to happen if your teeth and gums are in poor condition.

Having a catheter or other medical devices inserted through your skin, especially for long periods, also can allow bacteria to enter your bloodstream. People who use intravenous (IV) drugs also are at risk for infections due to germs on needles and syringes.

Bacteria also may spread to the blood and heart from infections in other parts of the body, such as the gut, skin, or genitals.

Endocarditis Complications

As the bacteria or other germs multiply in your heart, they form clumps with other cells and matter found in the blood. These clumps are called vegetations.

As IE worsens, pieces of the vegetations can break off and travel to almost any other organ or tissue in the body. There, the pieces can block blood flow or cause a new infection. As a result, IE can cause a wide range of complications.

Heart Complications

Heart problems are the most common complication of IE. They occur in one third to one half of all people who have the infection. These problems may include a new heart murmur, heart failure, heart valve damage, heart block, or, rarely, a heart attack.

Central Nervous System Complications

These complications occur in as many as 20 to 40 percent of people who have IE. Central nervous system complications most often occur when bits of the vegetation, called emboli, break away and lodge in the brain.

There, they can cause local infections (called brain abscesses) or a more widespread brain infection (called meningitis).

Emboli also can cause a stroke or seizures. This happens if they block blood vessels or affect the brain's electrical signals. These complications can cause long-lasting damage to the brain and may even be fatal.

Complications in Other Organs

IE also can affect other organs in the body, such as the lungs, kidneys, and spleen.

Lungs: The lungs are especially at risk when IE affects the right side of the heart. This is called right-sided infective endocarditis. A vegetation or blood clot going to the lungs can cause a pulmonary embolism and lung damage. Other lung complications include pneumonia and a buildup of fluid or pus around the lungs.

Kidneys: IE can cause kidney abscesses and kidney damage. IE also can cause inflammation of the internal filtering structures of the kidneys. Signs and symptoms of kidney complications include back or side pain, blood in the urine, or a change in the color or amount of urine. In a small number of people, IE can cause kidney failure.

Spleen: The spleen is an organ located in the left upper part of the abdomen near the stomach. In as many as 25 to 60 percent of people who have IE, the spleen enlarges (especially in people who have long-term IE). Sometimes, emboli also can damage the spleen. Signs and symptoms of spleen problems include pain or discomfort in the upper left abdomen and/or left shoulder, a feeling of fullness or the inability to eat large meals, and hiccups.

Risk for Endocarditis

Infective endocarditis (IE) is an uncommon condition that can affect both children and adults. It's more common in men than women.

IE typically affects people who have abnormal hearts or other conditions that make them more likely to get the infection. In some cases, IE does affect people who were healthy before the infection.

Major Risk Factors

The germs that cause IE tend to attach and multiply on damaged, malformed, or artificial heart valves and implanted medical devices. Certain conditions put you at higher risk for IE. These include the following:

- Congenital heart defects (defects that are present at birth), such as a malformed heart or abnormal heart valves

- Artificial heart valves; an implanted medical device in the heart, such as a pacemaker wire; or an intravenous (IV) catheter in a blood vessel for a long time

- Heart valves damaged by rheumatic fever or calcium deposits that cause age-related valve thickening (Scars in the heart from a previous case of IE also can damage heart valves.)

- IV drug use, especially if needles are shared or reused, contaminated substances are injected, or the skin isn't properly cleaned before injection

Signs and Symptoms of Endocarditis

Infective endocarditis (IE) can cause a range of signs and symptoms that can vary from person to person. Signs and symptoms also can vary over time in the same person.

Signs and symptoms differ depending on whether you have an underlying heart problem, the type of germ causing the infection, and whether you have acute or subacute IE.

Signs and symptoms of IE may include the following:

- Flu-like symptoms, such as fever, chills, fatigue (tiredness), aching muscles and joints, night sweats, and headache
- Shortness of breath or a cough that won't go away
- A new heart murmur or a change in an existing heart murmur
- Skin changes such as the following:
  - Overall paleness
  - Small, painful, red or purplish bumps under the skin on the fingers or toes
  - Small, dark, painless, flat spots on the palms of the hands or the soles of the feet
  - Tiny spots under the fingernails, on the whites of the eyes, on the roof of the mouth and inside of the cheeks, or on the chest from broken blood vessels
- Nausea (feeling sick to your stomach), vomiting, a decrease in appetite, a sense of fullness with discomfort on the upper left side of the abdomen, or weight loss with or without a change in appetite
- Blood in the urine
- Swelling in the feet, legs, or abdomen

Treating Endocarditis

Infective endocarditis (IE) is treated with antibiotics and sometimes with heart surgery.

Chapter 22

Pericarditis

Pericarditis is a condition in which the membrane, or sac, around your heart is inflamed. This sac is called the pericardium.

The pericardium holds the heart in place and helps it work properly. The sac is made of two thin layers of tissue that enclose your heart. Between the two layers is a small amount of fluid. This fluid keeps the layers from rubbing against each other and causing friction.

In pericarditis, the layers of tissue become inflamed and can rub against the heart. This causes chest pain—a common symptom of pericarditis.

The chest pain from pericarditis may feel like pain from a heart attack. If you have chest pain, you should call 911 right away, as you may be having a heart attack.

Overview

Many factors can cause pericarditis. Viruses and infections are common causes. Less often, pericarditis occurs after a heart attack or heart surgery. Lupus, scleroderma, rheumatoid arthritis, or other autoimmune disorders also can cause the condition. In about half of all cases, the cause is unknown. Pericarditis can be acute or chronic. Acute means that it occurs suddenly and usually doesn't last long. Chronic means that it develops over time and may take longer to treat.

Excerpted from text by the National Heart, Lung, and Blood Institute (NHLBI, www.nhlbi.nih.gov), part of the National Institutes of Health, March 2008.

Both acute and chronic pericarditis can disrupt your heart's normal function and possibly (although rarely) lead to death. However, most cases of pericarditis are mild and clear up on their own or with rest and simple treatment. Other times, more intense treatment is needed to prevent complications.

Treatment may include medicines and, less often, procedures and/ or surgery.

Outlook

It may take from a few days to weeks or even months to recover from pericarditis. With proper and prompt treatment, such as rest and ongoing care, most people fully recover from pericarditis. These measures also can help reduce the chances of getting the condition again.

Other Names for Pericarditis

- Idiopathic pericarditis (pericarditis with no known cause)
- Acute pericarditis
- Chronic pericarditis
- Chronic effusive pericarditis (form of chronic pericarditis)
- Chronic constrictive pericarditis (form of chronic pericarditis)

Causes of Pericarditis

The cause of about half of all pericarditis cases (both acute and chronic) is unknown.

Viral infections are likely the most common cause of acute pericarditis, but the virus may never be found. Pericarditis often occurs after a respiratory infection. Bacterial, fungal, and other infections also can cause pericarditis.

Less often, pericarditis is caused by the following:

- Autoimmune disorders, such as lupus, scleroderma, and rheumatoid arthritis
- Heart attack and heart surgery
- Kidney failure, HIV/AIDS [human immunodeficiency virus/acquired immunodeficiency syndrome], cancer, tuberculosis, and other health problems
- Injury from accidents or radiation therapy

- Certain medicines, like phenytoin (an antiseizure medicine), warfarin and heparin (blood-thinning medicines), and procainamide (a medicine to treat abnormal heartbeats)

The causes of acute and chronic pericarditis are the same.

Risk for Pericarditis

Pericarditis occurs in people of all ages. However, men between the ages of 20 and 50 are more likely to get it.

People who are treated for acute pericarditis may get it again. This may happen in 15 to 30 percent of people who have the condition. A small number of these people go on to develop chronic pericarditis.

Signs and Symptoms of Pericarditis

Sharp, stabbing chest pain is a common symptom of acute pericarditis. The pain usually comes on quickly. It often is felt in the middle or the left side of the chest.

The pain tends to ease when you sit up and lean forward. Lying down and deep breathing worsens it. For some people, the pain feels like a dull ache or pressure in their chests.

The chest pain may feel like pain from a heart attack. If you have chest pain, you should call 911 right away, as you may be having a heart attack.

Fever is another common symptom of acute pericarditis. Other symptoms are weakness, trouble breathing, and coughing.

Chronic pericarditis often causes tiredness, coughing, and shortness of breath. Chest pain is often absent in this type of pericarditis. Severe cases of chronic pericarditis can lead to swelling in the stomach and legs and low blood pressure (hypotension).

Complications of Pericarditis

Two serious complications of pericarditis are cardiac tamponade and chronic constrictive pericarditis.

Cardiac tamponade occurs when too much fluid collects in the pericardium (the sac around the heart). The extra fluid puts pressure on the heart. This prevents the heart from properly filling with blood. As a result, less blood leaves the heart. This causes a sharp drop in blood pressure. If left untreated, cardiac tamponade can cause death.

Chronic constrictive pericarditis is a rare disease that develops over time. It leads to scar-like tissue throughout the pericardium. The sac becomes stiff and can't move properly. In time, the scarred tissue compresses the heart and prevents it from working correctly.

Treatment of Pericarditis

Most cases of pericarditis are mild and clear up on their own or with rest and simple treatment. Other times, more intense treatment is needed to prevent complications. Treatment may include medicines and, less often, procedures and/or surgery.

The goals of treatment are to do the following:

- Reduce pain and inflammation
- Treat the underlying cause, if it's known
- Check for complications

Specific Types of Treatment

As a first step in your treatment, your doctor may advise you to rest until you feel better and have no fever.

He or she may tell you to take over-the-counter, anti-inflammatory medicines, such as aspirin or ibuprofen, to reduce pain and inflammation. You may need stronger medicine if your pain is severe.

If your pain continues to be severe, your doctor may prescribe a medicine called colchicine and, possibly, prednisone (a steroid medicine).

If an infection is causing your pericarditis, your doctor will prescribe an antibiotic or other appropriate medicine to treat the infection.

You may need to stay in the hospital during treatment so your doctor can check you for complications.

The symptoms of acute pericarditis can last from a few days to 3 weeks. Chronic cases may last several months.

Other Types of Treatment

If you have complications of pericarditis, you'll need treatment for those problems. Two serious complications of pericarditis are cardiac tamponade and chronic constrictive pericarditis.

Cardiac tamponade is treated with a procedure called pericardiocentesis. A needle or tube (called a catheter) is inserted into the chest wall to remove excess fluid that has collected inside the pericardium. This relieves pressure on the heart.

If time allows, the fluid may be removed with a special catheter or tube put through a small cut in the chest.

The only cure for chronic constrictive pericarditis is surgery to remove the pericardium. This is known as a pericardiectomy.

The treatments for these complications require hospital stays.

Chapter 23

Cardiac Tumor

An atrial myxoma is a noncancerous tumor in the upper left or right side of the heart. It grows on the wall (atrial septum) that separates the two sides of the heart.

Causes

A myxoma is a primary heart (cardiac) tumor. This means that the tumor started within the heart. Most heart tumors start somewhere else.

Primary cardiac tumors are rare. Myxomas are the most common type of these rare tumors. About 75% of myxomas occur in the left atrium of the heart, usually beginning in the wall that divides the two upper chambers of the heart. The rest are in the right atrium. Right atrial myxomas are sometimes associated with tricuspid stenosis and atrial fibrillation.

Myxomas are more common in women. About 10% of myxomas are passed down through families (inherited). Such tumors are called familial myxomas. They tend to occur in more than one part of the heart at a time, and often cause symptoms at a younger age than other myxomas.

Symptoms

Symptoms may occur at any time, but most often they accompany a change of body position. Symptoms may include:

"Atrial myxoma," © 2009 A.D.A.M., Inc. Reprinted with permission.

- breathing difficulty when lying flat;
- breathing difficulty when asleep;
- chest pain or tightness;
- dizziness;
- fainting;
- sensation of feeling your heart beat (palpitations);
- shortness of breath with activity.

The symptoms and signs of left atrial myxomas often mimic mitral stenosis. General symptoms may also be present, such as:

- blueness of skin, especially the fingers (Raynaud phenomenon);
- cough;
- curvature of nails accompanied with soft tissue enlargement (clubbing) of the fingers;
- fever;
- fingers that change color upon pressure or with cold or stress;
- general discomfort (malaise);
- involuntary weight loss;
- joint pain;
- swelling—any part of the body.

These general symptoms may also mimic those of infective endocarditis.

Exams and Tests

The health care provider will listen to the heart with stethoscope. A "tumor plop" (a sound related to movement of the tumor), abnormal heart sounds, or murmur may be heard. These sounds may change when the patient changes position.

Right atrial myxomas rarely produce symptoms until they have grown to be at least 13 cm (about 5 inches) wide.

Imaging tests may include:

- chest x-ray;
- CT [computed tomography] scan of chest;
- ECG [electrocardiogram];
- echocardiogram;

- Doppler study
- heart MRI [magnetic resonance imaging];
- left heart angiography;
- right heart angiography.

Blood tests: A complete blood count may show anemia and increased white blood cells. The erythrocyte sedimentation rate (ESR) is increased.

Treatment

The tumor must be surgically removed. Some patients will also need their mitral valve replaced. This can be done during the same surgery.

Myxomas may come back if surgery did not remove all of the tumor cells.

Outlook (Prognosis)

Although a myxoma is not cancer, complications are common. Untreated, a myxoma can lead to an embolism (tumor cells breaking off and traveling within the bloodstream), which can block blood flow or cause the myxoma to grow in another part of the body. Myxoma fragments can move to the brain, eye, or limbs.

If the tumor grows inside the heart, it can block blood flow through the mitral valve and cause symptoms of mitral stenosis. This may require emergency surgery to prevent sudden death.

Possible Complications

- Arrhythmias
- Pulmonary edema
- Peripheral emboli
- Spread (metastasis) of the tumor
- Blockage of the mitral heart valve

When to Contact a Medical Professional

Tell your health care provider if there is any family history of myxomas or if you have symptoms of atrial myxoma.

Updated by: Larry A. Weinrauch, MD, Assistant Professor of Medicine, Harvard Medical School, and Private practice specializing in

Cardiovascular Disease, Watertown, MA. Review provided by VeriMed Healthcare Network. Also reviewed by David Zieve, MD, MHA, Medical Director, A.D.A.M., Inc.

Part Three

Blood Vessel Disease

Chapter 24

Atherosclerosis

Atherosclerosis is a disease in which plaque builds up on the insides of your arteries. Arteries are blood vessels that carry oxygen-rich blood to your heart and other parts of your body.

Plaque is made up of fat, cholesterol, calcium, and other substances found in the blood. Over time, plaque hardens and narrows your arteries. The flow of oxygen-rich blood to your organs and other parts of your body is reduced. This can lead to serious problems, including heart attack, stroke, or even death.

Overview

Atherosclerosis can affect any artery in the body, including arteries in the heart, brain, arms, legs, and pelvis. As a result, different diseases may develop based on which arteries are affected.

- **Coronary artery disease (CAD):** This is when plaque builds up in the coronary arteries. These arteries supply oxygen-rich blood to your heart. When blood flow to your heart is reduced or blocked, it can lead to chest pain and heart attack. CAD also is called heart disease, and it's the leading cause of death in the United States.

- **Carotid artery disease:** This happens when plaque builds up in the carotid arteries. These arteries supply oxygen-rich blood

Excerpted from text by the National Heart, Lung, and Blood Institute (NHLBI, www.nhlbi.nih.gov), part of the National Institutes of Health, November 11, 2007.

to your brain. When blood flow to your brain is reduced or blocked, it can lead to stroke.

- **Peripheral arterial disease (PAD):** This occurs when plaque builds up in the major arteries that supply oxygen-rich blood to the legs, arms, and pelvis. When blood flow to these parts of your body is reduced or blocked, it can lead to numbness, pain, and sometimes dangerous infections.

Some people with atherosclerosis have no signs or symptoms. They may not be diagnosed until after a heart attack or stroke.

The main treatment for atherosclerosis is lifestyle changes. You also may need medicines and medical procedures. These, along with ongoing medical care, can help you live a healthier life.

The cause of atherosclerosis isn't known. However, certain conditions may raise your chances of developing it. These conditions are known as risk factors. You can control some risk factors, such as lack of physical activity, smoking, and unhealthy eating. Others you can't control, such as age and family history of heart disease.

Outlook

Better treatments have reduced the number of deaths from atherosclerosis-related diseases. These treatments also have improved the quality of life for people with these diseases. Still, the number of people diagnosed with atherosclerosis remains high.

You may be able to prevent or delay atherosclerosis and the diseases it can cause, mainly by maintaining a healthy lifestyle. This, along with ongoing medical care, can help you avoid the problems of atherosclerosis and live a long, healthy life.

Other Names for Atherosclerosis

- Arteriosclerosis
- Hardening of the arteries

Causes of Atherosclerosis

The exact cause of atherosclerosis isn't known. However, studies show that atherosclerosis is a slow, complex disease that may start in childhood. It develops faster as you age.

Atherosclerosis may start when certain factors damage the inner layers of the arteries. These factors include the following:

- Smoking
- High amounts of certain fats and cholesterol in the blood
- High blood pressure
- High amounts of sugar in the blood due to insulin resistance or diabetes

When damage occurs, your body starts a healing process. Fatty tissues release compounds that promote this process. This healing causes plaque to build up where the arteries are damaged.

Over time, the plaque may crack. Blood cells called platelets clump together to form blood clots where the cracks are. This narrows the arteries more and worsens angina (chest pain) or causes a heart attack.

Researchers continue to look at why atherosclerosis develops. They hope to find answers to the following questions:

- Why and how do the arteries become damaged?
- How does plaque develop and change over time?
- Why does plaque break open and lead to clots?

Risk for Atherosclerosis

Coronary artery disease (atherosclerosis of the coronary arteries) is the leading cause of death in the United States.

The exact cause of atherosclerosis isn't known. However, certain traits, conditions, or habits may raise your chance of developing it. These conditions are known as risk factors. Your chances of developing atherosclerosis increase with the number of risk factors you have.

You can control most risk factors and help prevent or delay atherosclerosis. Other risk factors can't be controlled.

Major Risk Factors

- **Unhealthy blood cholesterol levels:** This includes high LDL [low-density lipoprotein] cholesterol (sometimes called bad cholesterol) and low HDL [high-density lipoprotein] cholesterol (sometimes called good cholesterol).
- **High blood pressure:** Blood pressure is considered high if it stays at or above 140/90 mmHg [millimeters of mercury] over a period of time.

- **Smoking:** This can damage and tighten blood vessels, raise cholesterol levels, and raise blood pressure. Smoking also doesn't allow enough oxygen to reach the body's tissues.

- **Insulin resistance:** This condition occurs when the body can't use its own insulin properly. Insulin is a hormone that helps move blood sugar into cells where it's used.

- **Diabetes:** This is a disease in which the body's blood sugar level is high because the body doesn't make enough insulin or doesn't use its insulin properly.

- **Overweight or obesity:** Overweight is having extra body weight from muscle, bone, fat, and/or water. Obesity is having a high amount of extra body fat.

- **Lack of physical activity:** Lack of activity can worsen other risk factors for atherosclerosis.

- **Age:** As you get older, your risk for atherosclerosis increases. Genetic or lifestyle factors cause plaque to build in your arteries as you age. By the time you're middle-aged or older, enough plaque has built up to cause signs or symptoms. In men, the risk increases after age 45. In women, the risk increases after age 55.

- **Family history of early heart disease:** Your risk for atherosclerosis increases if your father or a brother was diagnosed with heart disease before 55 years of age, or if your mother or a sister was diagnosed with heart disease before 65 years of age.

Although age and a family history of early heart disease are risk factors, it doesn't mean that you will develop atherosclerosis if you have one or both.

Making lifestyle changes and/or taking medicines to treat other risk factors can often lessen genetic influences and prevent atherosclerosis from developing, even in older adults.

Emerging Risk Factors

Scientists continue to study other possible risk factors for atherosclerosis.

High levels of a protein called C-reactive protein (CRP) in the blood may raise the risk for atherosclerosis and heart attack. High levels of CRP are proof of inflammation in the body. Inflammation is the body's response to injury or infection. Damage to the arteries' inner walls seems to trigger inflammation and help plaque grow.

People with low CRP levels may get atherosclerosis at a slower rate than people with high CRP levels. Research is under way to find out whether reducing inflammation and lowering CRP levels also can reduce the risk of atherosclerosis.

High levels of fats called triglycerides in the blood also may raise the risk of atherosclerosis, particularly in women.

Other Factors That Affect Atherosclerosis

Other risk factors also may raise your risk for developing atherosclerosis. These include the following:

- **Sleep apnea:** Sleep apnea is a disorder in which your breathing stops or gets very shallow while you're sleeping. Untreated sleep apnea can raise your chances of having high blood pressure, diabetes, and even a heart attack or stroke.

- **Stress:** Research shows that the most commonly reported "trigger" for a heart attack is an emotionally upsetting event—particularly one involving anger.

- **Alcohol:** Heavy drinking can damage the heart muscle and worsen other risk factors for atherosclerosis. Men should have no more than two drinks containing alcohol a day. Women should have no more than one drink containing alcohol a day.

Signs and Symptoms of Atherosclerosis

Atherosclerosis usually doesn't cause signs and symptoms until it severely narrows or totally blocks an artery. Many people don't know they have the disease until they have a medical emergency, such as a heart attack or stroke.

Some people may have other signs and symptoms of the disease. These depend on which arteries are severely narrowed or blocked.

The coronary arteries supply oxygen-rich blood to your heart. When plaque narrows or blocks these arteries (a condition called coronary artery disease, or CAD), a common symptom is angina.

Angina is chest pain or discomfort that occurs when your heart muscle doesn't get enough oxygen-rich blood. Angina may feel like pressure or a squeezing pain in your chest. You also may feel it in your shoulders, arms, neck, jaw, or back.

This pain tends to get worse with activity and go away when you rest. Emotional stress also can trigger the pain.

Other symptoms of CAD are shortness of breath and arrhythmias (irregular heartbeats).

The carotid arteries supply oxygen-rich blood to your brain. When plaque narrows or blocks these arteries (a condition called carotid artery disease), you may have symptoms of a stroke. These symptoms include sudden numbness, weakness, and dizziness.

Plaque also can build up in the major arteries that supply oxygen-rich blood to the legs, arms, and pelvis (a condition called peripheral arterial disease). When these arteries are narrowed or blocked, it can lead to numbness, pain, and sometimes dangerous infections.

Diagnosing Atherosclerosis

Your doctor will diagnose atherosclerosis based on the following:

- Your medical and family histories
- Your risk factors
- The results of a physical exam and diagnostic tests

Specialists Involved

If you have atherosclerosis, a doctor, internist, or general practitioner may handle your care. Your doctor may send you to other health care specialists if you need expert care. These specialists may include the following:

- **A cardiologist** (a doctor who specializes in treating people with heart problems): You may see a cardiologist if you have coronary artery disease (CAD).

- **A vascular specialist** (a doctor who specializes in treating people with blood vessel problems): You may see a vascular specialist if you have peripheral arterial disease (PAD).

- **A neurologist** (a doctor who specializes in treating people with disorders of the nervous system): You may see a neurologist if you've had a stroke due to carotid artery disease.

Physical Exam

During the physical exam, your doctor may listen to your arteries for an abnormal whooshing sound called a bruit. Your doctor can hear a bruit when placing a stethoscope over an affected artery. A bruit may indicate poor blood flow due to plaque.

Your doctor also may check to see whether any of your pulses (for example, in the leg or foot) are weak or absent. A weak or absent pulse can be a sign of a blocked artery.

Diagnostic Tests and Procedures

Your doctor may order one or more tests to diagnose atherosclerosis. These tests also can help your doctor learn the extent of your disease and plan the best treatment.

Blood Tests

Blood tests check the levels of certain fats, cholesterol, sugar, and proteins in your blood. Abnormal levels may show that you have risk factors for atherosclerosis.

EKG (electrocardiogram): An EKG is a simple test that detects and records the electrical activity of your heart. An EKG shows how fast your heart is beating and whether it has a regular rhythm. It also shows the strength and timing of electrical signals as they pass through each part of your heart.

Certain electrical patterns that the EKG detects can suggest whether CAD is likely. An EKG also can show signs of a previous or current heart attack.

Chest x-ray: A chest x-ray takes a picture of the organs and structures inside the chest, including your heart, lungs, and blood vessels.

A chest x-ray can reveal signs of heart failure.

Ankle/brachial index: This test compares the blood pressure in your ankle with the blood pressure in your arm to see how well your blood is flowing. This test can help diagnose PAD.

Echocardiography: This test uses sound waves to create a moving picture of your heart. Echocardiography provides information about the size and shape of your heart and how well your heart chambers and valves are working.

The test also can identify areas of poor blood flow to the heart, areas of heart muscle that aren't contracting normally, and previous injury to the heart muscle caused by poor blood flow.

Computed tomography scan: A computed tomography, or CT, scan creates computer-generated images of the heart, brain, or other

227

areas of the body. The test can often show hardening and narrowing of large arteries.

Stress testing: During stress testing, you exercise to make your heart work hard and beat fast while heart tests are performed. If you can't exercise, you're given medicine to speed up your heart rate.

When your heart is beating fast and working hard, it needs more blood and oxygen. Arteries narrowed by plaque can't supply enough oxygen-rich blood to meet your heart's needs. A stress test can show possible signs of CAD, such as the following:

- Abnormal changes in your heart rate or blood pressure
- Symptoms such as shortness of breath or chest pain
- Abnormal changes in your heart rhythm or your heart's electrical activity

During the stress test, if you can't exercise for as long as what's considered normal for someone your age, it may be a sign that not enough blood is flowing to your heart. But other factors besides CAD can prevent you from exercising long enough (for example, lung diseases, anemia, or poor general fitness).

Some stress tests use a radioactive dye, sound waves, positron emission tomography (PET), or cardiac magnetic resonance imaging (MRI) to take pictures of your heart when it's working hard and when it's at rest.

These imaging stress tests can show how well blood is flowing in the different parts of your heart. They also can show how well your heart pumps blood when it beats.

Angiography: Angiography is a test that uses dye and special x-rays to show the insides of your arteries. This test can show whether plaque is blocking your arteries and how severe the plaque is.

A thin, flexible tube called a catheter is put into a blood vessel in your arm, groin (upper thigh), or neck. A dye that can be seen on x-ray is then injected into the arteries. By looking at the x-ray picture, your doctor can see the flow of blood through your arteries.

Treating Atherosclerosis

Treatments for atherosclerosis may include lifestyle changes, medicines, and medical procedures or surgery.

Goals of Treatment

The goals of treatment are to do the following:

- Relieve symptoms
- Reduce risk factors in an effort to slow, stop, or reverse the buildup of plaque
- Lower the risk of blood clots forming
- Widen or bypass clogged arteries
- Prevent diseases related to atherosclerosis

Lifestyle Changes

- Making lifestyle changes can often help prevent or treat atherosclerosis. For some people, these changes may be the only treatment needed.
- Follow a healthy eating plan to prevent or reduce high blood pressure and high blood cholesterol and to maintain a healthy weight.
- Increase your physical activity. Check with your doctor first to find out how much and what kinds of activity are safe for you.
- Lose weight, if you're overweight or obese.
- Quit smoking, if you smoke. Avoid exposure to secondhand smoke.
- Reduce stress.

Medicines

To help slow or reverse atherosclerosis, your doctor may prescribe medicines to help lower your cholesterol or blood pressure or prevent blood clots from forming.

For successful treatment, take all medicines as your doctor prescribes.

Medical Procedures and Surgery

If you have severe atherosclerosis, your doctor may recommend one of several procedures or surgeries.

Angioplasty is a procedure to open blocked or narrowed coronary (heart) arteries. Angioplasty can improve blood flow to the heart, relieve chest pain, and possibly prevent a heart attack. Sometimes a small mesh tube called a stent is placed in the artery to keep it open after the procedure.

Coronary artery bypass grafting (CABG) is a type of surgery. In CABG, arteries or veins from other areas in your body are used to bypass (that is, go around) your narrowed coronary arteries. CABG can improve blood flow to your heart, relieve chest pain, and possibly prevent a heart attack.

Bypass grafting also can be used for leg arteries. In this surgery, a healthy blood vessel is used to bypass a narrowed or blocked blood vessel in one of your legs. The healthy blood vessel redirects blood around the artery, improving blood flow to the leg.

Carotid artery surgery removes plaque buildup from the carotid arteries in the neck. This opens the arteries and improves blood flow to the brain. Carotid artery surgery can help prevent a stroke.

Preventing or Delaying Atherosclerosis

Taking action to control your risk factors can help prevent or delay atherosclerosis and its related diseases. Your chance of developing atherosclerosis goes up with the number of risk factors you have.

Making lifestyle changes and taking prescribed medicines are important steps.

Know your family history of health problems related to atherosclerosis. If you or someone in your family has this disease, be sure to tell your doctor. Also, let your doctor know if you smoke.

Chapter 25

Carotid Artery Disease

Carotid artery disease is a condition in which a fatty material called plaque builds up inside the carotid arteries. You have two common carotid arteries—one on each side of your neck—that divide into internal and external carotid arteries.

The internal carotid arteries supply oxygen-rich blood to your brain. The external carotid arteries supply oxygen-rich blood to your face, scalp, and neck.

Carotid artery disease can be very serious because it can cause a stroke, or "brain attack." A stroke occurs when blood flow to your brain is cut off.

If blood flow is cut off for more than a few minutes, the cells in your brain start to die. This impairs the parts of the body that the brain cells control. A stroke can cause lasting brain damage, long-term disability, paralysis (an inability to move), or death.

Overview

When plaque builds up in arteries, the condition is called atherosclerosis. Over time, plaque hardens and narrows the arteries. This limits the flow of oxygen-rich blood to your organs and other parts of your body.

Atherosclerosis can affect any artery in the body. For example, when plaque builds up in the coronary (heart) arteries, a heart attack can

Excerpted from text by the National Heart, Lung, and Blood Institute (NHLBI, www.nhlbi.nih.gov), part of the National Institutes of Health, March 2008.

occur. When plaque builds up in the carotid arteries, a stroke can occur.

A stroke also can occur if blood clots form in the carotid arteries. This can happen if, over time, the plaque in an artery cracks or ruptures. Blood cells called platelets stick to the site of the injury and may clump together to form blood clots. Blood clots can partly or fully block a carotid artery.

Also, a piece of plaque or a blood clot can break away from the wall of the carotid artery. It can travel through the bloodstream and get stuck in one of the brain's smaller arteries. This can block blood flow in the artery and cause a stroke.

Carotid artery disease may not cause signs or symptoms until the carotid arteries are severely narrowed or blocked. For some people, a stroke is the first sign of the disease.

Outlook

Carotid artery disease causes more than half of the strokes that occur in the United States. Other conditions, such as certain heart problems and bleeding in the brain, also can cause strokes.

Lifestyle changes, medicines, and/or medical procedures can help prevent or treat carotid artery disease and may reduce the risk for stroke.

If you think you're having a stroke, you need urgent treatment. Call 911 right away if you have symptoms of a stroke (don't drive yourself to the hospital). Getting care within 1 hour of having symptoms is important.

You have the best chance for full recovery if treatment to open a blocked artery is given within 6 hours of symptom onset. Ideally, treatment should be given within 3 hours of symptom onset.

Causes of Carotid Artery Disease

Carotid artery disease appears to start when damage occurs to the inner layers of the carotid arteries. Major factors that contribute to damage include the following:

- Smoking
- High amounts of certain fats and cholesterol in the blood
- High blood pressure
- High amounts of sugar in the blood due to insulin resistance or diabetes

When damage occurs, your body starts a healing process. The healing may cause plaque to build up where the arteries are damaged.

Over time, the plaque may crack. Blood cells called platelets stick to the injured lining of the artery and may clump together to form blood clots.

The buildup of plaque or blood clots can severely narrow or block the carotid arteries. This limits the flow of oxygen-rich blood to your brain and can cause a stroke.

Risk for Carotid Artery Disease

Certain traits, conditions, or habits may raise your risk for carotid artery disease. These conditions are known as risk factors. The more risk factors you have, the more likely you are to get the disease. You can control some, but not all, risk factors.

The major risk factors for carotid artery disease that follow also are the major risk factors for coronary artery disease (CAD) and heart disease.

- **Unhealthy blood cholesterol levels:** This includes high LDL [low-density lipoprotein] cholesterol (sometimes called bad cholesterol) and low HDL [high-density lipoprotein] cholesterol (sometimes called good cholesterol).

- **High blood pressure:** Blood pressure is considered high if it stays at or above 140/90 mmHg over time.

- **Smoking:** This can damage and tighten blood vessels, raise cholesterol levels, and raise blood pressure. Smoking also can limit how much oxygen reaches the body's tissues.

- **Older age:** As you get older, your risk for carotid artery disease goes up. About 1 percent of adults aged 50 to 59 have major plaque buildup in the carotid arteries. In contrast, 10 percent of adults aged 80 to 89 have this problem. Before age 75, the risk is greater in men than women. However, after age 75, the risk is higher in women.

- **Insulin resistance:** This condition occurs when the body can't use its own insulin properly. Insulin is a hormone that helps move blood sugar into cells where it's used. Insulin resistance may lead to diabetes.

- **Diabetes:** With this disease, the body's blood sugar level is high because the body doesn't make enough insulin or doesn't use its insulin properly. People who have diabetes are four times more likely to have carotid artery disease than people who don't have diabetes.

- **Overweight or obesity:** The most useful measure of overweight and obesity is the body mass index (BMI). BMI measures your weight in relation to your height and gives an estimate of your total body fat. A BMI between 25 and 29 is considered overweight. A BMI of 30 or more is considered obese. You can check your BMI using the National Heart, Lung, and Blood Institute's online BMI calculator, or your doctor can check your BMI.

- **Metabolic syndrome:** Metabolic syndrome is the name for a group of risk factors that raise your risk for stroke and other health problems, such as diabetes and heart disease.

- **Lack of physical activity:** Lack of activity can worsen other risk factors for carotid artery disease.

- **Family history of atherosclerosis:** If a family member has had atherosclerosis, it increases your risk.

Having any of these risk factors doesn't mean that you will get carotid artery disease. However, if you have one or more risk factors, you can take steps to help prevent the disease.

Steps include following a healthy lifestyle and taking any medicines your doctor prescribes.

The amount of plaque buildup in the carotid arteries also may suggest plaque buildup in other arteries. Doctors can predict the degree of atherosclerosis in other arteries based on the thickness of the carotid arteries. Thus, people who have carotid artery disease also are more likely to have CAD.

Signs and Symptoms of Carotid Artery Disease

Carotid artery disease may not cause signs or symptoms until it severely narrows or blocks the carotid arteries. Signs and symptoms may include a bruit, a transient ischemic attack (TIA), or a stroke.

Bruit

During a physical exam, your doctor may listen to your carotid arteries with a stethoscope. He or she may hear a whooshing sound called a bruit. This sound may suggest changed or reduced blood flow due to plaque. To find out more, your doctor may order tests.

Not all people who have carotid artery disease have bruits.

Transient Ischemic Attack

For some people, having a TIA, or "mini-stroke," is the first sign of carotid artery disease. During a mini-stroke, you may have some or all of the symptoms of a stroke. However, the symptoms usually go away on their own within 24 hours.

The symptoms may include the following:

• Sudden weakness or numbness in the face or limbs, often on just one side of the body

• The inability to move one or more of your limbs

• Trouble speaking and understanding

• Sudden trouble seeing in one or both eyes

• Dizziness or loss of balance

• A sudden, severe headache with no known cause

Even if the symptoms stop quickly, you should see a doctor right away. Call 911 (don't drive yourself to the hospital). It's important to get checked and to get treatment started within 1 hour of having symptoms.

A mini-stroke is a warning sign that you're at high risk of having a stroke. You shouldn't ignore these symptoms. About one third of people who have mini-strokes will have strokes if they don't get treatment.

Although a mini-stroke may warn of a stroke, it doesn't predict when a stroke will happen. A stroke may occur days, weeks, or even months after a mini-stroke. In about half of the cases of strokes that follow a TIA, the stroke occurs within 1 year.

Stroke

Most people who have carotid artery disease don't have mini-strokes before they have strokes. The symptoms of stroke are the same as those of mini-stroke, but the results are not. A stroke can cause lasting brain damage, long-term disability, paralysis (an inability to move), or even death.

Getting treatment for a stroke right away is very important. You have the best chance for full recovery if treatment to open a blocked artery is given within 6 hours of symptom onset. Ideally, treatment should be given within 3 hours of symptom onset.

Call 911 as soon as symptoms occur (don't drive yourself to the hospital). It's very important to get checked and to get treatment started within 1 hour of having symptoms.

Make those close to you aware of stroke symptoms and the need for urgent action. Learning the signs and symptoms of a stroke will allow you to help yourself or someone close to you lower the risk for damage or death from a stroke.

Diagnosing Carotid Artery Disease

Your doctor will diagnose carotid artery disease based on your medical history and the results from a physical exam and tests.

Medical History

Your doctor will find out whether you have any of the major risk factors for carotid artery disease. He or she also will ask whether you've had any signs or symptoms of a mini-stroke or stroke.

Physical Exam

To check your carotid arteries, your doctor will listen to them with a stethoscope. He or she will listen for a whooshing sound called a bruit. This sound may indicate changed or reduced blood flow due to plaque. To find out more, your doctor may order tests.

Diagnostic Tests

The following tests are common for diagnosing carotid artery disease. If you have symptoms of a mini-stroke or stroke, your doctor may use other tests as well.

Carotid ultrasound: Carotid ultrasound (also called sonography) is the most common test for diagnosing carotid artery disease. It's a painless, harmless test that uses sound waves to create pictures of the insides of your carotid arteries. This test can show whether plaque has narrowed your carotid arteries and how narrow they are.

A standard carotid ultrasound shows the structure of your carotid arteries. A Doppler carotid ultrasound shows how blood moves through your blood vessels.

Carotid angiography: Carotid angiography is a special type of x-ray. This test may be used if the ultrasound results are unclear or don't give your doctor enough information. For this test, your doctor will inject a special substance (called contrast dye) into a vein, most often in your leg. The dye travels to your carotid arteries and highlights them on x-ray pictures.

Magnetic resonance angiography: Magnetic resonance angiography (MRA) uses a large magnet and radio waves to take pictures of your carotid arteries. Your doctor can see these pictures on a computer screen.

For this test, your doctor may give you contrast dye to highlight your carotid arteries on the pictures.

Computed tomography angiography: Computed tomography, or CT, angiography takes x-ray pictures of the body from many angles. A computer combines the pictures into two- and three-dimensional images.

For this test, your doctor may give you contrast dye to highlight your carotid arteries on the pictures.

Treating Carotid Artery Disease

Treatments for carotid artery disease may include lifestyle changes, medicines, and medical procedures. The goals of treatment are to stop the disease from getting worse and to prevent a stroke.

Your treatment will depend on your symptoms, how severe the disease is, and your age and overall health.

Chapter 26

Coronary Microvascular Disease

Coronary microvascular disease (MVD) affects the heart's smallest coronary arteries. Coronary MVD occurs in the heart's tiny arteries when the following process takes place:

- Plaque forms in the arteries. Plaque is made up of fat, cholesterol, calcium, and other substances found in the blood. It narrows the coronary arteries and reduces blood flow to the heart muscle. As a result, the heart doesn't get the oxygen it needs. This is known as ischemic heart disease, or heart disease. In coronary MVD, plaque can scatter, spread out evenly, or build up into blockages in the tiny coronary arteries.

- The arteries spasm (tighten). Spasms of the small coronary arteries also can prevent enough oxygen-rich blood from moving through the arteries. This too can cause ischemic heart disease.

- The walls of the arteries are damaged or diseased. Changes in the arteries' cells and the surrounding muscle tissues may, over time, damage the arteries' walls.

Coronary MVD is a new concept. It's different from traditional coronary artery disease (CAD). In CAD, plaque builds up in the heart's large arteries. This buildup can lead to blockages that limit or prevent oxygen-rich blood from reaching the heart muscle.

Excerpted from text by the National Heart, Lung, and Blood Institute (NHLBI, www.nhlbi.nih.gov), part of the National Institutes of Health, September 2007.

In coronary MVD, however, the heart's smallest arteries are affected. Plaque doesn't always create blockages as it does in CAD. For this reason, coronary MVD also is called nonobstructive CAD.

No one knows whether coronary MVD is the same as MVD linked to other diseases, such as diabetes.

Overview

Death rates from heart disease have dropped quite a bit in the last 30 years. This is due to improved treatments for conditions such as blocked coronary arteries, heart attack, and heart failure.

However, death rates haven't improved as much in women as they have in men. Heart disease in men and women may differ. Many researchers think that a drop in estrogen levels in women at menopause combined with traditional risk factors for heart disease causes coronary MVD. Therefore, coronary MVD is being studied as a possible cause of heart disease in women.

Diagnosing coronary MVD has been a challenge for doctors. Most of the research on heart disease has been done on men.

Standard tests used to diagnose heart disease have been useful in finding blockages in the coronary arteries. However, these same tests used in women with symptoms of heart disease—such as chest pain—often show that they have "clear" arteries.

This is because standard tests for CAD don't always detect coronary MVD in women. Standard tests look for blockages that affect blood flow in the large coronary arteries. However, these tests can't detect plaque that forms, scatters, or builds up in the smallest coronary arteries.

The standard tests also can't detect when the arteries spasm (tighten) or when the walls of the arteries are damaged or diseased.

As a result, women are often thought to be at low risk for heart disease.

Outlook

Coronary MVD is thought to affect up to 3 million women with heart disease in the United States.

Most of the information known about coronary MVD comes from the National Heart, Lung, and Blood Institute's WISE study (Women's Ischemia Syndrome Evaluation). The WISE study began in 1996. Its goal was to learn more about how heart disease develops in women.

The role of hormones in heart disease has been studied, as well as how to improve the diagnosis of coronary MVD. Further studies are under way to learn more about the disease, how to treat it, and its outcomes.

Causes of Coronary Microvascular Disease

The same cluster of risk factors that causes atherosclerosis may cause coronary microvascular disease (MVD) in women. Atherosclerosis is when the arteries harden and narrow due to the buildup plaque on their inner walls. It's one of the key causes of heart disease.

Risk factors for atherosclerosis include the following:

- **Unhealthy cholesterol levels:** This includes high LDL [low-density lipoprotein] cholesterol (sometimes called bad cholesterol), low HDL [high-density lipoprotein] cholesterol (sometimes called good cholesterol), and high triglycerides (another type of fat in the blood).

- **High blood pressure:** Blood pressure is considered high if it stays at or above 140/90 mmHg [millimeters of mercury] over a period of time.

- **Smoking:** This can damage and tighten blood vessels, increase cholesterol levels, and increase blood pressure. Smoking also doesn't allow enough oxygen to reach the body's tissues.

- **Insulin resistance:** This condition occurs when the body can't use its own insulin properly. Insulin is a hormone that helps the body convert food to energy.

- **Diabetes:** This is a disease in which the body's blood sugar level is high because the body doesn't make enough insulin or doesn't use its insulin properly.

- **Overweight or obesity:** Overweight is having extra body weight from muscle, bone, fat, and/or water. Obesity is having a high amount of extra body fat.

- **Lack of physical activity:** Lack of activity can worsen other risk factors for atherosclerosis.

- **Age:** As you get older, your risk for atherosclerosis increases. Genetic or lifestyle factors cause plaque to build in arteries as you age. By the time you are middle-aged or older, enough plaque has built up to cause signs or symptoms. In men, the risk increases after age 45. In women, the risk increases after age 55.

- **Family history of early heart disease:** Your risk for atherosclerosis increases if your father or a brother was diagnosed with heart disease before 55 years of age, or if your mother or a sister was diagnosed with heart disease before 65 years of age.

Coronary MVD may be linked to low estrogen levels occurring before or after menopause. It also may be linked to anemia or conditions that affect blood clotting. Anemia is thought to slow the growth of cells needed to repair damaged blood vessels.

It's not yet known whether coronary MVD is the same as MVD linked to other diseases, such as diabetes.

Risk for Coronary Microvascular Disease

Women at high risk for coronary microvascular disease (MVD) often have multiple risk factors for atherosclerosis.

Women may be at risk for coronary MVD if they have low levels of estrogen at any point in their adult lives. (This refers to the estrogen that the ovaries produce, not the estrogen used in hormone replacement therapy.)

After menopause, women tend to have more of the traditional risk factors for atherosclerosis, putting them at higher risk for coronary MVD.

Lower than normal estrogen levels in women before menopause also can put younger women at higher risk for coronary MVD. One cause of low estrogen levels in younger women is mental stress. Another is a problem with the function of the ovaries.

Women who have high blood pressure before menopause, especially high systolic blood pressure, are at higher risk for coronary MVD. (Systolic blood pressure is the top or first number of a blood pressure measurement).

Women with heart disease have an increased risk for a worse outcome, such as a heart attack, if they also have anemia. Anemia is thought to slow the growth of cells needed to repair damaged blood vessels.

Signs and Symptoms of Coronary Microvascular Disease

Signs and symptoms of coronary microvascular disease (MVD) often differ from signs and symptoms of traditional coronary artery disease (CAD).

Many women with coronary MVD have angina (chest pain), but it may or may not be the "typical" chest pain seen in CAD. Typical signs and symptoms of CAD include angina, feeling pressure or squeezing in the chest, shortness of breath, heavy sweating, and arm or shoulder pain.

These signs and symptoms often first appear while a person is being physically active—such as while jogging, walking on a treadmill, or going up stairs. Typical angina is more frequent in women older than 65.

Other signs and symptoms of coronary MVD in women are shortness of breath, sleep problems, fatigue (tiredness), and lack of energy.

In women, coronary MVD symptoms are often first noticed during routine daily activities (such as shopping, cooking, cleaning, and going to work) and during times of mental stress. It's less likely that women will notice these symptoms during physical activity (such as jogging or walking fast).

Treating Coronary Microvascular Disease

Women who have coronary microvascular disease (MVD) are mainly treated to control their risk factors for heart disease and symptoms. Treatments may include the following medicines:

- Statins to improve cholesterol levels

- Angiotensin-converting enzyme (ACE) inhibitors and beta-blockers to lower blood pressure and decrease the heart's workload

- Aspirin to help prevent blood clots or control inflammation

- Nitroglycerin to relax blood vessels, improve blood flow to the heart muscle, and treat chest pain (if this medicine has helped the patient with past symptoms)

Women diagnosed with coronary MVD who also have anemia may benefit from treatment for that condition, because anemia slows repair of damaged blood vessels.

Women who are diagnosed and treated for coronary MVD should be checked regularly by their doctors.

Research is ongoing to find the best treatments for coronary MVD.

Chapter 27

Stroke

A stroke occurs when the blood supply to part of the brain is suddenly interrupted or when a blood vessel in the brain bursts, spilling blood into the spaces surrounding brain cells. In the same way that a person suffering a loss of blood flow to the heart is said to be having a heart attack, a person with a loss of blood flow to the brain or sudden bleeding in the brain can be said to be having a "brain attack."

Brain cells die when they no longer receive oxygen and nutrients from the blood or when they are damaged by sudden bleeding into or around the brain. Ischemia is the term used to describe the loss of oxygen and nutrients for brain cells when there is inadequate blood flow. Ischemia ultimately leads to infarction, the death of brain cells which are eventually replaced by a fluid-filled cavity (or infarct) in the injured brain.

When blood flow to the brain is interrupted, some brain cells die immediately, while others remain at risk for death. These damaged cells make up the ischemic penumbra and can linger in a compromised state for several hours. With timely treatment these cells can be saved.

Even though a stroke occurs in the unseen reaches of the brain, the symptoms of a stroke are easy to spot. They include sudden numbness or weakness, especially on one side of the body; sudden confusion or trouble speaking or understanding speech; sudden trouble

Excerpted from "Stroke: Hope Through Research," by the National Institute on Neurological Disorders and Stroke (NINDS, www.ninds.nih.gov), part of the National Institutes of Health, May 15, 2009.

seeing in one or both eyes; sudden trouble walking, dizziness, or loss of balance or coordination; or sudden severe headache with no known cause. All of the symptoms of stroke appear suddenly, and often there is more than one symptom at the same time. Therefore stroke can usually be distinguished from other causes of dizziness or headache. These symptoms may indicate that a stroke has occurred and that medical attention is needed immediately.

There are two forms of stroke: ischemic—blockage of a blood vessel supplying the brain, and hemorrhagic—bleeding into or around the brain. The following text describes these forms in detail.

Ischemic Stroke

An ischemic stroke occurs when an artery supplying the brain with blood becomes blocked, suddenly decreasing or stopping blood flow and ultimately causing a brain infarction. This type of stroke accounts for approximately 80 percent of all strokes. Blood clots are the most common cause of artery blockage and brain infarction. The process of clotting is necessary and beneficial throughout the body because it stops bleeding and allows repair of damaged areas of arteries or veins. However, when blood clots develop in the wrong place within an artery they can cause devastating injury by interfering with the normal flow of blood. Problems with clotting become more frequent as people age.

Blood clots can cause ischemia and infarction in two ways. A clot that forms in a part of the body other than the brain can travel through blood vessels and become wedged in a brain artery. This free-roaming clot is called an embolus and often forms in the heart. A stroke caused by an embolus is called an embolic stroke. The second kind of ischemic stroke, called a thrombotic stroke, is caused by thrombosis, the formation of a blood clot in one of the cerebral arteries that stays attached to the artery wall until it grows large enough to block blood flow.

Ischemic strokes can also be caused by stenosis, or a narrowing of the artery due to the buildup of plaque (a mixture of fatty substances, including cholesterol and other lipids) and blood clots along the artery wall. Stenosis can occur in large arteries and small arteries and is therefore called large vessel disease or small vessel disease, respectively. When a stroke occurs due to small vessel disease, a very small infarction results, sometimes called a lacunar infarction.

The most common blood vessel disease that causes stenosis is atherosclerosis. In atherosclerosis, deposits of plaque build up along the inner walls of large- and medium-sized arteries, causing thickening, hardening, and loss of elasticity of artery walls and decreased blood flow.

Hemorrhagic Stroke

In a healthy, functioning brain, neurons do not come into direct contact with blood. The vital oxygen and nutrients the neurons need from the blood come to the neurons across the thin walls of the cerebral capillaries. The glia (nervous system cells that support and protect neurons) form a blood-brain barrier, an elaborate meshwork that surrounds blood vessels and capillaries and regulates which elements of the blood can pass through to the neurons.

When an artery in the brain bursts, blood spews out into the surrounding tissue and upsets not only the blood supply but the delicate chemical balance neurons require to function. This is called a hemorrhagic stroke. Such strokes account for approximately 20 percent of all strokes.

Hemorrhage can occur in several ways. One common cause is a bleeding aneurysm, a weak or thin spot on an artery wall. Over time, these weak spots stretch or balloon out under high arterial pressure. The thin walls of these ballooning aneurysms can rupture and spill blood into the space surrounding brain cells.

Hemorrhage also occurs when arterial walls break open. Plaque-encrusted artery walls eventually lose their elasticity and become brittle and thin, prone to cracking. Hypertension, or high blood pressure, increases the risk that a brittle artery wall will give way and release blood into the surrounding brain tissue.

A person with an arteriovenous malformation (AVM) also has an increased risk of hemorrhagic stroke. AVMs are a tangle of defective blood vessels and capillaries within the brain that have thin walls and can therefore rupture.

Bleeding from ruptured brain arteries can either go into the substance of the brain or into the various spaces surrounding the brain. Intracerebral hemorrhage occurs when a vessel within the brain leaks blood into the brain itself. Subarachnoid hemorrhage is bleeding under the meninges, or outer membranes, of the brain into the thin fluid-filled space that surrounds the brain.

The subarachnoid space separates the arachnoid membrane from the underlying pia mater membrane. It contains a clear fluid (cerebrospinal fluid or CSF) as well as the small blood vessels that supply the outer surface of the brain. In a subarachnoid hemorrhage, one of the small arteries within the subarachnoid space bursts, flooding the area with blood and contaminating the cerebrospinal fluid. Since the CSF flows throughout the cranium, within the spaces of the brain, subarachnoid hemorrhage can lead to extensive damage throughout the brain. In fact, subarachnoid hemorrhage is the most deadly of all strokes.

Transient Ischemic Attacks

A transient ischemic attack (TIA), sometimes called a mini-stroke, starts just like a stroke but then resolves leaving no noticeable symptoms or deficits. The occurrence of a TIA is a warning that the person is at risk for a more serious and debilitating stroke. Of the approximately 50,000 Americans who have a TIA each year, about one third will have an acute stroke sometime in the future. The addition of other risk factors compounds a person's risk for a recurrent stroke.

The average duration of a TIA is a few minutes. For almost all TIAs, the symptoms go away within an hour. There is no way to tell whether symptoms will be just a TIA or persist and lead to death or disability. The patient should assume that all stroke symptoms signal an emergency and should not wait to see if they go away.

Recurrent Stroke

Recurrent stroke is frequent; about 25 percent of people who recover from their first stroke will have another stroke within 5 years. Recurrent stroke is a major contributor to stroke disability and death, with the risk of severe disability or death from stroke increasing with each stroke recurrence. The risk of a recurrent stroke is greatest right after a stroke, with the risk decreasing with time. About 3 percent of stroke patients will have another stroke within 30 days of their first stroke and one third of recurrent strokes take place within 2 years of the first stroke.

Research on Stroke

The NINDS is the leading supporter of stroke research in the United States and sponsors a wide range of experimental research studies, from investigations of basic biological mechanisms to studies with animal models and clinical trials.

Currently, NINDS researchers are studying the mechanisms of stroke risk factors and the process of brain damage that results from stroke. Some of this brain damage may be secondary to the initial death of brain cells caused by the lack of blood flow to the brain tissue. This secondary wave of brain injury is a result of a toxic reaction to the primary damage and mainly involves the excitatory neurochemical, glutamate. Glutamate in the normal brain functions as a chemical messenger between brain cells, allowing them to communicate. But an excess amount of glutamate in the brain causes too much activity and brain cells quickly "burn out" from too much excitement, releasing more toxic chemicals, such as caspases, cytokines, monocytes, and oxygen-free radicals. These substances poison the chemical environment of surrounding cells, initiating a cascade of degeneration and programmed cell death, called apoptosis. NINDS researchers are studying the mechanisms underlying this secondary insult, which consists mainly of inflammation, toxicity, and a breakdown of the blood vessels that provide blood to the brain. Researchers are also looking for ways to prevent secondary injury to the brain by providing different types of neuroprotection for salvageable cells that prevent inflammation and block some of the toxic chemicals created by dying brain cells. From this research, scientists hope to develop neuroprotective agents to prevent secondary damage.

Basic research has also focused on the genetics of stroke and stroke risk factors. One area of research involving genetics is gene therapy. Gene therapy involves putting a gene for a desired protein in certain cells of the body. The inserted gene will then "program" the cell to produce the desired protein. If enough cells in the right areas produce enough protein, then the protein could be therapeutic. Scientists must find ways to deliver the therapeutic DNA [deoxyribonucleic acid] to the appropriate cells and must learn how to deliver enough DNA to enough cells so that the tissues produce a therapeutic amount of protein. Gene therapy is in the very early stages of development and there are many problems to overcome, including learning how to penetrate the highly impermeable blood-brain barrier and how to halt the host's immune reaction to the virus that carries the gene to the cells. Some of the proteins used for stroke therapy could include neuroprotective proteins, anti-inflammatory proteins, and DNA/cellular repair proteins, among others.

The NINDS supports and conducts a wide variety of studies in animals, from genetics research on zebrafish to rehabilitation research on primates. Much of the Institute's animal research involves rodents, specifically mice and rats. For example, one study of hypertension and stroke uses rats that have been bred to be hypertensive and therefore stroke-prone. By studying stroke in rats, scientists hope to get a better picture of what might be happening in human stroke patients.

Scientists can also use animal models to test promising therapeutic interventions for stroke. If a therapy proves to be beneficial to animals, then scientists can consider testing the therapy in human subjects.

One promising area of stroke animal research involves hibernation. The dramatic decrease of blood flow to the brain in hibernating animals is extensive—extensive enough that it would kill a non-hibernating animal. During hibernation, an animal's metabolism slows down, body temperature drops, and energy and oxygen requirements of brain cells decrease. If scientists can discover how animals hibernate without experiencing brain damage, then maybe they can discover ways to stop the brain damage associated with decreased blood flow in stroke patients. Other studies are looking at the role of hypothermia, or decreased body temperature, on metabolism and neuroprotection.

Both hibernation and hypothermia have a relationship to hypoxia and edema. Hypoxia, or anoxia, occurs when there is not enough oxygen available for brain cells to function properly. Since brain cells require large amounts of oxygen for energy requirements, they are especially vulnerable to hypoxia. Edema occurs when the chemical balance of brain tissue is disturbed and water or fluids flow into the brain cells, making them swell and burst, releasing their toxic contents into the surrounding tissues. Edema is one cause of general brain tissue swelling and contributes to the secondary injury associated with stroke.

The basic and animal studies discussed above do not involve people and fall under the category of preclinical research; clinical research involves people. One area of investigation that has made the transition from animal models to clinical research is the study of the mechanisms underlying brain plasticity and the neuronal rewiring that occurs after a stroke.

New advances in imaging and rehabilitation have shown that the brain can compensate for function lost as a result of stroke. When cells in an area of the brain responsible for a particular function die after a stroke, the patient becomes unable to perform that function. For example, a stroke patient with an infarct in the area of the brain responsible for facial recognition becomes unable to recognize faces, a syndrome called facial agnosia. But, in time, the person may come to recognize faces again, even though the area of the brain originally programmed to perform that function remains dead. The plasticity of the brain and the rewiring of the neural connections make it possible for one part of the brain to change functions and take up the more important functions of a disabled part. This rewiring of the brain and restoration of function, which the brain tries to do automatically, can be helped with therapy. Scientists are working to develop new and better ways to help the brain repair itself to restore important functions to the stroke patient.

One example of a therapy resulting from this research is the use of transcranial magnetic stimulation (TMS) in stroke rehabilitation. Some evidence suggests that TMS, in which a small magnetic current is delivered to an area of the brain, may possibly increase brain plasticity and speed up recovery of function after a stroke. The TMS device is a small coil which is held outside of the head, over the part of the brain needing stimulation. Currently, several studies at the NINDS are testing whether TMS has any value in increasing motor function and improving functional recovery.

Chapter 28

Aneurysm

An aneurysm is a balloon-like bulge in an artery. Arteries are blood vessels that carry oxygen-rich blood from your heart to your body.

Arteries have thick walls to withstand normal blood pressure. However, certain medical problems, genetic conditions, and trauma can damage or injure artery walls. The force of blood pushing against the weakened or injured walls can cause an aneurysm.

An aneurysm can grow large and burst (rupture) or cause a dissection. Rupture causes dangerous bleeding inside the body. A dissection is a split in one or more layers of the artery wall. The split causes bleeding into and along the layers of the artery wall.

Both conditions are often fatal.

Overview

Most aneurysms occur in the aorta—the main artery that carries blood from the heart to the rest of the body. The aorta goes through the chest and abdomen.

An aneurysm that occurs in the part of the aorta that's in the chest is called a thoracic aortic aneurysm. An aneurysm that occurs in the part of the aorta that's in the abdomen is called an abdominal aortic aneurysm.

Excerpted from text by the National Heart, Lung, and Blood Institute (NHLBI, www.nhlbi.nih.gov), part of the National Institutes of Health, April 2009.

Aneurysms also can occur in other arteries, but these types of aneurysm are less common. This article will focus on aortic aneurysms.

About 14,000 Americans die each year from aortic aneurysms. Most of the deaths result from rupture or dissection.

Early diagnosis and medical treatment can help prevent many cases of rupture and dissection. However, aneurysms can develop and become large before causing any symptoms. Thus, people who are at high risk for aneurysms can benefit from early, routine screening.

Outlook

When found in time, aortic aneurysms often can be successfully treated with medicines or surgery. Medicines may be given to lower blood pressure, relax blood vessels, and reduce the risk of rupture.

Large aortic aneurysms often can be repaired with surgery. During surgery, the weak or damaged portion of the aorta is replaced or reinforced.

Types of Aneurysm

Aortic Aneurysms

The two types of aortic aneurysm are abdominal aortic aneurysm (AAA) and thoracic aortic aneurysm (TAA).

Abdominal aortic aneurysms: An aneurysm that occurs in the part of the aorta that's located in the abdomen is called an abdominal aortic aneurysm. AAAs account for three in four aortic aneurysms. They're found more often now than in the past because of computed tomography, or CT, scans done for other medical problems.

Small AAAs rarely rupture. However, an AAA can grow very large without causing symptoms. Thus, routine checkups and treatment for an AAA are important to prevent growth and rupture.

Thoracic aortic aneurysms: An aneurysm that occurs in the part of the aorta that's located in the chest and above the diaphragm is called a thoracic aortic aneurysm. TAAs account for one in four aortic aneurysms.

TAAs don't always cause symptoms, even when they're large. Only half of all people who have TAAs notice any symptoms. TAAs are found more often now than in the past because of chest CT scans done for other medical problems.

With a common type of TAA, the walls of the aorta weaken, and a section close to the heart enlarges. As a result, the valve between the heart and the aorta can't close properly. This allows blood to leak back into the heart.

A less common type of TAA can develop in the upper back, away from the heart. A TAA in this location may result from an injury to the chest, such as from a car crash.

Other Types of Aneurysms

Brain aneurysms: When an aneurysm occurs in an artery in the brain, it's called a cerebral aneurysm or brain aneurysm. Brain aneurysms also are sometimes called berry aneurysms because they're often the size of a small berry.

Most brain aneurysms cause no symptoms until they become large, begin to leak blood, or rupture. A ruptured brain aneurysm causes a stroke.

Peripheral aneurysms: Aneurysms that occur in arteries other than the aorta and the brain arteries are called peripheral aneurysms. Common locations for peripheral aneurysms include the popliteal, femoral, and carotid arteries.

The popliteal arteries run down the back of the thighs, behind the knees. The femoral arteries are the main arteries in the groin. The carotid arteries are the two main arteries on each side of your neck.

Peripheral aneurysms aren't as likely to rupture or dissect as aortic aneurysms. However, blood clots can form in peripheral aneurysms. If a blood clot breaks away from the aneurysm, it can block blood flow through the artery.

If a peripheral aneurysm is large, it can press on a nearby nerve or vein and cause pain, numbness, or swelling.

Other Names for Aneurysm

- Abdominal aortic aneurysm
- Aortic aneurysm
- Berry aneurysm
- Brain aneurysm
- Cerebral aneurysm

- Peripheral aneurysm
- Thoracic aortic aneurysm

Causes of Aneurysm

The force of blood pushing against the walls of an artery combined with damage or injury to the artery's walls can cause an aneurysm.

A number of factors can damage and weaken the walls of the aorta and cause aortic aneurysms.

Aging, smoking, high blood pressure, and atherosclerosis are all factors that can damage or weaken the walls of the aorta. Atherosclerosis is the hardening and narrowing of the arteries due to the buildup of a fatty material called plaque.

Rarely, infections, such as untreated syphilis (a sexually transmitted infection), can cause aortic aneurysms. Aortic aneurysms also can occur as a result of diseases that inflame the blood vessels, such as vasculitis.

Family history also may play a role in causing aortic aneurysms.

In addition to the factors above, certain genetic conditions may cause thoracic aortic aneurysms (TAAs). Examples include Marfan syndrome, Loeys-Dietz syndrome, and Ehlers-Danlos syndrome (the vascular type).

These conditions can weaken the body's connective tissues and damage the aorta. People who have these conditions tend to develop aneurysms at a younger age and are at higher risk for rupture or dissection.

Trauma, such as a car accident, also can damage the aorta walls and lead to TAAs.

Researchers continue to look for other causes of aortic aneurysms. For example, they're looking for genetic mutations that may contribute to or cause aneurysms.

Risk for Aneurysm

Certain factors put you at higher risk for an aortic aneurysm. These include the following:

- **Male gender:** Men are more likely than women to have abdominal aortic aneurysms (AAAs)—the most common type of aneurysm.

- **Age:** The risk for AAAs increases as you get older. These aneurysms are more likely to occur in people who are 65 or older.

- **Smoking:** Smoking can damage and weaken the walls of the aorta.

- **Family history of aortic aneurysm:** People who have family histories of aortic aneurysm are at higher risk of having one, and they may have aneurysms before the age of 65.

Certain diseases and conditions that weaken the walls of the aorta and car accidents or trauma also can injure the arteries and increase your risk for an aneurysm.

If you have any of these risk factors, talk with your doctor about whether you need to be screened for aneurysms.

Signs and Symptoms of Aneurysm

The signs and symptoms of an aortic aneurysm depend on the type of aneurysm, its location, and whether it has ruptured or is affecting other parts of the body.

Aneurysms can develop and grow for years without causing any signs or symptoms. They often don't cause signs or symptoms until they rupture, grow large enough to press on nearby parts of the body, or block blood flow.

Abdominal aortic aneurysms: Most abdominal aortic aneurysms (AAAs) develop slowly over years. They often don't have signs or symptoms unless they rupture. If you have an AAA, your doctor may feel a throbbing mass while checking your abdomen.

When symptoms are present, they can include the following:

- A throbbing feeling in the abdomen
- Deep pain in your back or the side of your abdomen
- Steady, gnawing pain in your abdomen that lasts for hours or days

If an AAA ruptures, symptoms can include sudden, severe pain in your lower abdomen and back; nausea (feeling sick to your stomach) and vomiting; clammy, sweaty skin; lightheadedness; and a rapid heart rate when standing up.

Internal bleeding from a ruptured AAA can send you into shock. This is a life-threatening situation that requires emergency treatment.

Thoracic aortic aneurysms: A thoracic aortic aneurysm (TAA) may not cause symptoms until it dissects or grows large. Then, symptoms may include pain in your jaw, neck, back, or chest and coughing, hoarseness, or trouble breathing or swallowing.

A dissection is a split in one or more layers of the artery wall. The split causes bleeding into and along the layers of the artery wall.

If a TAA ruptures or dissects, you may feel sudden, severe pain starting in your upper back and moving down into your abdomen. You may have pain in your chest and arms, and you can quickly go into shock. Shock is a life-threatening condition in which the body's organs don't get enough blood flow.

If you have any symptoms of TAA or aortic dissection, call 911. If left untreated, these conditions may lead to organ damage or death.

Treating Aneurysm

Aortic aneurysms are treated with medicines and surgery. A small aneurysm that's found early and isn't causing symptoms may not need treatment. Other aneurysms need to be treated.

The goals of treatment are to do the following:

- Prevent the aneurysm from growing
- Prevent or reverse damage to other body structures
- Prevent or treat a rupture or dissection
- Allow you to continue to do your normal daily activities

Treatment for aortic aneurysms is based on the size of the aneurysm. Your doctor may recommend routine testing to make sure an aneurysm isn't getting bigger. This method usually is used for aneurysms that are smaller than 5 centimeters (about 2 inches) across.

How often you need testing (for example, every few months or every year) will be based on the size of the aneurysm and how fast it's growing. The larger it is and the faster it's growing, the more often you may need to be checked.

Medicines

If you have an aortic aneurysm, your doctor may prescribe medicines before surgery or instead of surgery. Medicines are used to lower blood pressure, relax blood vessels, and reduce the risk of rupture. Beta-blockers and calcium channel blockers are the medicines most commonly used.

Surgery

Your doctor may recommend surgery if your aneurysm is growing quickly or if it reaches a size linked with an increased risk of rupture or dissection.

The two main types of surgery to repair aortic aneurysms are open abdominal or open chest repair and endovascular repair.

Open abdominal or open chest repair: The standard and most common type of surgery for aortic aneurysms is open abdominal or open chest repair. It involves a major incision (cut) in the abdomen or chest. General anesthesia is used for this procedure—that is, you will be temporarily put to sleep so you don't feel pain during the surgery.

The aneurysm is removed, and the section of aorta is replaced with a graft made of material such as Dacron® or Teflon.® The surgery takes 3 to 6 hours, and you will remain in the hospital for 5 to 8 days.

It often takes a month to recover from open abdominal or open chest surgery and return to full activity. Most patients make a full recovery.

Endovascular repair: In endovascular repair, the aneurysm isn't removed. Instead, a graft is inserted into the aorta to strengthen it. This type of surgery is done using catheters (tubes) inserted into the arteries; it doesn't require surgically opening the chest or abdomen.

The surgeon first inserts a catheter into an artery in the groin (upper thigh) and threads it to the aneurysm. Then, using an x-ray to see the artery, the surgeon threads the graft (also called a stent graft) into the aorta to the aneurysm.

The graft is then expanded inside the aorta and fastened in place to form a stable channel for blood flow. The graft reinforces the weakened section of the aorta to prevent the aneurysm from rupturing.

Endovascular repair reduces recovery time to a few days and greatly reduces time in the hospital. However, doctors can't repair all aortic aneurysms with this procedure. The location or size of the aneurysm may prevent a stent graft from being safely or reliably placed inside the aneurysm.

Chapter 29

Peripheral Arterial Disease

Peripheral arterial disease (PAD) occurs when plaque builds up in the arteries that carry blood to your head, organs, and limbs. Plaque is made up of fat, cholesterol, calcium, fibrous tissue, and other substances in the blood.

When plaque builds up in arteries, the condition is called atherosclerosis. Over time, plaque can harden and narrow the arteries. This limits the flow of oxygen-rich blood to your organs and other parts of your body.

PAD usually affects the legs, but also can affect the arteries that carry blood from your heart to your head, arms, kidneys, and stomach. This text focuses on PAD that affects blood flow to the legs.

Overview

Blocked blood flow to your legs can cause pain and numbness. It also can raise your risk of getting an infection in the affected limbs. It may be hard for your body to fight the infection.

If severe enough, blocked blood flow can cause tissue death (gangrene). In very serious cases, this can lead to leg amputation.

If you have leg pain when you walk or climb stairs, talk to your doctor. Sometimes older people think that leg pain is just a symptom of aging. However, the cause for the pain could be PAD. Tell your doctor

Excerpted from text by the National Heart, Lung, and Blood Institute (NHLBI, www.nhlbi.nih.gov), part of the National Institutes of Health, September 2008.

261

if you're feeling pain in your legs and discuss whether you should be tested for PAD.

Smoking is the main risk factor for PAD. If you smoke or have a history of smoking, your risk for PAD increases four times. Other factors, such as age and having certain diseases or conditions, also increase your risk.

Outlook

If you have PAD, your risk for coronary artery disease, heart attack, stroke, and transient ischemic attack ("mini-stroke") is six to seven times greater than the risk for people who don't have PAD. If you have heart disease, you have a one in three chance of having blocked leg arteries.

Although PAD is serious, it's treatable. If you have the disease, it's important to see your doctor regularly and treat the underlying atherosclerosis.

PAD treatment may slow or stop disease progress and reduce the risk of complications. Treatments include lifestyle changes, medicines, and surgery or procedures. Researchers continue to explore new therapies for PAD.

Other Names for Peripheral Arterial Disease

- Atherosclerotic peripheral arterial disease
- Peripheral vascular disease
- Vascular disease
- Hardening of the arteries
- Claudication
- Poor circulation
- Leg cramps from poor circulation

Causes of Peripheral Arterial Disease

The most common cause of peripheral arterial disease (PAD) is atherosclerosis. The exact cause of atherosclerosis isn't known.

The disease may start when certain factors damage the inner layers of the arteries. These factors include the following:

- Smoking
- High amounts of certain fats and cholesterol in the blood

- High blood pressure
- High amounts of sugar in the blood due to insulin resistance or diabetes

When damage occurs, your body starts a healing process. The healing may cause plaque to build up where the arteries are damaged.

Over time, the plaque may crack. Blood cell fragments called platelets stick to the injured lining of the artery and may clump together to form blood clots.

The buildup of plaque or blood clots can severely narrow or block the arteries and limit the flow of oxygen-rich blood to your body.

Risk for Peripheral Arterial Disease

Peripheral arterial disease (PAD) affects 8 to 12 million people in the United States. African Americans are more than twice as likely as Caucasians to have PAD.

The major risk factors for PAD are smoking, age, and having certain diseases or conditions.

Smoking

Smoking is more closely related to getting PAD than any other risk factor. Your risk for PAD increases four times if you smoke or have a history of smoking. On average, smokers who develop PAD have symptoms 10 years earlier than nonsmokers who develop PAD.

Quitting smoking slows the progress of PAD. Smoking even one or two cigarettes a day can interfere with PAD treatments. Smokers and people who have diabetes are at highest risk for PAD complications, including gangrene (tissue death) in the leg from decreased blood flow.

Age

As you get older, your risk for PAD increases. Genetic or lifestyle factors cause plaque to build in your arteries as you age.

About 5 percent of U.S. adults who are older than 50 have PAD. Among adults aged 65 and older, 12 to 20 percent may have PAD. Older age combined with other risk factors, such as smoking or diabetes, also puts you at higher risk.

Diseases and Conditions

A number of diseases and conditions can raise your risk for PAD. These include the following:

- Diabetes (One in three people who has diabetes and is older than 50 is likely to have PAD.)
- High blood pressure or a family history of it
- High blood cholesterol or a family history of it
- Heart disease or a family history of it
- Stroke or a family history of it

Signs and Symptoms of Peripheral Arterial Disease

At least half of the people who have peripheral arterial disease (PAD) don't have any signs or symptoms of it. Others may have a number of signs and symptoms.

Even if you don't have signs or symptoms, discuss with your doctor whether you should get checked for PAD if you're aged 70 or older, aged 50 or older and have a history of smoking or diabetes, or younger than 50 and have diabetes and one or more risk factors for atherosclerosis.

Intermittent Claudication

People who have PAD may have symptoms when walking or climbing stairs. These may include pain, numbness, aching, or heaviness in the leg muscles. Symptoms also may include cramping in the affected leg(s) and in the buttocks, thighs, calves, and feet. Symptoms may ease after resting.

These symptoms are called intermittent claudication. During physical activity, your muscles need increased blood flow. If your blood vessels are narrowed or blocked, your muscles won't get enough blood. When resting, the muscles need less blood flow, so the pain goes away.

About 10 percent of people who have PAD have claudication. This symptom is more likely in people who also have atherosclerosis in other arteries.

Other Signs and Symptoms

Other signs and symptoms of PAD include the following:

- Weak or absent pulses in the legs or feet
- Sores or wounds on the toes, feet, or legs that heal slowly, poorly, or not at all
- A pale or bluish color to the skin

- A lower temperature in one leg compared to the other leg
- Poor nail growth on the toes and decreased hair growth on the legs
- Erectile dysfunction, especially among men who have diabetes

Diagnosing Peripheral Arterial Disease

Peripheral arterial disease (PAD) is diagnosed based on your medical and family histories, a physical exam, and results from tests.

PAD often is diagnosed after symptoms are reported. An accurate diagnosis is important, because people who have PAD are at increased risk for coronary artery disease (CAD), heart attack, stroke, and transient ischemic attack (mini-stroke). If you have PAD, your doctor also may want to look for signs of these conditions.

Treating Peripheral Arterial Disease

Treatments for peripheral arterial disease (PAD) include lifestyle changes, medicines, and surgery or procedures.

The overall goals of treating PAD are to reduce symptoms, improve quality of life, and prevent complications. Treatment is based on your signs and symptoms, risk factors, and results from a physical exam and tests.

Lifestyle Changes

Treatment often includes making long-lasting lifestyle changes, such as the following:

- **Quitting smoking:** Your risk for PAD increases four times if you smoke. Smoking also raises your risk for other diseases, such as coronary artery disease (CAD). Talk to your doctor about programs and products that can help you quit smoking.
- **Lowering blood pressure:** This lifestyle change can help you avoid the risk of stroke, heart attack, heart failure, and kidney disease.
- **Lowering high blood cholesterol levels:** Lowering cholesterol can delay or even reverse the buildup of plaque in the arteries.
- **Lowering blood glucose levels if you have diabetes:** A hemoglobin A1C test can show how well you have controlled your blood sugar level over the past 3 months.

- **Getting regular physical activity:** Talk with your doctor about taking part in a supervised exercise program. This type of program has been shown to reduce PAD symptoms.

- **Follow a healthy eating plan that's low in total fat, saturated fat, trans fat, cholesterol, and sodium (salt):** Eat more fruits, vegetables, and low-fat dairy products. If you're overweight or obese, work with your doctor to create a reasonable weight-loss plan.

Medicines

Your doctor may prescribe medicines to do the following:

- Lower high blood cholesterol levels and high blood pressure
- Thin the blood to prevent clots from forming due to low blood flow
- Help ease leg pain that occurs when you walk or climb stairs

Surgery or Procedures

Bypass grafting: Your doctor may recommend bypass grafting surgery if blood flow in your limb is blocked or nearly blocked. For this surgery, your doctor uses a blood vessel from another part of your body or a man-made tube to make a graft.

This graft bypasses (goes around) the blocked part of the artery, which allows blood to flow around the blockage. This surgery doesn't cure PAD, but it may increase blood flow to the affected limb.

Angioplasty: Your doctor may recommend angioplasty to restore blood flow through a narrowed or blocked artery.

During this procedure, a catheter with a balloon or other device on the end is inserted into a blocked artery. The balloon is then inflated, which pushes the plaque outward against the wall of the artery. This widens the artery and restores blood flow.

A stent (a small mesh tube) may be placed in the artery during angioplasty. A stent helps keep the artery open after angioplasty is done. Some stents are coated with medicine to help prevent blockages in the artery.

Other types of treatment: Researchers are studying cell and gene therapies to treat PAD. However, these treatments aren't yet available outside of clinical trials.

Chapter 30

Raynaud Syndrome

Raynaud is a rare disorder that affects the arteries. Arteries are blood vessels that carry blood from your heart to different parts of your body.

Raynaud is sometimes called a disease, syndrome, or phenomenon. The disorder is marked by brief episodes of vasospasm (narrowing of the blood vessels).

Vasospasm of the arteries reduces blood flow to the fingers and toes. In people who have Raynaud, the disorder usually affects the fingers. In about 40 percent of people who have Raynaud, it affects the toes. Rarely, the disorder affects the nose, ears, nipples, and lips.

Overview

In most cases, the cause of Raynaud isn't known. This type of Raynaud is called Raynaud disease or primary Raynaud.

Sometimes, a disease, condition, or other factor causes Raynaud. This type of Raynaud is known as Raynaud phenomenon or secondary Raynaud. Primary Raynaud is more common and tends to be less severe than secondary Raynaud.

If you have primary or secondary Raynaud, cold temperatures or stressful emotions can trigger "Raynaud attacks." During an attack, little or no blood flows to affected body parts.

Excerpted from "Raynaud's," by the National Heart, Lung, and Blood Institute (NHLBI, www.nhlbi.nih.gov), part of the National Institutes of Health, February 2009.

As a result, the skin may turn white and then blue for a short time. As blood flow returns, the affected areas may turn red and may throb, tingle, burn, or feel numb.

In both types of Raynaud, even mild or brief changes in temperature can cause attacks. For example, taking something out of the freezer or being exposed to temperatures below 60 degrees Fahrenheit can cause your fingers to turn blue.

Most people who have Raynaud have no long-term tissue damage or disability. However, people who have severe Raynaud can develop skin sores or gangrene from prolonged or repeated Raynaud attacks. Gangrene refers to the death or decay of body tissues.

Outlook

About 5 percent of the U.S. population has Raynaud. For most people who have primary Raynaud, the disorder is more of a bother than a serious illness. They usually can manage the condition with minor lifestyle changes.

Secondary Raynaud may be harder to manage. However, several types of treatments are available to help prevent or relieve symptoms. With secondary Raynaud, it's important to treat the underlying disease or condition that's causing it.

Researchers continue to look for better ways to diagnose and treat Raynaud.

Causes of Raynaud

In most cases, the cause of Raynaud isn't known. This type of Raynaud is called Raynaud disease or primary Raynaud.

Sometimes a disease, condition, or other factor causes Raynaud. This type of Raynaud is called Raynaud phenomenon or secondary Raynaud.

Causes of Secondary Raynaud

A number of different things can cause secondary Raynaud:

- Diseases and conditions that directly damage the arteries or damage the nerves that control the arteries in the hands and feet
- Repetitive actions that damage the nerves that control the arteries in the hands and feet
- Injuries to the hands and feet

- Exposure to certain chemicals
- Medicines that narrow the arteries or affect blood pressure

Diseases and conditions: Secondary Raynaud is linked to diseases and conditions that directly damage the arteries or damage the nerves that control the arteries in the hands and feet.

Scleroderma and lupus are two examples of conditions that are linked to Raynaud. About nine out of 10 people who have scleroderma have Raynaud. About one out of three people who has lupus has Raynaud.

Other examples of diseases and conditions linked to Raynaud include the following:

- Rheumatoid arthritis
- Atherosclerosis
- Blood disorders, such as cryoglobulinemia and polycythemia
- Sjögren syndrome, dermatomyositis, and polymyositis
- Buerger disease

Raynaud also has been linked to thyroid problems and pulmonary hypertension.

Repetitive actions: Repetitive actions that damage the arteries or the nerves that control the arteries in the hands and feet may lead to Raynaud.

Typing, playing the piano, or doing other similar movements repeatedly over long periods may lead to secondary Raynaud. Using vibrating tools, such as jackhammers and drills, also may raise your risk for Raynaud.

Hand or foot injuries: Injuries to the hands or feet from accidents, frostbite, surgery, or other causes can lead to Raynaud.

Chemicals: Exposure to certain workplace chemicals can cause a scleroderma-like illness that's linked to Raynaud. An example of such a chemical is vinyl chloride. This chemical is used in the plastics industry.

The nicotine in cigarettes also can raise your risk for Raynaud.

Medicines: Several medicines are linked to secondary Raynaud, including the following:

- Migraine headache medicines that contain ergotamine are linked to Raynaud. This substance causes the arteries to narrow.

- Certain cancer medicines, such as cisplatin and vinblastine, can cause Raynaud.

- Some over-the-counter cold and allergy medicines and diet aids are linked to Raynaud. Some of these medicines can narrow your arteries.

- Beta-blockers, which slow your heart rate and lower your blood pressure, can cause Raynaud.

- Birth control pills can affect blood flow and are linked to Raynaud.

Risk for Raynaud

The risk factors for primary Raynaud (Raynaud disease) and secondary Raynaud (Raynaud phenomenon) are different.

The risk factors for primary Raynaud include the following:

- Gender: About 80 percent of people who have primary Raynaud are women.

- Age: Primary Raynaud usually develops before the age of 30.

- Family history: Primary Raynaud may occur in members of the same family.

- Living in a cold climate: Cold temperatures can trigger Raynaud attacks.

The risk factors for secondary Raynaud include the following:

- Age (Secondary Raynaud usually develops after the age of 30.)

- Certain diseases and conditions (For example, diseases that directly damage the arteries or damage the nerves that control the arteries in the hands and feet may cause secondary Raynaud.)

- Injuries to the hands or feet

- Exposure to certain workplace chemicals, such as vinyl chloride (used in the plastics industry)

- Repetitive actions with the hands, such as typing or using vibrating tools

- Certain medicines, such as migraine, cancer, cold/allergy, or blood pressure medicines

- Smoking

- Living in a cold climate

Signs and Symptoms of Raynaud

People who have primary Raynaud (Raynaud disease) or secondary Raynaud (Raynaud phenomenon) can have attacks in response to cold temperatures or emotional stress.

Raynaud attacks usually affect the fingers and toes. Rarely, the attacks affect the nose, ears, nipples, or lips.

During a Raynaud attack, the arteries become very narrow for a brief period. As a result, little or no blood flows to affected body parts. This may cause these areas to do the following:

- Turn pale or white and then blue

- Feel numb, cold, or painful

- Turn red, throb, tingle, burn, or feel numb as blood flow returns to the affected areas

Raynaud attacks can last less than a minute or as long as several hours. Attacks can occur daily or weekly.

Attacks often begin in one finger or toe and move on to other fingers or toes. Sometimes only one or two fingers or toes are affected. Different areas may be affected at different times.

Severe cases of secondary Raynaud can cause skin sores or gangrene. Gangrene refers to the death or decay of body tissues. Fortunately, severe Raynaud is rare.

Diagnosing Raynaud

Your doctor will diagnose primary Raynaud (Raynaud disease) or secondary Raynaud (Raynaud phenomenon) based on your medical history, a physical exam, and the results from tests.

Treating Raynaud

Primary Raynaud (Raynaud disease) and secondary Raynaud (Raynaud phenomenon) have no cure. However, treatments can reduce the number and severity of Raynaud attacks. Treatments include lifestyle changes, medicines, and, rarely, surgery.

Most people who have primary Raynaud can manage the condition with lifestyle changes. People who have secondary Raynaud may need medicines in addition to lifestyle changes. Rarely, they may need surgery or shots.

If you have Raynaud and develop sores on your fingers, toes, or other parts of your body, see your doctor right away. Timely treatment can help prevent permanent damage to these areas.

Chapter 31

Vasculitis

Vasculitis is a condition that involves inflammation in the blood vessels. The condition occurs if your immune system attacks your blood vessels by mistake. This may happen as the result of an infection, a medicine, or another disease or condition.

The inflammation can lead to serious problems. Complications depend on which blood vessels, organs, or other body systems are affected.

Outlook

There are many types of vasculitis, but overall the condition is rare. If you have vasculitis, the outlook depends on the following:

- The type of vasculitis you have
- Which organs are affected
- How quickly the condition worsens
- How severe the condition is

Treatment often works well if the condition is diagnosed and treated early. In some cases, vasculitis may go into remission. "Remission"

Excerpted from text by the National Heart, Lung, and Blood Institute (NHLBI, www.nhlbi.nih.gov), part of the National Institutes of Health, March 2009.

means the condition isn't active, but it can come back, or "flare," at any time.

Some cases of vasculitis are chronic (ongoing) and never go into remission. Long-term treatment with medicines often can control the signs and symptoms of chronic vasculitis.

Rarely, vasculitis doesn't respond well to treatment. This can lead to disability and even death.

Much is still unknown about vasculitis. However, researchers continue to learn more about the condition and its various types, causes, and treatments.

Types of Vasculitis

There are many types of vasculitis. Each type involves inflamed blood vessels. However, most types differ in whom they affect and the organs that are involved.

The types of vasculitis often are grouped based on the size of the blood vessels they affect.

Mostly Large Vessel Vasculitis

These types of vasculitis usually, but not always, affect the larger blood vessels.

Behçet disease: Behçet disease can cause recurrent, painful ulcers in the mouth, ulcers on the genitals, acne-like skin lesions, and eye inflammation called uveitis.

The disease occurs most often in people aged 20 to 40. Men are more likely to get it, but it also can affect women. It's more common in people of Mediterranean, Middle Eastern, and Far Eastern descent, although it rarely affects Blacks.

Researchers believe that a gene called the HLA-B51 [human leukocyte antigen B51] gene may play a role in Behçet disease. However, not everyone who has the gene gets the disease.

Cogan syndrome: Cogan syndrome can occur in people who have a systemic vasculitis that affects the large vessels, especially the aorta and aortic valve. The aorta is the main artery that carries oxygen-rich blood from the heart to the body. A systemic vasculitis is a type of vasculitis that affects you in a general or overall way.

Cogan syndrome can lead to eye inflammation called interstitial keratitis. It also can cause hearing changes, including sudden deafness.

Giant cell arteritis: Giant cell arteritis usually affects the temporal artery, an artery on the side of your head. This condition also is called temporal arteritis. Symptoms of this condition can include headache, scalp tenderness, jaw pain, blurred vision, double vision, and acute (sudden) vision loss.

Giant cell arteritis is the most common form of vasculitis in adults older than 50. It's more likely to occur in people of Scandinavian origin, but it can affect people of any race.

Polymyalgia rheumatica: Polymyalgia rheumatica, or PMR, commonly affects the large joints in the body, such as the shoulders and hips. PMR typically causes stiffness and pain in the muscles of the neck, shoulders, lower back, hips, and thighs.

Most often, PMR occurs by itself, but 10–20 percent of people who have PMR also develop giant cell arteritis. Also, about half of the people who have giant cell arteritis also can have PMR.

Takayasu arteritis: Takayasu arteritis affects medium- and large-sized arteries, particularly the aorta and its branches. The condition is sometimes called aortic arch syndrome.

Though rare, Takayasu arteritis occurs mostly in teenage girls and young women. The condition is more common in Asians, but it can affect people of all races and occur throughout the world.

Takayasu arteritis is a systemic disease. A systemic disease is one that affects you in a general or overall way. Symptoms of Takayasu arteritis may include tiredness and a sense of feeling unwell, fever, night sweats, sore joints, loss of appetite, and weight loss. These symptoms usually occur before other signs develop that point to arteritis.

Mostly Medium Vessel Vasculitis

These types of vasculitis usually, but not always, affect the medium-sized blood vessels.

Buerger disease: Buerger disease, also known as thromboangiitis obliterans, typically affects blood flow to the hands and feet. In this disease, the blood vessels in the hands and feet tighten or become blocked. This causes less blood to flow to the affected tissues, which can lead to pain and tissue damage.

Rarely, Buerger disease also can affect blood vessels in the brain, abdomen, and heart. The disease usually affects men aged 20 to 40 of

Asian or Eastern European descent. The disease is strongly linked to cigarette smoking.

Symptoms of Buerger disease include pain in the calves or feet when walking, or pain in the forearms and hands with activity. Other symptoms include blood clots in the surface veins of the limbs and Raynaud phenomenon.

In severe cases, ulcers may develop on the fingers and toes, leading to gangrene. The term "gangrene" refers to the death or decay of body tissues.

Surgical bypass of the blood vessels may help restore blood flow to some areas. Medicines generally aren't effective treatments. The best treatment is to stop using tobacco of any kind.

Central nervous system vasculitis: Central nervous system (CNS) vasculitis usually occurs as a result of a systemic vasculitis. A systemic vasculitis is one that affects you in a general or overall way.

Very rarely, vasculitis affects only the brain and/or spinal cord. When it does, the condition is called isolated vasculitis of the CNS or primary angiitis of the CNS.

Symptoms of CNS vasculitis are headache, problems thinking clearly or changes in mental function, or stroke-like symptoms, such as muscle weakness and paralysis (an inability to move).

Kawasaki disease: Kawasaki disease is a rare childhood disease in which the walls of the blood vessels throughout the body become inflamed. The disease can affect any blood vessel in the body, including arteries, veins, and capillaries. Kawasaki disease also is known as mucocutaneous lymph node syndrome.

Sometimes the disease affects the coronary arteries, which carry oxygen-rich blood to the heart. As a result, a small number of children who have Kawasaki disease may develop serious heart problems.

Polyarteritis nodosa: Polyarteritis nodosa can affect many parts of the body. It often affects the kidneys, the digestive tract, the nerves, and the skin.

Symptoms often include fever, a general feeling of being unwell, weight loss, and muscle and joint aches, including pain in the calf muscles that develops over weeks or months. Other signs and symptoms include anemia (a low red blood cell count), a lace- or web-like rash, bumps under the skin, and abdominal pain after eating.

Researchers believe that this type of vasculitis is very rare, although the symptoms can be similar to those of other types of vasculitis. Some cases of polyarteritis nodosa seem to be linked to hepatitis B or C infections.

Mostly Small Vessel Vasculitis

These types of vasculitis usually, but not always, affect the small blood vessels.

Churg-Strauss syndrome: Churg-Strauss syndrome is a very rare disorder that causes blood vessel inflammation. It's also known as allergic angiitis and granulomatosis.

This disorder can affect many organs, including the lungs, skin, kidneys, nervous system, and heart. Symptoms can vary widely. They may include asthma, higher than normal levels of white blood cells in the blood and tissues, and tissue formations known as granulomas.

Essential mixed cryoglobulinemia: Essential mixed cryoglobulinemia can occur alone, or it may be linked to a systemic vasculitis. A systemic vasculitis is one that affects the body in a general or overall way.

Symptoms often include joint aches; weakness; nerve changes, such as numbness, tingling, and pain in the limbs; kidney inflammation; and a raised, bumpy, reddish-purple skin rash known as palpable purpura.

While essential mixed cryoglobulinemia can occur with other conditions, it most often is linked to chronic hepatitis C infection.

Henoch-Schönlein purpura: Henoch-Schönlein purpura (HSP) is a type of vasculitis that affects the smallest blood vessels—the capillaries—in the skin, joints, intestines, and kidneys.

Symptoms often include abdominal pain, aching and swollen joints, and signs of kidney damage, such as blood in the urine. Another symptom is a bruise-like rash that mostly shows up as reddish-purple blotches on the lower legs and buttocks (although it can appear anywhere on the body).

HSP is more common in children, but it also can affect teens and adults. In children, about half of all cases follow a viral or bacterial upper respiratory infection. Most people get better in a few weeks and have no lasting problems.

Hypersensitivity vasculitis: Hypersensitivity vasculitis affects the skin. This condition also is known as allergic vasculitis, cutaneous vasculitis, or leukocytoclastic vasculitis.

A common symptom is red spots on the skin, usually on the lower legs. For people who are bedridden, the rash appears on the lower back.

An allergic reaction to a medicine or infection often causes this type of vasculitis. Stopping the medicine or treating the infection usually clears up the vasculitis. However, some people may need to take anti-inflammatory medicines, such as corticosteroids, for a short time. These medicines help reduce inflammation.

Microscopic polyangiitis: Microscopic polyangiitis affects small vessels, particularly those in the kidneys and the lungs. This disease mainly occurs in middle-aged people; it affects men slightly more often than women.

The symptoms often aren't specific, and they can begin gradually with fever, weight loss, and muscle aches. In some cases, the symptoms come on suddenly and progress quickly, leading to kidney failure.

If the lungs are involved, the first symptom may be coughing up blood. In some cases, the disease occurs along with a vasculitis that affects the intestinal tract, the skin, and the nervous system.

The signs and symptoms of microscopic polyangiitis are similar to those of the vasculitis condition called Wegener granulomatosis. However, microscopic polyangiitis usually doesn't affect the nose and sinuses or cause abnormal tissue formations in the lungs and kidneys.

The results of certain blood tests can suggest inflammation. These results include a higher than normal erythrocyte sedimentation rate (ESR); lower than normal hemoglobin and hematocrit levels (which suggest anemia); and higher than normal white blood cell and platelet counts.

Also, more than half of the people with microscopic polyangiitis have certain antibodies called antineutrophil cytoplasmic autoantibodies (ANCA) in their blood. These antibodies also are seen in people who have Wegener granulomatosis.

Testing for ANCA can't be used to diagnose either of these two types of vasculitis. However, testing can help evaluate people who have vasculitis-like symptoms.

Wegener granulomatosis: Wegener granulomatosis is a rare vasculitis. It affects men and women equally, but occurs more often in Whites than in African Americans. This type of vasculitis can occur at any age, but it is more common in middle-aged people.

Wegener granulomatosis typically affects the sinuses, nose, and throat; the lungs; and the kidneys. Other organs also can be involved.

In addition to inflamed blood vessels, the affected tissues also develop abnormal formations called granulomas. If granulomas develop in the lungs, they can destroy the lung tissue. The damage can be mistaken for pneumonia or even lung cancer.

Symptoms of Wegener granulomatosis often are not specific and can begin gradually with fever, weight loss, and muscle aches. Sometimes, the symptoms come on suddenly and progress rapidly, leading to kidney failure. If the lungs are involved, the first symptom may be coughing up blood.

The results of certain blood tests can suggest inflammation. These results include a higher than normal ESR; lower than normal hemoglobin and hematocrit levels (which suggest anemia); and higher than normal white blood cell and platelet counts.

Another test looks for antiproteinase-3 (an antineutrophil cytoplasmic autoantibody) in the blood. Most people who have active Wegener granulomatosis will have this antibody. A small portion may have another ANCA known as antimyeloperoxidase-specific ANCA.

Having either ANCA antibody isn't enough on its own to make a diagnosis of Wegener granulomatosis. However, testing for the antibodies can help support the diagnosis in patients who have other signs and symptoms of the condition.

A biopsy of an affected organ is the best way for your doctor to make a firm diagnosis. A biopsy is a procedure in which your doctor takes a small sample of your body tissue to examine under a microscope.

Other Names for Vasculitis

- Angiitis
- Arteritis

Causes of Vasculitis

Vasculitis occurs when your immune system attacks your own blood vessels by mistake. What causes this to happen isn't fully known.

A recent or chronic (ongoing) infection may prompt the attack. Your body also may attack its own blood vessels in reaction to a medicine.

Sometimes an autoimmune disorder triggers vasculitis. Autoimmune disorders occur when the immune system makes antibodies (proteins) that attack and damage the body's own tissues or cells. Examples of such autoimmune disorders include lupus, rheumatoid arthritis, and scleroderma. You can have these disorders for years before developing vasculitis.

Vasculitis also may be linked to certain blood cancers, such as leukemia and lymphoma.

Risk for Vasculitis

Vasculitis can affect people of all ages and races and both genders. Some types of vasculitis seem to occur more often in people who have or do the following:

- Certain medical conditions, such as chronic hepatitis B or C infection
- Certain autoimmune diseases, such as lupus
- Smoke

Signs and Symptoms of Vasculitis

The signs and symptoms of vasculitis vary. They depend on the type of vasculitis you have, the organs involved, and how severe the condition is. Some people may have few signs and symptoms. Other people may become very sick.

Sometimes, the signs and symptoms develop gradually over months. Other times, the signs and symptoms develop faster, over days or weeks.

Systemic Signs and Symptoms

Systemic signs and symptoms are those that affect you in a general, or overall, way. Common systemic signs and symptoms of vasculitis include the following:

- Fever
- Loss of appetite
- Weight loss
- Fatigue (tiredness)
- General aches and pains

Organ- or Body System-Specific Signs and Symptoms

Vasculitis can affect specific organs and body systems, causing a range of signs and symptoms.

Skin: If the condition affects your skin, you may notice a number of skin changes. For example, you may notice purple or red spots or bumps, clusters of small dots, splotches, bruises, or hives. Your skin also may itch.

Joints: If the condition affects your joints, you may ache or develop arthritis in one or more joints.

Lungs: If the condition affects your lungs, you may feel short of breath. You may even cough up blood. The results from a chest x-ray may show signs of pneumonia, even though that isn't what you have.

Gastrointestinal tract: If the condition affects your gastrointestinal tract, you may get ulcers in your mouth or have abdominal pain.

In severe cases, blood flow to the intestines can be blocked. This can cause the wall of the intestines to weaken and possibly rupture. A rupture can lead to serious problems or even death.

Sinuses, nose, throat, and ears: If the condition affects your sinuses, nose, throat, and ears, you may have sinus or chronic (ongoing) middle ear infections.

Other symptoms include ulcers in the nose and, in some cases, hearing loss.

Eyes: If vasculitis affects your eyes, you may develop red, itchy, burning eyes. Your eyes also may become sensitive to light, and your vision may become blurry. In rare cases, certain types of vasculitis may cause blindness.

Brain: If vasculitis affects your brain, symptoms may include headache, problems thinking clearly or changes in mental function, or stroke-like symptoms, such as muscle weakness and paralysis (an inability to move).

Nerves: If the condition affects your nerves, you may have numbness, tingling, and weakness in various parts of your body. You also may have a loss of feeling or strength in your hands and feet and shooting pains in your arms and legs.

Diagnosing Vasculitis

Your doctor will diagnose vasculitis based on your signs and symptoms, your medical history, a physical exam, and the results from tests.

Treating Vasculitis

Treatment for vasculitis will depend on the type of vasculitis you have, which organs are affected, and how severe the condition is.

People who have severe vasculitis are treated with prescription medicines. Rarely, surgery may be done. People who have mild vasculitis may find relief with over-the-counter pain medicines, such as acetaminophen, aspirin, ibuprofen, or naproxen.

Goals of Treatment

The main goal of vasculitis treatment is to reduce inflammation in the affected blood vessels. This usually is done by reducing or stopping the immune response that caused the inflammation.

Types of Treatment

Common prescription medicines used to treat vasculitis include corticosteroid and cytotoxic medicines.

Corticosteroids help reduce inflammation in your blood vessels. Examples of corticosteroids are prednisone, prednisolone, and methylprednisolone.

Cytotoxic medicines may be prescribed if vasculitis is severe or if corticosteroids don't work well. Cytotoxic medicines kill the cells that are causing the inflammation. Examples of these medicines are azathioprine, methotrexate, and cyclophosphamide.

Your doctor may prescribe both corticosteroids and cytotoxic medicines.

Other treatments may be used for certain types of vasculitis. For example, the standard treatment for Kawasaki disease is high-dose aspirin and immune globulin. Immune globulin is a medicine given intravenously (injected into a vein).

Certain types of vasculitis may require surgery to remove aneurysms that have formed as a result of the condition. (An aneurysm is an abnormal bulge in the wall of a blood vessel.)

Chapter 32

Deep Vein Thrombosis

Deep vein thrombosis, or DVT, is a blood clot that forms in a vein deep in the body. Blood clots occur when blood thickens and clumps together.

Most deep vein blood clots occur in the lower leg or thigh. They also can occur in other parts of the body.

A blood clot in a deep vein can break off and travel through the bloodstream. The loose clot is called an embolus. When the clot travels to the lungs and blocks blood flow, the condition is called pulmonary embolism, or PE.

PE is a very serious condition. It can damage the lungs and other organs in the body and cause death.

Blood clots in the thigh are more likely to break off and cause PE than blood clots in the lower leg or other parts of the body.

Blood clots also can form in the veins closer to the skin's surface. However, these clots won't break off and cause PE.

Other Names for Deep Vein Thrombosis

- Blood clot in the legs
- Venous thrombosis
- Venous thromboembolism (VTE; used for both deep vein thrombosis and pulmonary embolism)

Excerpted from text by the National Heart, Lung, and Blood Institute (NHLBI, www.nhlbi.nih.gov), part of the National Institutes of Health, November 2007.

Causes of Deep Vein Thrombosis

Blood clots can form in your body's deep veins. The following situations may contribute to DVT:

- **Damage occurs to a vein's inner lining:** This damage may result from injuries caused by physical, chemical, and biological factors. Such factors include surgery, serious injury, inflammation, or an immune response.

- **Blood flow is sluggish or slow:** Lack of motion can cause sluggish or slowed blood flow. This may occur after surgery, if you're ill and in bed for a long time, or if you're traveling for a long time.

- **Your blood is thicker or more likely to clot than usual:** Certain inherited conditions (such as factor V Leiden) increase blood's tendency to clot. This also is true of treatment with hormone replacement therapy or birth control pills.

Risk for Deep Vein Thrombosis

Many factors increase your risk for deep vein thrombosis (DVT). They include the following:

- A history of DVT
- Injury to a deep vein from surgery, a broken bone, or other trauma
- Slow blood flow in a deep vein from lack of movement
- Pregnancy and the first 6 weeks after giving birth
- Recent or ongoing treatment for cancer
- A central venous catheter (a tube placed in vein to allow easy access to the bloodstream for medical treatment)
- Being older than 60 (although DVT can occur in any age group)
- Being overweight or obese

Disorders or factors that make your blood thicker or more likely to clot than normal can also increase your risk for DVT. Certain inherited blood disorders (such as factor V Leiden) will do this. This also is true of treatment with hormone replacement therapy or using birth control pills.

Your risk for DVT increases if you have more than one of the risk factors listed above.

Signs and Symptoms of Deep Vein Thrombosis

The signs and symptoms of deep vein thrombosis (DVT) may be related to DVT itself or to pulmonary embolism (PE). See your doctor right away if you have symptoms of either. Both DVT and PE can cause serious, possibly life-threatening complications if not treated.

Deep Vein Thrombosis

Only about half of the people with DVT have symptoms. These symptoms occur in the leg affected by the deep vein clot. They include the following:

- Swelling of the leg or along a vein in the leg
- Pain or tenderness in the leg, which you may feel only when standing or walking
- Increased warmth in the area of the leg that's swollen or in pain
- Red or discolored skin on the leg

Pulmonary Embolism

Some people don't know they have DVT until they have signs or symptoms of PE. Symptoms of PE include the following:

- Unexplained shortness of breath
- Pain with deep breathing
- Coughing up blood

Rapid breathing and a fast heart rate also may be signs of PE.

Diagnosing Deep Vein Thrombosis

Your doctor will diagnose deep vein thrombosis (DVT) based on your medical history, a physical exam, and the results from tests. He or she will identify your risk factors and rule out other causes for your symptoms.

Medical History

To learn about your medical history, your doctor may ask about the following:

- Your overall health

- Any prescription medicines you're taking
- Any recent surgeries or injuries you've had
- Whether you've been treated for cancer

Physical Exam

During the physical exam, your doctor will check your legs for signs of DVT. He or she also will check your blood pressure and your heart and lungs.

Diagnostic Tests

You may need one or more tests to find out whether you have DVT. The most common tests used to diagnose DVT are the following:

- **Ultrasound:** This is the most common test for diagnosing deep vein blood clots. It uses sound waves to create pictures of blood flowing through the arteries and veins in the affected leg.

- **A D-dimer test:** This test measures a substance in the blood that's released when a blood clot dissolves. If the test shows high levels of the substance, you may have a deep vein blood clot. If your test is normal and you have few risk factors, DVT isn't likely.

- **Venography:** This test is used if ultrasound doesn't provide a clear diagnosis. Dye is injected into a vein, and then an x-ray is taken of the leg. The dye makes the vein visible on the x-ray. The x-ray will show whether blood flow is slow in the vein. This may indicate a blood clot.

Other less common tests used to diagnose DVT include magnetic resonance imaging (MRI) and computed tomography (CT) scanning. These tests provide pictures of the inside of the body.

You may need blood tests to check whether you have an inherited blood clotting disorder that can cause DVT. You may have this type of disorder if you have repeated blood clots that can't be linked to another cause, or if you develop a blood clot in an unusual location, such as a vein in the liver, kidney, or brain.

If your doctor thinks that you have pulmonary embolism (PE), he or she may order extra tests, such as a ventilation perfusion scan (V/Q scan). The V/Q scan uses a radioactive material to show how well oxygen and blood are flowing to all areas of the lungs.

Treating Deep Vein Thrombosis

Goals of Treatment

The main goals of treating deep vein thrombosis (DVT) are to do the following:

- Stop the blood clot from getting bigger

- Prevent the blood clot from breaking off and moving to your lungs

- Reduce your chance of having another blood clot

Medicines

Medicines are used to prevent and treat DVT.

Anticoagulants: Anticoagulants are the most common medicines for treating DVT. They're also known as blood thinners.

These medicines decrease your blood's ability to clot. They also stop existing blood clots from getting bigger. However, blood thinners can't break up blood clots that have already formed. (The body dissolves most blood clots with time.)

Blood thinners can be taken as either a pill, an injection under the skin, or through a needle or tube inserted into a vein (called intravenous, or IV, injection).

Warfarin and heparin are two blood thinners used to treat DVT. Warfarin is given in pill form. (Coumadin® is a common brand name for warfarin.) Heparin is given as an injection or through an IV tube. There are different types of heparin. Your doctor will discuss the options with you.

Your doctor may treat you with both heparin and warfarin at the same time. Heparin acts quickly. Warfarin takes 2 to 3 days before it starts to work. Once the warfarin starts to work, the heparin is stopped.

Pregnant women usually are treated with heparin only, because warfarin is dangerous during pregnancy.

Treatment for DVT with blood thinners usually lasts from 3 to 6 months. The following situations may change the length of treatment.

- If your blood clot occurred after a short-term risk (for example, surgery), your treatment time may be shorter.

- If you've had blood clots before, your treatment time may last longer.

- If you have certain other illnesses, such as cancer, you may need to take blood thinners for as long as you have the illness.

The most common side effect of blood thinners is bleeding. This happens if the medicine thins your blood too much. This side effect can be life threatening.

Sometimes, the bleeding is internal (inside your body). People treated with blood thinners usually receive regular blood tests to measure their blood's ability to clot. These blood tests are called PT and PTT tests.

These tests also help your doctor make sure you're taking the right amount of medicine. Call your doctor right away if you have easy bruising or bleeding. This may be a sign that your medicines have thinned your blood too much.

Thrombin inhibitors: These medicines interfere with the blood clotting process. They're used to treat blood clots in patients who can't take heparin.

Thrombolytics: These medicines are given to quickly dissolve a blood clot. They're used to treat large blood clots that cause severe symptoms.

Because thrombolytics can cause sudden bleeding, they're used only in life-threatening situations.

Other Types of Treatment

Vena cava filter: A vena cava filter is used if you can't take blood thinners or if you're taking blood thinners and still developing blood clots.

The filter is inserted inside a large vein called the vena cava. The filter catches blood clots that break off in a vein before they move to the lungs. This prevents pulmonary embolism. However, it doesn't stop new blood clots from forming.

Graduated compression stockings: These stockings can reduce the swelling that may occur after a blood clot has developed in your leg. Graduated compression stockings are worn on the legs from the arch of the foot to just above or below the knee.

These stockings are tight at the ankle and become looser as they go up the leg. This creates gentle pressure up the leg.

The pressure keeps blood from pooling and clotting. These stockings should be worn for at least a year after DVT is diagnosed.

Preventing Deep Vein Thrombosis

You can take steps to prevent deep vein thrombosis (DVT).

If you're at risk for DVT or pulmonary embolism (PE), you can help prevent the condition by doing the following:

- See your doctor for regular checkups.

- Take all medicines your doctor prescribes.

- Get out of bed and move around as soon as possible after surgery or illness. This lowers your chance of developing a blood clot.

- Exercise your lower leg muscles during long trips. This helps prevent a blood clot from forming.

If you've had DVT or PE before, you can help prevent future blood clots by following the above steps as well as the following:

- Take all medicines your doctor prescribes to prevent or treat blood clots.

- Follow up with your doctor for tests and treatment.

- Use compression stockings as your doctor directs to prevent swelling in your legs from DVT.

Contact your doctor at once if you have any signs or symptoms of DVT or PE.

Travel Tips

Your risk of developing DVT while traveling is small. The risk increases if the travel time is longer than 4 hours, or if you have other risk factors for DVT.

During long trips, it may help to do the following:

- Walk up and down the aisles of the bus, train, or airplane.

- If traveling by car, stop about every hour and walk around.

- Move your legs and flex and stretch your feet to encourage blood flow in your calves.

- Wear loose and comfortable clothing.

- Drink plenty of fluids and avoid alcohol.

If you're at increased risk for DVT, your doctor may recommend wearing compression stockings during travel or taking a blood-thinning medicine before traveling.

Living with Deep Vein Thrombosis

Medicines that thin your blood and prevent blood clots are used to treat DVT. These medicines can thin your blood too much and cause bleeding (sometimes inside the body). This side effect can be life threatening.

Bleeding may occur in the digestive system or the brain. Signs and symptoms of bleeding in the digestive system include the following:

• Bright red vomit or vomit that looks like coffee grounds

• Bright red blood in your stools or black, tarry stools

• Pain in your abdomen

Signs and symptoms of bleeding in the brain include the following:

• Severe pain in your head

• Sudden changes in your vision

• Sudden loss of movement in your arms or legs

• Memory loss or confusion

If you have any of these signs or symptoms, get treatment right away.

You also should seek treatment right away if you have a lot of bleeding after a fall or injury. This could be a sign that your DVT medicines have thinned your blood too much.

Talk to your doctor before taking any medicines other than your DVT medicines. This includes over-the-counter medicines. Aspirin, for example, also can thin your blood. Taking two medicines that thin your blood may raise your risk for bleeding.

Ask your doctor about how your diet affects these medicines. Foods that contain vitamin K can change how warfarin (a blood-thinning medicine used to treat DVT) works. Vitamin K is found in green, leafy vegetables and some oils, like canola and soybean oil. Your doctor can help you plan a balanced and healthy diet.

Discuss with your doctor whether drinking alcohol will interfere with your medicines. Your doctor can tell you what amount of alcohol is safe for you.

Chapter 33

Other Vein Problems

Chapter Contents

Section 33.1

Chronic Venous Insufficiency

"Venous insufficiency," © 2009 A.D.A.M., Inc.
Reprinted with permission.

Venous insufficiency is a condition in which the veins have problems sending blood from the legs back to the heart.

Causes

Venous insufficiency is caused by problems in one or more deeper leg veins. Normally, valves in your veins keep your blood flowing back towards the heart so it does not collect in one place. But the valves in varicose veins are either damaged or missing. This causes the veins to remain filled with blood, especially when you are standing.

The condition may also be caused by a blockage in a vein from a clot (deep vein thrombosis).

Chronic venous insufficiency is a long-term condition. It occurs because of partial vein blockage or blood leakage around the valves of the veins.

Risk factors for venous insufficiency include:

- history of deep vein thrombosis in the legs;
- age;
- being female (related to levels of the hormone progesterone);
- being tall;
- genetic factors;
- obesity;
- pregnancy;
- prolonged sitting or standing.

Symptoms

- Dull aching, heaviness, or cramping in legs

- Itching and tingling
- Pain that gets worse when standing
- Pain that gets better when legs are raised
- Swelling of the legs

People with chronic venous insufficiency may also have:

- redness of the legs and ankles;
- skin color changes around the ankles;
- varicose veins on the surface (superficial);
- thickening of the skin on the legs and ankles;
- ulcers on the legs and ankles.

Treatment

Take the following steps to help manage venous insufficiency:

- Use compression stockings to decrease chronic swelling.
- Avoid long periods of sitting or standing. Even moving your legs slightly will help the blood in your veins return to your heart.
- Care for wounds aggressively if any skin breakdown or infection occurs.

Surgery (varicose vein stripping) may be recommended.

Section 33.2

Varicose and Spider Veins

Excerpted from "Varicose Veins and Spider Veins," by the Office of Women's Health (www.womenshealth.gov), December 1, 2005.

What are varicose veins and spider veins?

Varicose veins are enlarged veins that can be flesh colored, dark purple, or blue. They often look like cords and appear twisted and bulging. They are swollen and raised above the surface of the skin. Varicose veins are commonly found on the backs of the calves or on the inside of the leg. During pregnancy, varicose veins called hemorrhoids can form in the vagina or around the anus.

Spider veins are similar to varicose veins, but they are smaller. They are often red or blue and are closer to the surface of the skin than varicose veins. They can look like tree branches or spider webs with their short jagged lines. Spider veins can be found on the legs and face. They can cover either a very small or very large area of skin.

What causes varicose veins and spider veins?

The heart pumps blood filled with oxygen and nutrients to the whole body. Arteries carry blood from the heart toward the body parts.

Veins carry oxygen-poor blood from the body back to the heart. The squeezing of leg muscles pumps blood back to the heart from the lower body. Veins have valves that act as one-way flaps. These valves prevent the blood from flowing backward as it moves up the legs. If the one-way valves become weak, blood can leak back into the vein and collect there. This problem is called venous insufficiency. Pooled blood enlarges the vein and it becomes varicose. Spider veins can also be caused by the backup of blood. Hormone changes, inherited factors, and exposure to the sun can also cause spider veins.

How common are abnormal leg veins?

About 50 to 55% of American women and 40 to 45% of American men suffer from some form of vein problem. Varicose veins affect one out of two people age 50 and older.

Who usually has varicose veins and spider veins?

Many factors increase a person's chances of developing varicose or spider veins.

- Increasing age can increase the risk of varicose veins.

- Having family members with vein problems or being born with weak vein valves can increase the risk of varicose veins.

- Hormonal changes can increase risk. These occur during puberty, pregnancy, and menopause. Taking birth control pills and other medicines containing estrogen and progesterone also increase the risk of varicose or spider veins.

- Pregnancy can increase risk. During pregnancy there is a huge increase in the amount of blood in the body. This can cause veins to enlarge. The expanding uterus also puts pressure on the veins. Varicose veins usually improve within 3 months after delivery. A growing number of abnormal veins usually appear with each additional pregnancy.

- Obesity, leg injury, prolonged standing, and other things that weaken vein valves can increase the risk of varicose or spider veins.

- Sun exposure can cause spider veins on the cheeks or nose of a fair-skinned person.

Why do varicose veins and spider veins usually appear in the legs?

The force of gravity, the pressure of body weight, and the task of carrying blood from the bottom of the body up to the heart make legs the primary location for varicose and spider veins. Compared with other veins in the body, leg veins have the toughest job of carrying blood back to the heart. They endure the most pressure. This pressure can be stronger than the veins' one-way valves.

Are varicose veins and spider veins painful or dangerous?

Spider veins usually do not need medical treatment. But varicose veins usually enlarge and worsen over time. Severe varicose veins can cause health problems.

- Severe venous insufficiency can be caused by varicose veins. This severe pooling of blood in the veins slows the return of blood to the heart. This condition can cause blood clots and severe infections. Blood clots can be very dangerous because they can move from leg veins and travel to the lungs. Blood clots in the lungs are life-threatening because they can block the heart and lungs from functioning.

- Sores or skin ulcers can occur on skin tissue around varicose veins.

- Ongoing irritation, swelling, and painful rashes of the legs can occur due to varicose veins.

What are the signs of varicose veins?

Some common symptoms of varicose veins include the following:

- Aching pain
- Easily tired legs
- Leg heaviness
- Swelling in the legs
- Darkening of the skin (in severe cases)
- Numbness in the legs
- Itching or irritated rash in the legs

How can I prevent varicose veins and spider veins?

Not all varicose and spider veins can be prevented. But some things can reduce your chances of getting new varicose and spider veins. These same things can help ease discomfort from the ones you already have:

- Wear sunscreen to protect your skin from the sun and to limit spider veins on the face.

- Exercise regularly to improve your leg strength, circulation, and vein strength. Focus on exercises that work your legs, such as walking or running.

- Control your weight to avoid placing too much pressure on your legs.

- Do not cross your legs when sitting.

- Elevate your legs when resting as much as possible.

- Do not stand or sit for long periods of time. If you must stand for a long time, shift your weight from one leg to the other every few minutes. If you must sit for long periods of time, stand up and move around or take a short walk every 30 minutes.

- Wear elastic support stockings and avoid tight clothing that constricts your waist, groin, or legs.

- Eat a low-salt diet rich in high-fiber foods. Eating fiber reduces the chances of constipation, which can contribute to varicose veins. High fiber foods include fresh fruits and vegetables and whole grains, like bran. Eating too much salt can cause you to retain water or swell.

Should I see a doctor about varicose veins?

Remember these important questions when deciding whether to see your doctor:

Has the varicose vein become swollen, red, or very tender or warm to the touch?

- If yes, see your doctor.

- If no, are there sores or a rash on the leg or near the ankle with the varicose vein, or do you think there may be circulation problems in your feet?

  - If yes, see your doctor.

  - If no, continue to follow the self-care tips above.

How are varicose and spider veins treated?

Besides a physical exam, your doctor can take x-rays or ultrasound pictures of the vein to find the cause and severity of the problem. You may want to speak with a doctor who specializes in vein diseases or phlebology. Talk to your doctor about what treatment options are best for your condition and lifestyle. Not all cases of varicose veins are the same.

Some available treatments include the following.

Sclerotherapy: This is the most common treatment for both spider veins and varicose veins. The doctor injects a solution into the vein that causes the vein walls to swell, stick together, and seal shut. This stops the flow of blood and the vein turns into scar tissue. In a few weeks, the vein should fade. The same vein may need to be treated more than once.

This treatment is very effective if done the right way. Most patients can expect a 50% to 90% improvement. Microsclerotherapy uses special solutions and injection techniques that increase the success rate for removal of spider veins. Sclerotherapy does not require anesthesia, and can be done in the doctor's office.

Possible side effects include the following:

- Temporary stinging or painful cramps where the injection was made

- Temporary red raised patches of skin where the injection was made

- Temporary small skin sores where the injection was made

- Temporary bruises where the injection was made

- Spots around the treated vein that usually disappear

- Brown lines around the treated vein that usually disappear

- Groups of fine red blood vessels around the treated vein that usually disappear

The treated vein can also become inflamed or develop lumps of clotted blood. This is not dangerous. Applying heat and taking aspirin or antibiotics can relieve inflammation. Lumps of coagulated blood can be drained.

Laser surgery: New technology in laser treatments can effectively treat spider veins in the legs. Laser surgery sends very strong bursts of light onto the vein. This can makes the vein slowly fade and disappear. Lasers are very direct and accurate. So the proper laser controlled by a skilled doctor will usually only damage the area being treated. Most skin types and colors can be safely treated with lasers.

Laser surgery is more appealing to some patients because it does not use needles or incisions. Still, when the laser hits the skin, the patient feels a heat sensation that can be quite painful. Cooling helps reduce the pain. Laser treatments last for 15 to 20 minutes. Depending on the severity of the veins, two to five treatments are generally needed to remove spider veins in the legs. Patients can return to normal activity right after treatment, just as with sclerotherapy. For spider veins larger than 3 mm, laser therapy is not very practical.

Possible side effects of laser surgery include the following:

- Redness or swelling of the skin right after the treatment that disappears within a few days may occur.

- Discolored skin that will disappear within 1 to 2 months may occur.

- Rarely burns and scars result from poorly performed laser surgery.

Endovenous techniques (radiofrequency and laser): These methods for treating the deeper varicose veins of the legs (the saphenous veins) have been a huge breakthrough. They have replaced surgery for the vast majority of patients with severe varicose veins. This technique is not very invasive and can be done in a doctor's office.

The doctor puts a very small tube called a catheter into the vein. Once inside, the catheter sends out radiofrequency or laser energy that shrinks and seals the vein wall. Healthy veins around the closed vein restore the normal flow of blood. As this happens, symptoms from the varicose vein improve. Veins on the surface of the skin that are connected to the treated varicose vein will also usually shrink after treatment. When needed, these connected varicose veins can be treated with sclerotherapy or other techniques.

Possible side effects include slight bruising.

Surgery: Surgery is used mostly to treat very large varicose veins. Types of surgery for varicose veins include:

- **Surgical ligation and stripping:** With this treatment, problematic veins are tied shut and completely removed from the leg. Removing the veins does not affect the circulation of blood in the leg. Veins deeper in the leg take care of the larger volumes of blood. Most varicose veins removed by surgery are surface veins and collect blood only from the skin. This surgery requires either local or general anesthesia and must be done in an operating room on an outpatient basis. Serious side effects or problems from this surgery are uncommon.

  - With general anesthesia, there is a risk of heart and breathing problems.

  - Bleeding and congestion of blood can be a problem. But the collected blood usually settles on its own and does not require any further treatment.

  - Wound infection, inflammation, swelling, and redness may occur.

  - Permanent scars may occur.

- Damage of nerve tissue around the treated vein may occur. It is hard to avoid harming small nerve branches when veins are removed. This damage can cause numbness, burning, or a change in sensation around the surgical scar.

- A deep vein blood clot may occur. These clots can travel to the lungs and heart. Injections of heparin, a medicine that reduces blood clotting, reduce the chance of these dangerous blood clots. But, heparin also can increase the normal amount of bleeding and bruising after surgery.

- Significant pain in the leg and recovery time of 1 to 4 weeks depending on the extent of surgery is typical after surgery.

- **Ambulatory phlebectomy:** With this surgery, a special light source marks the location of the vein. Tiny cuts are made in the skin, and surgical hooks pull the vein out of the leg. This surgery requires local or regional anesthesia. The vein usually is removed in one treatment. Very large varicose veins can be removed with this treatment while leaving only very small scars. Patients can return to normal activity the day after treatment. Possible side effects include slight bruising and temporary numbness.

- **Endoscopic vein surgery:** With this surgery, a small video camera is used to see inside the veins. Then varicose veins are removed through small cuts. People who have this surgery must have some kind of anesthesia including epidural, spinal, or general anesthesia. Patients can return to normal activity within a few weeks.

Can varicose and spider veins return even after treatment?

Current treatments for varicose veins and spider veins have very high success rates compared to traditional surgical treatments. Over a period of years, however, more abnormal veins can develop. The major reason for this is that there is no cure for weak vein valves.

So with time, pressure gradually builds up in the leg veins. Ultrasound can be used to keep track of how badly the valves are leaking (venous insufficiency). Ongoing treatment can help keep this problem under control.

The single most important thing a person can do to slow down the development of new varicose veins is to wear graduated compression support stockings as much as possible during the day.

Part Four

Cardiovascular Disorders in Specific Populations

Chapter 34

Cardiovascular Disorders in Women

Chapter Contents

Section 34.1

Cardiovascular Disease: The Number One Killer of Women in the United States

Excerpted from "Research on Cardiovascular Disease in Women," by the Agency for Healthcare Research and Quality (AHRQ, www.ahrq.gov), May 2009.

Cardiovascular disease (CVD) is the number one killer of women in the United States. Long thought of as primarily affecting men, we now know that CVD—including heart disease, hypertension, and stroke—also affects a substantial number of women. Experts estimate that one in two women will die of heart disease or stroke, compared with one in 25 women who will die of breast cancer.

Recent statistics show significant differences between men and women in survival following a heart attack. For example, 42 percent of women who have heart attacks die within 1 year compared with 24 percent of men. The reasons for these differences are not well understood. We know that women tend to get heart disease about 10 years later in life than men, and they are more likely to have coexisting chronic conditions. Research also has shown that women may not be diagnosed or treated as aggressively as men, and their symptoms may be very different from those of men who are having a heart attack.

Process-of-care variables may explain some of the male-female differences in cardiovascular disease outcomes. Researchers analyzed seven cardiovascular disease quality of care indicators in a national sample of managed care plans and found inadequate lipid control in both men and women, with a lower rate of control in women. Also, women with diabetes were 19 percent less likely than men to have their LDL [low-density lipoprotein] cholesterol controlled; women with a history of CVD were 28 percent less likely than men to have their LDL cholesterol controlled. More women than men had their blood pressure controlled, although the difference was small (2 percent).

Commercial health plans show disparities between women and men in cardiovascular care. Researchers evaluated plan-level performance of seven quality of care measures for CVD and found that over half of the plans showed a disparity of 5 percent or more in favor of men for cholesterol control measures among people with diabetes, a recent CVD procedure, or heart attack. The greatest disparity (9.3 percent in favor of men) was among those with recent acute cardiac events; none of the plans showed disparities in favor of women. Disparities between women and men were even greater among Medicare managed care plans.

Among heart disease patients, women are less likely than men to use low-dose aspirin therapy. Use of a low-dose aspirin regimen reduces the risk of heart attack, stroke, and other vascular events and reduces heart disease deaths. Although daily aspirin is recommended for all patients with cardiovascular disease unless contraindicated, women with heart disease are less likely than men with heart disease to use aspirin regularly, according to this study. Researchers examined data on 1,869 men and women aged 40 or older who reported heart disease prior to a heart attack. After adjusting for demographic, socioeconomic, and clinical characteristics, 62 percent of women reported regular aspirin use, compared with 76 percent of men.

Women continue to fare worse than men in treatment for heart attack and congestive heart failure. According to this study of gender disparities among adults age 65 and older, women with acute myocardial infarction (AMI) or congestive heart failure (CHF) do not receive the same care as men. Also, women or men who have other medical conditions associated with AMI or CHF—such as diabetes, hypertension, or end-stage renal disease—do not receive better quality of cardiovascular care than those who have only the heart conditions.

Immunosuppression related to transfusion may explain women's increased risk of dying after CABG surgery. A study of more than 9,000 Michigan Medicare patients found that women undergoing coronary artery bypass graft (CABG) surgery were 3.4 times as likely as men to have received blood transfusions and generally received more units of blood, after accounting for age, coexisting conditions, and other factors. Patients who received a transfusion were more than three times as likely to develop an infection as those who did not, and they were 5.6 times as likely to die within 100 days after surgery. The presence of foreign leukocytes in donor blood may suppress the immune system of the recipient and thus increase the risk of postoperative infection, note the researchers.

Women with atherosclerosis and high cholesterol receive less intense cholesterol management than men. The researchers examined cholesterol management of 243 primary care patients from one academic medical center. The patients had coronary heart disease, cerebrovascular disease, or peripheral vascular disease and high (over 130 mg/dl) low-density (bad) cholesterol. Cholesterol management by either medication adjustments or LDL monitoring occurred at 31.2 percent of women's visits and 38.5 percent of men's visits. Women were 23 percent less likely than men to have their cholesterol managed.

Management of chest pain differs by sex and race. Researchers analyzed the care of 72,508 people with hypertension who were treated at about 50 primary care practices in the Southeastern United States. More men than women received definitive diagnoses of angina, while more women than men were diagnosed with vague chest pain. Also, women and blacks received fewer cardiovascular medications than men and whites.

Section 34.2

Heart Disease Deaths Decline in American Women

Excerpted from "Heart Disease Deaths Continue to Decline in American Women," by the National Institutes of Health (NIH, www.nih.gov), February 1, 2008.

Heart disease deaths in American women continued to decline in 2005, and for the first time, have declined 6 years consecutively, covering the years 2000–2005, according to data announced by the National Heart, Lung, and Blood Institute (NHLBI) of the National Institutes of Health. NHLBI experts analyzed preliminary data for 2005, the most recent year for which data are available. The analysis shows that women are living longer and healthier lives, and dying of heart disease at much later ages than in the past years.

"Considerable progress continues to be made in the fight against heart disease in women," said Elizabeth G. Nabel, M.D., director of NHLBI.

But serious challenges remain—one in four women dies from heart disease. Women of color have higher rates of some risk factors for heart disease and are more likely to die of the disease.

"Unfortunately, many women still do not take heart disease seriously and personally," said Dr. Nabel. "Millions of women still have one or more risk factors for heart disease, dramatically increasing their risk of developing heart disease. In fact, having just one risk factor increases a woman's chance of developing heart disease twofold."

Heart disease is largely preventable. In fact, just by leading a healthy lifestyle—such as following a heart healthy eating plan, getting regular physical activity, maintaining a healthy weight, and not smoking—Americans can lower their risk by as much as 82 percent. Risk factors for heart disease include the following:

- Age (55 or older for women)
- A family history of early heart disease
- High blood pressure

- High blood cholesterol
- Diabetes
- Smoking
- Being overweight or obese
- Being physically inactive

Section 34.3

Birth Control, Menopausal Hormone Therapy, and Heart Disease

Excerpted from "Heart Disease: Frequently Asked Questions,"
by the Office of Women's Health (www.womenshealth.gov), part of the
U.S. Department of Health and Human Services, February 2, 2008.

Do women need to worry about heart disease?

Yes. Among all U.S. women who die each year, one in four dies of heart disease. In 2004, nearly 60 percent more women died of cardiovascular disease (both heart disease and stroke) than from all cancers combined. The older a woman gets, the more likely she is to get heart disease. But women of all ages should be concerned about heart disease. All women should take steps to prevent heart disease.

Both men and women have heart attacks, but more women who have heart attacks die from them. Treatments can limit heart damage but they must be given as soon as possible after a heart attack starts. Ideally, treatment should start within 1 hour of the first symptoms.

If you think you're having a heart attack, call 911 right away. Tell the operator your symptoms and that you think you're having a heart attack.

Do women of color need to worry about heart disease?

Yes. African American and Hispanic American/Latina women should be concerned about getting heart disease because they tend to have more risk factors than white women. These risk factors include obesity, lack of physical activity, high blood pressure, and diabetes. If you're a woman of color, take steps to reduce your risk factors.

How do I know if I have heart disease?

Heart disease often has no symptoms. But, there are some signs to watch for. Chest or arm pain or discomfort can be a symptom of heart disease and a warning sign of a heart attack. Shortness of breath (feeling like you can't get enough air), dizziness, nausea (feeling sick to your stomach), abnormal heartbeats, or feeling very tired also are signs. Talk with your doctor if you're having any of these symptoms. Tell your doctor that you are concerned about your heart.

Your doctor will take a medical history, do a physical exam, and may order tests.

One of my family members had a heart attack. Does that mean I'll have one, too?

If your dad or brother had a heart attack before age 55, or if your mom or sister had one before age 65, you're more likely to develop heart disease. This does not mean you will have a heart attack. It means you should take extra good care of your heart to keep it healthy.

Does taking birth control pills increase my risk for heart disease?

Taking birth control pills is generally safe for young, healthy women if they do not smoke. But birth control pills can pose heart disease risks for some women, especially women older than 35; women with high blood pressure, diabetes, or high cholesterol; and women who smoke. Talk with your doctor if you have questions about the pill.

If you're taking birth control pills, watch for signs of trouble, including the following:

- Eye problems such as blurred or double vision
- Pain in the upper body or arm
- Bad headaches
- Problems breathing
- Spitting up blood
- Swelling or pain in the leg
- Yellowing of the skin or eyes

- Breast lumps
- Unusual (not normal) heavy bleeding from your vagina

If you have any of these symptoms, call 911.

Does using the birth control patch increase my risk for heart disease?

The patch is generally safe for young, healthy women. The patch can pose heart disease risks for some women, especially women older than 35; women with high blood pressure, diabetes, or high cholesterol; and women who smoke.

Recent studies show that women who use the patch may be exposed to more estrogen than women who use the birth control pill. Estrogen is the female hormone in birth control pills and the patch that keeps you from getting pregnant. Research is underway to see if the risk for blood clots is higher in patch users. Blood clots can lead to heart attack or stroke. Talk with your doctor if you have questions about the patch.

If you're using the patch, watch for signs of trouble, such as those listed in the previous answer. If you have any of these symptoms, call 911.

Does menopausal hormone therapy (MHT) increase a woman's risk for heart disease?

Menopausal hormone therapy (MHT) can help with some symptoms of menopause, including hot flashes, vaginal dryness, mood swings, and bone loss, but there are risks, too. For some women, taking hormones can increase their chances of having a heart attack or stroke. If you decide to use hormones, use them at the lowest dose that helps for the shortest time needed. Talk with your doctor if you have questions about MHT.

Chapter 35

Cardiovascular Disorders in Men

Chapter Contents

Section 35.1

Facts about Men and Cardiovascular Disease

Excerpted from "Facts on Men and Heart Disease," by the Centers for Disease Control and Prevention's Division for Heart Disease and Stroke Prevention (www.cdc.gov/dhdsp), updated September 2009.

- Heart disease is the leading cause of death for men in the United States. In 2006, 315,706 men died from it.

- Heart disease killed 26% of the men who died in 2006—more than one in every four.

- Heart disease is the leading cause of death for men of most racial/ethnic groups in the United States, including African Americans, American Indians or Alaska Natives, Hispanics, and whites. For Asian American men, heart disease is second only to cancer.

- In 2006, about 8.8% of all white men, 9.6% of black men, and 5.4% of Mexican American men were living with coronary heart disease.

- Half of the men who die suddenly of coronary heart disease have no previous symptoms. Even if you have no symptoms, you may still be at risk for heart disease.

- Between 70% and 89% of sudden cardiac events occur in men.

Heart disease refers to several different types of heart conditions. In the United States, the most common type is coronary artery disease, also known as coronary heart disease.

Nine out of 10 heart disease patients have at least one risk factor. Several medical conditions and lifestyle choices can put men at a higher risk for heart disease, including the following:

- High cholesterol
- High blood pressure
- Diabetes

- Cigarette smoking
- Overweight and obesity
- Poor diet
- Physical inactivity
- Alcohol use

Section 35.2

Developmental Changes in Adolescence Raise Men's Heart Disease Risk

Study Highlights

- The risks and protection from cardiovascular disease appear to emerge during adolescence.

- Boys had a rapid increase in insulin resistance and cardiovascular risk and girls had a decrease—despite boys' decreasing body fat and girls' increasing body fat, although the reasons are unclear.

- The study followed children transitioning through adolescence to adulthood, while previous studies have not followed this population over time.

Normal developmental changes during the teenage years leave young adult men at higher risk of heart disease than their female counterparts, researchers report in *Circulation: Journal of the American Heart Association.*

"Women's protective advantage against heart disease starts young," said Antoinette Moran, MD, lead author of the study and professor and division chief of pediatric endocrinology and diabetes at the University of Minnesota Children's Hospital in Minneapolis.

In adults, a constellation of factors increases the risk of heart disease. They include high blood pressure, smoking, obesity, physical inactivity, abnormal cholesterol levels, and insulin resistance (a prediabetic condition in which the body can't use insulin effectively).

To track the emergence of these risk factors, researchers followed 507 Minneapolis school children from ages 11 to 19, when they had all reached sexual maturity. Fifty-seven percent of the children were male, 80 percent were white, and 20 percent were black.

During the study, the researchers made 996 observations on the group, noting blood pressure, insulin sensitivity (opposite to insulin resistance), body mass index and other body composition measures, blood glucose, and cholesterol measurements.

"We wanted to see which risks emerge first and how they relate to one another in normal, healthy school kids without diabetes or other major illnesses," Moran said.

At age 11, boys and girls were similar in their body composition, lipid levels, and blood pressure, researchers said.

Boys and girls became heavier during adolescence, increasing in body mass index and waist size. As expected during puberty, changes in body composition differed sharply between genders, with percentage of body fat decreasing in boys and increasing in girls.

During the study, changes in several cardiovascular risk factors or risk markers differed significantly between boys and girls:

- Triglycerides (a type of fat in the blood) increased in males and decreased in females.

- High-density lipoprotein (HDL or "good") cholesterol decreased in males and increased in females.

- Systolic blood pressure (the first number in the blood pressure reading, measuring the pressure when the heart contracts) increased in both, but significantly more in the males.

- Insulin resistance, which had been lower in the boys at age 11, steadily increased until the young men at age 19 were more insulin resistant than the women.

Researchers found no gender difference in two other cardiovascular risk factors, total cholesterol and low-density lipoprotein (LDL or "bad") cholesterol.

"By age 19, the boys were at greater cardiovascular risk," Moran said. "This is particularly surprising because we usually think of body fat as associated with cardiovascular risk, and the increasing risk in boys happened at the time in normal development when they were gaining muscle mass and losing fat."

Although girls gained cardiovascular protection when their proportion of body fat was increasing, excess fat is still a cause for concern.

"Obesity trumps all of the other factors and erases any gender-protective effect," Moran said. "Obese boys and girls and men and women all have higher cardiovascular risk."

The researchers said further studies are needed to better understand the development of cardiovascular protection during adolescence.

"That the protection associated with female gender starts young is fascinating and something that we don't understand very well," Moran said. "That this protection emerges during puberty and disappears after menopause suggests that sex hormones give women a protective advantage. There's still a lot that needs to be sorted out in future studies—estrogen may be protective or testosterone may be harmful."

Moran noted that this is normal physiology and not something that is influenced by lifestyle factors.

Co-authors are: David R. Jacobs Jr., PhD; Julia Steinberger, MD, MS; Lyn M. Steffen, PhD; James S. Pankow, PhD; Ching-Ping Hong, MS; and Alan R. Sinaiko, MD.

The National Institutes of Health partly funded the study.

Section 35.3

Erectile Dysfunction Common among Men with Heart Disease

Reprinted with permission from the University of Michigan
Health System, (www.med.umich.edu). Copyright © 2005 Regents
of the University of Michigan.

Heart disease—a potentially lethal and often debilitating afflic-
tion—can affect much more than just the heart.

The most common cause of heart disease, a hardening of the arteries known as atherosclerosis, often causes erectile dysfunction in
men, says a cardiologist from the University of Michigan (U-M) Health
System. Indeed, he says, erectile dysfunction can be a sign that someone has heart disease and can be a predictor of the leading cause of
death in the United States.

"Erectile dysfunction is much more common in people who have cardiovascular risk factors," says Melvyn Rubenfire, MD, director of preventive cardiology at the U-M Health System and professor in the
Department of Internal Medicine at the U-M Medical School. "The critical message is that erectile dysfunction may be a very early sign of
atherosclerosis or a risk for heart attacks, strokes, and other problems."

Since the risk factors for heart disease also can lead to the artery
problems that cause erectile dysfunction, Rubenfire recommends that
men take action to prevent both conditions with changes in diet and
exercise.

"If you take a look at a population of men between 45 and 60, almost half of them may have erectile dysfunction. And if you look at
those who have erectile dysfunction, lack of exercise, a high-fat diet,
and hypertension are all very common," says Rubenfire. "Prevention
is the key."

Rubenfire encourages everyone, particularly men in this age group,
to practice a healthy lifestyle that includes regular exercise, adequate
rest, good hygiene (including dental hygiene), a reduction of fat in one's
diet, adequate amounts of fruits and vegetables, and receiving a regular health screening by one's physician.

He also notes that smokers have a much higher incidence of erectile dysfunction because smoking impairs the function of the small vessels, and the lining cells of the vessels that are responsible for the erection.

Several studies presented at the recent annual meeting of the American Urological Association found strong links between erectile dysfunction and heart disease, including a paper that noted a relationship between erectile dysfunction and high blood levels of homocysteine, an amino acid marker for heart disease.

This sort of evidence, Rubenfire says, confirms that people with recurring erectile dysfunction should treat it as a potentially serious medical problem. They should talk to their doctors rather than just seeking information from the internet, and they should never take medication from a friend or that they have bought online without a prescription.

"I think it's important that we think of erectile dysfunction as a medical problem and that we seek medical attention, just as we would for any other medical problem that seems to linger on," Rubenfire says.

Facts about Erectile Dysfunction and Heart Disease

- Heart disease is the leading cause of death for men and women in the United States.

- In 2005, heart disease is projected to cost $393 billion, including health care services, medications, and lost productivity, according to the American Heart Association.

- There are many possible causes of erectile dysfunction, including trouble with blood flow to the penis, eating or drinking too much, exhaustion, fear of failure at intercourse, loss of interest in sex, depression, diabetes, low levels of testosterone, problems after surgery for prostate cancer, and side effects of some medications.

- Many experts believe that 10 to 20 percent of erectile dysfunction cases are caused by psychological factors such as depression, anxiety, grief, low self-esteem, and stress, according to the National Kidney and Urologic Diseases Information Clearinghouse.

Chapter 36

Cardiovascular Disorders in Minorities

Chapter Contents

Section 36.1

Facts about Cardiovascular Disease in Minorities

From "Heart Disease Data/Statistics," by the Office of Minority Health (OMHRC, www.omhrc.gov), part of the U.S. Department of Health and Human Services, June 27, 2008.

Heart disease is the leading killer across most racial and ethnic minority communities in the United States, accounting for 27% of all deaths in 2005.

African American men are 30% more likely to die from heart disease than non-Hispanic white males. This occurs despite the fact that 10% of African Americans have heart disease versus 11% of whites. Some 32% of African Americans have hypertension compared to 22.5% of whites, in 2007.

Mexican Americans, who make up the largest share of the U.S. Hispanic population, suffer in greater percentages than whites from overweight and obesity, two of the leading risk factors for heart disease. Premature death was higher for Hispanics (23.5%) than non-Hispanics (16.5%). In 2005, in the Asian and Pacific Islander community, 29.5% of deaths are caused by heart disease. In 2001, the number of premature deaths (<65 years) from heart disease was greatest among American Indians or Alaska Natives (36%) and lowest among whites.

Quick Facts

*   African Americans are 1.5 times as likely as non-Hispanic whites to have high blood pressure.

*   American Indian/Alaska Native adults are 1.3 times as likely as white adults to have high blood pressure.

*   Overall, Asian/Pacific Islander adults are less likely than white adults to have heart disease and they are less likely to die from heart disease.

*   Mexican American women are 1.3 times more likely than non-Hispanic white women to be obese.

Section 36.2

African Americans and Cardiovascular Disease

Excerpted from "Heart Disease and African Americans,"
by the Office of Minority Health (www.omhrc.gov), July 2009.

African American adults are less likely to be diagnosed with coronary heart disease, however they are more likely to die from heart disease.

Although African American adults are 40% more likely to have high blood pressure, they are 10% less likely than their non-Hispanic white counterparts to have their blood pressure under control.

In 2005, African American men were 30% more likely to die from heart disease, as compared to non-Hispanic white men. African Americans were 1.5 times as likely as non-Hispanic whites to have high blood pressure. African American women were 1.7 times as likely as non-Hispanic white women to be obese.

Section 36.3

Heart Failure before Age Fifty More Common in Blacks

From "Heart Failure Before Age 50 Substantially More
Common in Blacks," by the National Institutes of Health (NIH,
www.nih.gov), March 18, 2009.

As many as one in 100 black men and women develop heart failure before the age of 50, 20 times the rate in whites in this age group, according to new findings from the National Heart, Lung, and Blood Institute (NHLBI) of the National Institutes of Health. In the study, heart failure developed in black participants at an average age of 39, often preceded by risk factors such as high blood pressure, obesity, and chronic kidney disease 10 to 20 years earlier.

Findings from the 20-year observational study Coronary Artery Risk Development in Young Adults study (CARDIA) are published in the March 19 [2009] issue of the *New England Journal of Medicine.*

By the tenth year of the study, when participants were between ages 28 and 40, 87 percent of black participants who later developed heart failure had untreated or poorly controlled high blood pressure. Black participants who developed heart failure were also more likely in their young adulthood to be obese and have diabetes and chronic kidney disease. Furthermore, 10 years before developing heart failure, they were more likely already to have some level of systolic dysfunction, or impairment in the ability of the heart muscle to contract, visible on echocardiograms.

"The disproportionate rate at which heart failure impacts relatively young African-Americans in this country underscores the importance of recognizing and treating risk factors for heart disease," said Elizabeth G. Nabel, MD, director, NHLBI.

With heart failure, the heart loses its ability to pump enough blood through the body. The life-threatening condition usually develops over several years. The leading causes of heart failure are coronary artery disease, high blood pressure, and diabetes. About 5 million people in the United States have heart failure, and it results in about 300,000 deaths each year.

CARDIA includes 5,115 black and white men and women (52 percent black, 55 percent women) who were age 18 to 30 at the start of the study in 1985 and 1986, recruited from Birmingham, Alabama, Chicago, Minneapolis, and Oakland, California. Participants were followed for 20 years, with physical exams conducted every few years and telephone interviews every 6 months. Twenty-seven men and women developed heart failure; all but one were black.

Higher blood pressure, greater body mass index, lower HDL (high density lipoprotein, or "good" cholesterol), and chronic kidney disease were all independent predictors at ages 18 to 30 of heart failure developing 15 years later.

"Through this long-term study, we saw the clear links between the development of risk factors and the onset of disease 1 to 2 decades later. Targeting these risk factors for screening and treatment during young adulthood could be important for heart failure prevention," said Kirsten Bibbins-Domingo, PhD, MD, study author, University of California, San Francisco.

The study found that each 10 mmHg increase in diastolic blood pressure among blacks in their 20s doubles the likelihood of developing heart failure 10 to 20 years later.

"This study shows how devastating high blood pressure in young adulthood, especially if uncontrolled, can be for developing heart failure later on. Unfortunately, we know from national data that younger adults with high blood pressure are often unaware that they have the condition, and even when they are aware, their blood pressure is often not controlled," said Gina Wei, MD, medical officer, CARDIA study, NHLBI.

Chapter 37

Cardiovascular Disease Diagnosed in Childhood and Adolescence

Chapter Contents

Section 37.1

Cardiac Disease in Children: Statistics

Thousands of infants born each year have congenital cardiovascular defects. Of those who have these defects:

- 4–10 percent have atrioventricular septal defect;
- 8–11 percent have coarctation of the aorta;
- 9–14 percent have tetralogy of Fallot;
- 10–11 percent have transposition of the great arteries;
- 14–16 percent have ventricular septal defects;
- 4–8 percent have hypoplastic left heart syndrome

Other children will develop acquired heart disease. This includes:

- Arrhythmias: The projected incidence estimate for supraventricular tachycardia alone is 1–4 per 1,000.
- Cardiomyopathies
- Kawasaki disease
- Rheumatic fever
- Familial hypercholesterolemia will affect the future of an unknown but probably large number of children.
- Acquired immune deficiency syndrome (AIDS) with its myocarditis

Section 37.2

Heart Murmurs

Excerpted from "Heart Murmur," by the National Heart,
Lung, and Blood Institute (NHLBI, www.nhlbi.nih.gov), part of
the National Institutes of Health, June 2008.

A heart murmur is an extra or unusual sound heard during a heartbeat. Murmurs range from very faint to very loud. They sometimes sound like a whooshing or swishing noise.

Normal heartbeats make a "lub-DUPP" or "lub-DUB" sound. This is the sound of the heart valves closing as blood moves through the heart. Doctors can hear these sounds and heart murmurs using a stethoscope.

Overview

There are two types of heart murmurs: innocent (harmless) and abnormal.

People who have innocent heart murmurs have normal hearts. They usually have no other signs or symptoms of heart problems. Innocent murmurs are common in healthy children. Many, if not most, children will have heart murmurs heard by their doctors at some time in their lives.

People who have abnormal murmurs may have other signs or symptoms of heart problems. Most abnormal murmurs in children are due to congenital heart defects. These are heart defects that are present at birth.

In adults, abnormal murmurs are most often due to heart valve problems caused by infection, disease, or aging.

Outlook

A heart murmur isn't a disease, and most murmurs are harmless. Innocent murmurs don't cause symptoms or require you to limit physical activity. Although an innocent murmur may be a lifelong condition, your heart is normal and you likely won't need treatment.

The outlook and treatment for abnormal heart murmurs depends on the type and severity of the heart problem causing them.

Other Names for Heart Murmurs

Innocent Heart Murmurs

- Normal heart murmurs
- Benign heart murmurs
- Functional heart murmurs
- Physiologic heart murmurs
- Still murmurs
- Flow murmurs

Abnormal Heart Murmurs

- Pathologic heart murmurs

Causes of Heart Murmur

Innocent Heart Murmurs

Innocent heart murmurs are sounds heard when blood flows through a normal heart. These murmurs may occur when blood flows faster than normal through the heart and its attached blood vessels. Illnesses or conditions that may cause this to happen include fever, anemia, and hyperthyroidism (too much thyroid hormone in the body).

Extra blood flow through the heart also may cause innocent heart murmurs. After childhood, the most common cause of extra blood flow through the heart is pregnancy. Most heart murmurs found in pregnant women are innocent. They're due to the extra blood that women's bodies make while they're pregnant.

Changes to the heart that result from heart surgery or aging also may cause some innocent heart murmurs.

Abnormal Heart Murmurs

The most common cause of abnormal murmurs in children is congenital heart defects. These are problems with the heart's structure that are present at birth.

These defects can involve the interior walls of the heart, the valves inside the heart, or the arteries and veins that carry blood to the heart or out to the body. Some babies are born with more than one heart defect. Congenital heart defects change the normal flow of blood through the heart.

Heart valve defects and septal defects (also called holes in the heart) are common heart defects that cause abnormal heart murmurs.

Valve defects may include narrow valves that limit blood flow or leaky valves that don't close properly.

Septal defects are holes in the wall that separates the right and left sides of the heart. This wall is called the septum.

A hole in the septum between the heart's two upper chambers is called an atrial septal defect (ASD). A hole in the septum between the heart's two lower chambers is called a ventricular septal defect (VSD). ASDs and VSDs account for more than half of all abnormal heart murmurs in children.

Conditions that damage heart valves or other structures of the heart also may cause abnormal heart murmurs. These include rheumatic fever, endocarditis, calcification, and mitral valve prolapse (MVP). Heart murmurs due to these problems are more common in adults.

Rheumatic fever: The bacteria that cause strep throat, scarlet fever, and, in some cases, impetigo also can cause rheumatic fever. This serious illness can develop if a person has an untreated or not fully treated strep infection.

Rheumatic fever can lead to permanent heart damage. If you or your child has strep throat, take all of the antibiotics prescribed, even if you feel better before the medicine runs out.

Endocarditis: Endocarditis is a serious infection of the heart valves or lining of the heart. A bacterial infection usually causes endocarditis, and it usually occurs in an abnormal heart. Endocarditis can lead to permanent heart damage and other health problems.

Calcification: Calcification occurs when the heart's valves get hard and thick as a result of aging. When this happens, the valves don't work as they should.

Mitral valve prolapse: MVP is a condition in which the heart's mitral valve doesn't work properly. In MVP, when the left ventricle contracts, one or both flaps of the mitral valve flop or bulge back (prolapse) into the left atrium. This can cause a heart murmur.

Signs and Symptoms of a Heart Murmur

Most people who have heart murmurs don't have any other signs or symptoms of heart problems. These murmurs usually are innocent (harmless).

Some people who have heart murmurs do have signs or symptoms of heart problems. The signs and symptoms may include the following:

- Blue coloring of the skin, especially on the fingertips and inside the mouth
- Poor eating and abnormal growth (in infants)
- Shortness of breath
- Excessive sweating
- Chest pain
- Dizziness or fainting
- Fatigue (feeling very tired)

Signs and symptoms depend on the problem causing the murmur and how severe that problem is.

Treating Heart Murmur

Innocent Heart Murmurs

Healthy children who have innocent heart murmurs don't need treatment because they have normal hearts. If your child has an innocent murmur, alert his or her doctor during regular checkups.

Pregnant women who have innocent heart murmurs due to extra blood volume also don't need treatment.

You may have an innocent heart murmur due to an illness or condition, such as anemia, hyperthyroidism, or fever. The murmur will go away once the illness or condition is treated.

Abnormal Heart Murmurs

Treatment for abnormal heart murmurs depends on the heart problems causing them. For example, treatment for a congenital heart defect depends on the type and severity of the defect. Treatment may include medicine or surgery.

When an infection or disease causes a heart murmur, treatment depends on the type, amount, and severity of the heart damage. Treatments may include medicine or surgery.

330

Section 37.3

Congenital Heart Defects

Excerpted from "Congenital Heart Defects," by the National
Heart, Lung, and Blood Institute (NHLBI, www.nhlbi.nih.gov), part
of the National Institutes of Health, December 2007.

Congenital heart defects are problems with the heart's structure
that are present at birth. These defects can involve the following:

- The interior walls of the heart
- The valves inside the heart
- The arteries and veins that carry blood to the heart or out to
  the body

Congenital heart defects change the normal flow of blood through
the heart.

There are many types of congenital heart defects. They range from
simple defects with no symptoms to complex defects with severe, life-
threatening symptoms.

Congenital heart defects are the most common type of birth defect.
They affect eight of every 1,000 newborns. Each year, more than
35,000 babies in the United States are born with congenital heart
defects.

Many of these defects are simple conditions that are easily fixed
or need no treatment. A small number of babies are born with complex congenital heart defects that require special medical care soon
after birth.

Over the past few decades, the diagnosis and treatment of these
complex defects has greatly improved. As a result, almost all children
who have complex heart defects survive to adulthood and can live
active, productive lives.

Most people who have complex heart defects continue to need special heart care throughout their lives. They may need to pay special
attention to how their condition may affect certain issues, such as
health insurance, employment, pregnancy and contraception, and
other health issues.

the United States, about 1 million adults are living with congeni-
heart defects.

Types of Congenital Heart Defects

Congenital heart defects change the normal flow of blood through
the heart. This is because some part of the heart didn't develop properly before birth.

There are many types of congenital heart defects. Some are simple,
such as a hole in the septum that allows blood from the left and right
sides of the heart to mix, or a narrowed valve that blocks blood flow
to the lungs or other parts of the body.

Other defects are more complex. These include combinations of
simple defects, problems with where the blood vessels leading to and
from the heart are located, and more serious problems with how the
heart develops.

Examples of Simple Congenital Heart Defects

Holes in the heart (septal defects): The septum is the wall that
separates the chambers on the left side of the heart from those on the
right. The wall prevents mixing of blood between the two sides of the
heart. Sometimes, a baby is born with a hole in the septum. The hole
allows blood to mix between the two sides of the heart.

- **Atrial septal defect (ASD):** An ASD is a hole in the part of
  the septum that separates the atria—the upper chambers of the
  heart. This heart defect allows oxygen-rich blood from the left
  atrium to flow into the right atrium instead of flowing to the left
  ventricle as it should. Many children who have ASDs have few, if
  any, symptoms. An ASD can be small or large. Small ASDs allow
  only a little blood to leak from one atrium to the other. Very small
  ASDs don't affect the way the heart works and don't require any
  treatment. Many small ASDs close on their own as the heart grows
  during childhood. Medium to large ASDs allow more blood to leak
  from one atrium to the other, and they're less likely to close on
  their own. Half of all ASDs close on their own or are so small that
  no treatment is needed. Medium to large ASDs that need treatment can be repaired using a catheter procedure or open-heart
  surgery.

- **Ventricular septal defect (VSD):** A VSD is a hole in the part
  of the septum that separates the ventricles—the lower chambers

of the heart. The hole allows oxygen-rich blood to flow from the left ventricle into the right ventricle instead of flowing into the aorta and out to the body as it should. A VSD can be small or large. A small VSD doesn't cause problems and may close on its own. Large VSDs cause the left side of the heart to work too hard. This increases blood pressure in the right side of the heart and the lungs because of the extra blood flow. The increased work of the heart can cause heart failure and poor growth. If the hole isn't closed, high blood pressure can scar the delicate arteries in the lungs. Open-heart surgery is used to repair VSDs.

Narrowed valves: Simple congenital heart defects also can involve the heart's valves. These valves control the flow of blood from the atria to the ventricles and from the ventricles into the two large arteries connected to the heart (the aorta and the pulmonary artery). Valves can have the following types of defects:

- **Stenosis:** This defect occurs if the flaps of a valve thicken, stiffen, or fuse together. This prevents the valve from fully opening. The heart has to work harder to pump blood through the valve.

- **Atresia:** This defect occurs if a valve doesn't form correctly and lacks a hole for blood to pass through. Atresia of a valve generally results in more complex congenital heart disease.

- **Regurgitation:** This is when the valve doesn't close completely, so blood leaks back through the valve.

The most common valve defect is called pulmonary valve stenosis, which is a narrowing of the pulmonary valve. This valve allows blood to flow from the right ventricle into the pulmonary artery. From there it flows to the lungs to pick up oxygen.

Pulmonary valve stenosis can range from mild to severe. Most children who have this defect have no signs or symptoms other than a heart murmur. (A heart murmur is an extra or unusual sound heard during a heartbeat.) Treatment isn't needed if the stenosis is mild.

In babies who have severe pulmonary valve stenosis, the right ventricle can get very overworked trying to pump blood to the pulmonary artery. These infants may have symptoms such as rapid or heavy breathing, fatigue (tiredness), or poor feeding.

If a baby also has an ASD or patent ductus arteriosus (PDA), oxygen-poor blood can flow from the right side of the heart to the left side. This can cause cyanosis. Cyanosis is a bluish tint to the skin, lips, and fingernails. It occurs because the oxygen level in the blood leaving the heart is below normal.

Older children who have severe pulmonary valve stenosis may have symptoms such as fatigue while exercising. Severe pulmonary valve stenosis is treated with a catheter procedure.

Example of a Complex Congenital Heart Defect

Complex congenital heart defects need to be repaired with surgery. Because of advances in diagnosis and treatment, doctors can now successfully repair even very complex congenital heart defects.

The most common complex heart defect is tetralogy of Fallot, a combination of four defects:

- Pulmonary valve stenosis

- A large VSD

- An overriding aorta (In this defect, the aorta sits above both the left and right ventricles over the VSD, rather than just over the left ventricle. As a result, oxygen-poor blood from the right ventricle can flow directly into the aorta instead of into the pulmonary artery to the lungs.)

- Right ventricular hypertrophy (In this defect, the muscle of the right ventricle is thicker than usual because of having to work harder than normal.)

Together, these four defects mean that not enough blood is able to reach the lungs to get oxygen, and oxygen-poor blood flows out to the body.

Babies and children who have tetralogy of Fallot have episodes of cyanosis, which can sometimes be severe. In the past, when this condition wasn't treated in infancy, older children would get very tired during exercise and could have fainting spells. Tetralogy of Fallot is now repaired in infancy to prevent these types of symptoms.

Tetralogy of Fallot must be repaired with open-heart surgery, either soon after birth or later in infancy. The timing of the surgery will depend on how much the pulmonary artery is narrowed.

Children who have had this heart defect repaired need lifelong medical care from a specialist to make sure they stay as healthy as possible.

Other Names for Congenital Heart Defects

- Congenital heart disease

- Heart defects
- Congenital cardiovascular malformations

Causes of Congenital Heart Defects

If you have a child who has a congenital heart defect, you may think you did something wrong during your pregnancy to cause the problem. However, most of the time doctors don't know why congenital heart defects develop.

Heredity may play a role in some heart defects. For example, a parent who has a congenital heart defect may be more likely than other people to have a child with the condition. In rare cases, more than one child in a family is born with a heart defect.

Children who have genetic disorders, such as Down syndrome, often have congenital heart defects. In fact, half of all babies who have Down syndrome have congenital heart defects.

Smoking during pregnancy also has been linked to several congenital heart defects, including septal defects. Scientists continue to search for the causes of congenital heart defects.

Signs and Symptoms of Congenital Heart Defects

Many congenital heart defects have few or no signs or symptoms. A doctor may not even detect signs of a heart defect during a physical exam.

Some heart defects do have signs and symptoms. They depend on the number, type, and severity of the defects. Severe defects can cause signs and symptoms, usually in newborns. These signs and symptoms may include the following:

- Rapid breathing
- Cyanosis (a bluish tint to the skin, lips, and fingernails)
- Fatigue (tiredness)
- Poor blood circulation

Congenital heart defects don't cause chest pain or other painful symptoms.

Heart defects can cause abnormal blood flow through the heart that will make a certain sound called a heart murmur. Your doctor can hear a heart murmur with a stethoscope. However, not all murmurs are signs of congenital heart defects. Many healthy children have heart murmurs.

Normal growth and development depend on a normal workload for the heart and normal flow of oxygen-rich blood to all parts of the body. Babies who have congenital heart defects may have cyanosis and/or tire easily when feeding. As a result, they may not gain weight or grow as they should.

Older children who have congenital heart defects may get tired easily or short of breath during physical activity.

Many types of congenital heart defects cause the heart to work harder than it should. In severe defects, this can lead to heart failure. Heart failure is a condition in which the heart can't pump enough blood to meet the body's needs. Symptoms of heart failure include the following:

• Fatigue with physical activity

• Shortness of breath

• A buildup of blood and fluid in the lungs

• A buildup of fluid in the feet, ankles, and legs

Treating Congenital Heart Defects

Although many children who have congenital heart defects don't need treatment, some do. Doctors repair congenital heart defects with catheter procedures or surgery.

The treatment your child receives depends on the type and severity of his or her heart defect. Other factors include your child's age, size, and general health.

Some children who have complex congenital heart defects may need several catheter or surgical procedures over a period of years, or they may need to take medicines for years.

Living with a Congenital Heart Defect

The outlook for a child who has a congenital heart defect is much better today than in the past. Advances in testing and treatment mean that most children who have heart defects survive to adulthood and are able to live active, productive lives.

Many of these children need only occasional checkups with a cardiologist (heart specialist) as they grow up and go through adult life.

Children who have complex heart defects need long-term, special care by trained specialists. This will help them stay as healthy as possible and maintain a good quality of life.

Part Five

Identifying Cardiovascular Disorders

Chapter 38

Blood Tests for Cardiovascular Disorders

Chapter Contents

Section 38.1

Overview of Blood Tests

From "Common Blood Tests," by the National Heart, Lung, and Blood Institute (NHLBI, www.nhlbi.nih.gov), part of the National Institutes of Health, December 2007.

Blood tests help doctors check for certain diseases and conditions. They also help check the function of your organs and show how well treatments are working.

Specifically, blood tests can help doctors do the following:

- Evaluate how well organs, like the kidneys, liver, and heart, are working

- Diagnose diseases like cancer, HIV/AIDS [human immunodeficiency virus/acquired immunodeficiency syndrome], diabetes, anemia, and heart disease

- Learn whether you have risk factors for heart disease

- Check whether medicines you're taking are working

Overview

Blood tests are very common. When you have routine checkups, your doctor often orders blood tests to see how your body is working.

Many blood tests don't require any special preparations. For some, you may need to fast (not eat any food) for 8 to 12 hours before the test. Your doctor will let you know whether this is necessary.

During a blood test, a small amount of blood is taken from your body. It's usually drawn from a vein in your arm using a thin needle. A finger prick also may be used. The procedure is usually quick and easy, although it may cause some short-term discomfort. Most people don't have serious reactions to having blood drawn.

Lab workers draw the blood and analyze it. They use either whole blood to count blood cells, or they separate the blood cells from the fluid that contains them. This fluid is called plasma or serum.

The fluid is used to measure different substances in the blood. The results can help detect health problems in early stages, when treatments or lifestyle changes may work best.

However, blood tests alone can't be used to diagnose or treat many diseases or medical problems. Your doctor may consider other factors, such as your signs and symptoms, your medical history, and results from other tests and procedures, to confirm a diagnosis.

Outlook

Blood tests have few risks. Most complications are minor and go away shortly after the tests are done.

Types of Blood Tests

Some of the most common blood tests that doctors order include the following:

- Complete blood count (CBC)
- Blood chemistry tests
- Blood enzyme tests
- Blood tests to assess heart disease risk

Complete Blood Count

The CBC is one of the most common types of blood test. It's often done as part of a routine checkup.

A CBC measures many different parts of your blood. This test can help detect blood diseases and disorders. These include anemia, infection, clotting problems, blood cancers, and immune system disorders.

Red blood cells: Red blood cells carry oxygen from your lungs to the rest of your body. Abnormal red blood cell levels may be a sign of anemia, dehydration (too little fluid in the body), bleeding, or another disorder.

White blood cells: White blood cells are part of your immune system, which fights infections and disease. Abnormal white blood cell levels may be a sign of infection, blood cancer, or an immune system disorder.

A CBC measures the overall number of white blood cells in your blood. A differential count looks at the amounts of different types of white blood cells in your blood.

341

Platelets: Platelets are blood cells that help your blood clot. They stick together to seal cuts or breaks and stop bleeding. Abnormal platelet levels may be a sign of a bleeding disorder (not enough clotting) or a thrombotic disorder (too much clotting).

Hemoglobin: Hemoglobin is an iron-rich protein in red blood cells that carries oxygen. Abnormal hemoglobin levels may be a sign of anemia, sickle cell anemia, thalassemia, or other blood disorders.

If you have diabetes, excess glucose in your blood can attach to hemoglobin and raise the level of hemoglobin A1C.

Hematocrit: Hematocrit is a measure of how much space red blood cells take up in your blood. A high hematocrit level might mean you're dehydrated. A low hematocrit level might mean you have anemia. Abnormal hematocrit levels also may be a sign of a blood or bone marrow disorder.

Mean corpuscular volume: Mean corpuscular volume (MCV) is a measure of the average size of your red blood cells. Abnormal MCV levels may be a sign of anemia or thalassemia.

Blood Chemistry Tests/Basic Metabolic Panel

The basic metabolic panel (BMP) is a group of tests that measure different chemicals in the blood. These tests usually are done on the fluid (plasma) part of blood. The tests can give doctors information about your muscles, including the heart; bones; and organs, such as the kidneys and liver.

The BMP includes blood glucose, calcium, electrolyte, and kidney tests. Some of these tests require you to fast (not eat any food) before the test, and others don't.

Blood glucose: Glucose is a type of sugar that the body uses for energy. Abnormal glucose levels in your blood may be a sign of diabetes.

For some blood glucose tests, you have to fast before your blood is drawn. Other blood glucose tests are done after a meal or at any time with no preparation.

Calcium: Calcium is one of the most important minerals in the body. Abnormal calcium levels in the blood may be a sign of kidney problems, bone disease, thyroid disease, cancer, malnutrition, or another disorder.

Electrolytes: Electrolytes are minerals that help maintain fluid levels and acid-base balance in the body. They include sodium, potassium, bicarbonate, and chloride.

Abnormal electrolyte levels may be a sign of dehydration, kidney disease, liver disease, heart failure, high blood pressure, or other disorders.

Kidneys: Kidney tests measure levels of blood urea nitrogen (BUN) and creatinine. Both of these are waste products that the kidneys filter out of the body. Abnormal BUN and creatinine levels may be signs of a kidney disease or disorder.

Blood Enzyme Tests

Enzymes are chemicals that help control different reactions in your body. There are many blood enzyme tests. This portion of text focuses on blood enzyme tests used to check for heart attack. These include creatine kinase (CK) and troponin tests.

Creatine kinase: When muscle or heart cells are injured, CK (a blood product) leaks out, and its levels in your blood rise. There are different types of CK. CK-MB is released when the heart muscle is damaged.

High CK levels can mean that you've had muscle damage in your body. High levels of CK-MB can mean that you've had a heart attack.

Doctors order CK tests (such as CK-MB) when patients have chest pain or other heart attack signs and symptoms.

Troponin: This is a muscle protein that helps your muscles contract. Blood levels of troponin rise when you have a heart attack.

For this reason, doctors often order troponin tests along with CK-MB tests when patients have chest pain or other heart attack signs and symptoms.

Blood Tests to Assess Heart Disease Risk

Abnormal levels of certain chemicals in the blood may mean that you're at higher risk for heart disease. Your doctor may want to test the levels of these chemicals to assess your risk and to suggest ways to reduce it.

Lipoprotein panel: This test can help show how high your risk is for coronary heart disease. A lipoprotein panel looks at substances in your blood that carry cholesterol.

The test gives information about the following:

- Total cholesterol

- LDL (low-density lipoprotein, or bad) cholesterol, the main source of cholesterol buildup and blockages in the arteries

- HDL (high-density lipoprotein, or good) cholesterol, the type of cholesterol that helps decrease blockages in the arteries

- Triglycerides, a form of fat in your blood

A lipoprotein panel measures the levels of HDL and LDL cholesterol and triglycerides in your blood. Abnormal cholesterol and triglyceride levels may be signs of increased risk for coronary heart disease.

Most people will need to fast for 9 to 12 hours before a lipoprotein panel.

High-sensitivity C-reactive protein (hs-CRP): This is a fairly new test for heart disease risk. It looks at blood levels of C-reactive protein (CRP). High CRP blood levels can be a sign of inflammation.

Doctors use standard CRP tests to check for inflammation and autoimmune diseases. Your doctor may order an hs-CRP test, along with other tests, to see whether you're at increased risk for heart disease.

However, CRP tests aren't routinely done, because it's still unclear how useful they are for showing heart disease risk.

Homocysteine: High levels of this chemical in the blood can mean that you're at higher risk for heart attack or stroke. This isn't a routine test for heart disease risk. But some doctors may use it, a long with other tests, if they think you're at increased risk.

What to Expect with Blood Tests

What to Expect before Blood Tests

Many blood tests don't require any special preparation and take only a few minutes.

Other blood tests require fasting (not eating any food) anywhere from 8 to 12 hours before the test. Your doctor will let you know whether you need to fast for your blood test(s).

What to Expect during Blood Tests

Blood usually is drawn from a vein in your arm or other part of your body using a thin needle. It also can be drawn using a finger prick.

The person who draws your blood might tie a band around the upper part of your arm or ask you to make a fist. These things can make the veins in your arm stick out more. This makes it easier to insert the needle.

The needle that goes into your vein is attached to a small test tube. The person who draws your blood removes the tube when it's full, and the tube seals on its own. The needle is then removed from your vein. If you're getting a few different blood tests, more than one test tube may be attached to the needle before it's withdrawn.

Some people get nervous about blood tests because they're afraid of the needle. Others may not want to see blood leaving their bodies.

If you're nervous or scared, it can help to look away or talk to someone to distract yourself. You might feel a slight sting when the needle goes in or comes out.

Drawing blood usually takes less than 3 minutes.

What to Expect after Blood Tests

Once the needle is withdrawn, you'll be asked to apply gentle pressure with a piece of gauze or bandage to the place where the needle went in. This helps stop bleeding. It also helps prevent swelling and bruising.

After a minute or two, you can remove the pressure. You may want to keep a bandage on for a few hours.

Usually, you don't need to do anything else after a blood test, except wait for the results. They can take anywhere from a few minutes to a few weeks to come back. Your doctor should get the results. It's important that you follow up with your doctor to discuss your test results.

Risks of Blood Tests

The main risks with blood tests are discomfort or bruising at the site where the needle goes in. These complications usually are minor and go away shortly after the tests are done.

What Blood Tests Show

Blood tests show whether the levels of different substances in your blood fall within a normal range.

For many blood substances, the normal range is the range of levels seen in 95 percent of healthy people in a particular group. For many tests, normal ranges are different depending on your age, gender, race, and other factors.

Many factors can cause your blood test levels to fall outside the normal range. Abnormal levels may be a sign of a disorder or disease. Other factors—such as diet, menstrual cycle, how much physical activity you do, how much alcohol you drink, and the medicines you take (both prescription and over-the-counter)—also can cause abnormal levels.

Your doctor should discuss any unusual or abnormal blood tests results with you. These results may or may not suggest a health problem.

Many diseases or medical problems can't be diagnosed with blood tests alone. However, they can help you and your doctor learn more about your health. Blood tests also can help find potential problems early, when treatments or lifestyle changes may work best.

Result Ranges for Common Blood Tests

This text presents the result ranges for some of the most common blood tests. All values in this section are for adults only. They don't apply to children. Talk to your child's doctor about values on blood tests for children.

Complete blood count: Table 38.1 shows some normal ranges for different components of the complete blood count (CBC). Some of the normal ranges are different for men and women. Other factors, such as age and race, also may affect normal ranges.

Your doctor should discuss your results with you. He or she will advise you further if your results are outside the normal range for your group.

Table 38.1. Complete Blood Count Results

Test	Normal Range Results*
Red blood cell (varies with altitude)	Male: 5 to 6 million cells/mcL; Female: 4 to 5 million cells/mcL
White blood cell	4,500 to 10,000 cells/mcL
Platelets	140,000 to 450,000 cells/mcL
Hemoglobin (varies with altitude)	Male: 14 to 17 gm/dL; Female: 12 to 15 gm/dL
Hematocrit (varies with altitude)	Male: 41 to 50%; Female: 36 to 44%
Mean corpuscular volume	80 to 95 femtoliter

*Cells/mcL = cells per microliter; gm/dL = grams per deciliter

Blood glucose: Table 38.2 shows the ranges for blood glucose levels after 8 to 12 hours of fasting (not eating). It shows the normal range and also the abnormal ranges that are a sign of prediabetes or diabetes.

Table 38.2. Blood Glucose Level Results

Plasma Glucose Results (mg/dL)	Diagnosis
99 and below	Normal
100 to 125	Prediabetes
126 and above	Diabetes**

*mg/dL = milligrams per deciliter.

**The test is repeated on another day to confirm the results.

Lipoprotein panel: Table 38.3 shows ranges for total cholesterol, LDL cholesterol, and HDL cholesterol levels after 9 to 12 hours of fasting. High blood cholesterol is a risk factor for coronary heart disease.

Your doctor should discuss your results with you. He or she will advise you further if your results are outside the desirable range.

Table 38.3. Lipoprotein Panel Results

Total Cholesterol Level	Total Cholesterol Category
Less than 200 mg/dL	Desirable
200–239 mg/dL	Borderline high
240 mg/dL and above	High
LDL Cholesterol Level	**LDL Cholesterol Category**
Less than 100 mg/dL	Optimal
100–129 mg/dL	Near optimal/above optimal
130–159 mg/dL	Borderline high
160–189 mg/dL	High
190 mg/dL and above	Very high
HDL Cholesterol Level	**HDL Cholesterol Category**
Less than 40 mg/dL	A major risk factor for heart disease
40–59 mg/dL	The higher, the better
60 mg/dL and above	Considered protective against heart disease

Section 38.2

Biomarkers to Predict
Cardiovascular Event Risk

From "Newer Biomarkers Predict Cardiovascular Risk but Offer Only Modest Improvement in Risk Prediction over Established Risk Factors," by the National Heart, Lung, and Blood Institute (NHLBI, www.nhlbi.nih .gov), part of the National Institutes of Health, December 20, 2006.

Results of a long-term Framingham Heart Study investigation of multiple biomarkers for the prediction of first major cardiovascular events and death are reported in the December 21 [2006] issue of the *New England Journal of Medicine* (NEJM).

In the study, scientists followed 3,209 participants in the Framingham Heart Study for 10 years and measured 10 of the most promising 'novel' biomarkers for predicting the risk of cardiovascular disease (CVD). The newer biomarkers such as natriuretic peptides, C-reactive protein, fibrinogen, urinary albumin, and homocysteine were compared with established risk factors such as high blood pressure, diabetes, and high cholesterol. Measuring several biomarkers simultaneously, referred to as the "multimarker" approach, enabled the scientists to stratify risk. They found that persons with high multimarker scores had a risk of death four times as great and a risk of major cardiovascular events almost two times as great as persons with low multimarker scores. However, the use of multiple biomarkers added only moderately to the overall prediction of risk based on conventional risk factors.

Section 38.3

C-Reactive Protein and Cardiovascular Disease Risk

Excerpted from "C-Reactive Protein: Basic and Clinical Research Needs Workshop," by the National Heart, Lung, and Blood Institute (NHLBI, www.nhlbi.nih.gov), July 2006. Complete references available online.

The relation between levels of C-reactive protein (CRP) and vascular disease risk has been investigated in several completed and ongoing projects from the Framingham Heart Study.

One research study assessed risk for stroke in the original cohort and found that elevated CRP levels were predictive of increased risk for ischemic cerebrovascular disease and the risk was increased for persons in the top quartile of CRP after multivariable adjustment.

Another study investigated the interaction between CRP and the metabolic syndrome and found that CRP levels were significantly related to the number of components of the metabolic syndrome that were present in both sexes. In a statistical model that predicted incident CVD events the top quartile of CRP and presence of the metabolic syndrome were both statistically associated with an increased risk for events.

In 2005, a research team estimated risk of vascular events according to level of CRP and found that CRP levels greater than 3.0 mg/L were associated with a significantly increased risk of major CHD [coronary heart disease] and major CVD [cardiovascular disease] events in age- and sex-adjusted models, but the CRP greater than 3.0 mg/L effects were no longer statistically significant for major CHD or major CVD in multivariable models.

Researchers also assessed the role of hs-CRP [high-sensitivity CRP] and homocysteine (Hcys) levels on cardiovascular disease (CVD) risk in 3090 Framingham Offspring participants followed for 12 years. Hard CHD (MI and CHD death), CHD (hard CHD and angina pectoris), and hard CVD (hard CHD and stroke) were increased for all outcomes in the category CRP greater than 3.0 mg/L. In a multivariable analysis of risk that also included age, sex, systolic blood pressure, total/HDL [high-density lipoprotein] cholesterol ratio, diabetes mellitus, current smoking, hypertension treatment, and homocysteine, a CRP level greater than 3.0 mg/L was associated with a 1.51 relative risk for developing CVD.

In another study, researchers examined the relation between CRP, other markers of inflammation, and risk of intermittent claudication for the Framingham Offspring with 8 years of follow up. The top tertile of CRP was associated with an increased risk of claudication in analyses that were adjusted by age and sex and also increased in models that were adjusted for sex and Framingham Risk Score.

In conclusion, these CRP results from Framingham Heart Study men and women show consistent but modestly greater relative risk for CVD and CHD events with increasing levels of CRP, but there is little evidence of improved discrimination, and there are stronger risks associated with incidence of cerebrovascular disease and intermittent claudication.

Section 38.4

Homocysteine Levels and Cardiovascular Disease

"Homocysteine, Folic Acid and Cardiovascular Disease,"
reprinted with permission. © 2009 American Heart Association, Inc.
(www.americanheart.org).

AHA Recommendation

The American Heart Association has not yet called hyperhomocysteinemia (high homocysteine level in the blood) a major risk factor for cardiovascular disease. We don't recommend widespread use of folic acid and B vitamin supplements to reduce the risk of heart disease and stroke. We advise a healthy, balanced diet that's rich in fruits and vegetables, whole grains, and fat-free or low-fat dairy products. For folic acid, the recommended daily value is 400 micrograms (mcg). Citrus fruits, tomatoes, vegetables, and grain products are good sources. Since January 1998, wheat flour has been fortified with folic acid to add an estimated 100 micrograms per day to the average diet. Supplements should only be used when the diet doesn't provide enough.

What is homocysteine, and how is it related to cardiovascular risk?

Homocysteine is an amino acid in the blood. Too much of it is related to a higher risk of coronary heart disease, stroke, and peripheral vascular disease (fatty deposits in peripheral arteries).

Evidence suggests that homocysteine may promote atherosclerosis (fatty deposits in blood vessels) by damaging the inner lining of arteries and promoting blood clots. However, a causal link hasn't been established.

How do folic acid and other B vitamins affect homocysteine levels?

Folic acid and other B vitamins help break down homocysteine in the body. Homocysteine levels in the blood are strongly influenced by diet and genetic factors. Dietary folic acid and vitamins B6 and B12 have the greatest effects. Several studies found that higher blood levels of B vitamins are related, at least in part, to lower concentrations of homocysteine. Other evidence shows that low blood levels of folic acid are linked with a higher risk of fatal coronary heart disease and stroke.

So far, no controlled treatment study has shown that folic acid supplements reduce the risk of atherosclerosis or that taking these vitamins affects the development or recurrence of cardiovascular disease. Researchers are trying to find out how much folic acid, B6, and/or B12 are needed to lower homocysteine levels. Screening for homocysteine levels in the blood may be useful in patients with a personal or family history of cardiovascular disease but who don't have the well-established risk factors (smoking, high blood cholesterol, high blood pressure, physical inactivity, obesity, and diabetes).

Although evidence for the benefit of lowering homocysteine levels is lacking, patients at high risk should be strongly advised to be sure to get enough folic acid and vitamins B6 and B12 in their diet. They should eat fruits and green, leafy vegetables daily.

This is just one possible risk factor. A physician taking any type of nutritional approach to reducing risk should consider a person's overall risk factor profile and total diet.

Chapter 39

Echocardiography

Echocardiography, or echo, is a painless test that uses sound waves to create pictures of your heart.

The test gives your doctor information about the size and shape of your heart and how well your heart's chambers and valves are working. Echo also can be done to detect heart problems in infants and children.

The test also can identify areas of heart muscle that aren't contracting normally due to poor blood flow or injury from a previous heart attack. In addition, a type of echo called Doppler ultrasound shows how well blood flows through the chambers and valves of your heart.

Echo can detect possible blood clots inside the heart, fluid buildup in the pericardium (the sac around the heart), and problems with the aorta. The aorta is the main artery that carries oxygen-rich blood from your heart to your body.

Who Needs Echocardiography?

Your doctor may recommend echocardiography (echo) if you have signs and symptoms of heart problems. For example, shortness of breath and swelling in the legs can be due to weakness of the heart (heart failure), which can be seen on an echocardiogram.

Excerpted from text by the National Heart, Lung, and Blood Institute (NHLBI, www.nhlbi.nih.gov), part of the National Institutes of Health, August 2009.

For more information about who needs echocardiography, see the What Echocardiography Shows portion of this text.

Types of Echocardiography

There are several types of echocardiography (echo)—all use sound waves to create pictures of your heart. This is the same technology that allows doctors to see an unborn baby inside a pregnant woman.

Unlike x-rays and some other tests, echo doesn't involve radiation.

Transthoracic Echocardiography

Transthoracic echo is the most common type of echocardiogram test. It's painless and noninvasive. Noninvasive means that no surgery is done and no instruments are inserted into your body.

This type of echo involves placing a device called a transducer on your chest. The device sends special sound waves, called ultrasound, through your chest wall to your heart. The human ear can't hear ultrasound waves.

As the ultrasound waves bounce off the structures of your heart, a computer in the echo machine converts them into pictures on a screen.

Stress Echocardiography

Stress echo is done as part of a stress test. During a stress test, you exercise or take medicine (given by your doctor) to make your heart work hard and beat fast. A technician will take pictures of your heart using echo before you exercise and as soon as you finish.

Some heart problems, such as coronary heart disease, are easier to diagnose when the heart is working hard and beating fast.

Transesophageal Echocardiography

With standard transthoracic echo, it can be hard to see the aorta and other parts of your heart. If your doctor needs a better look at these areas, he or she may recommend transesophageal echo (TEE).

During this test, the transducer is attached to the end of a flexible tube. The tube is guided down your throat and into your esophagus (the passage leading from your mouth to your stomach). This allows your doctor to get more detailed pictures of your heart.

Fetal Echocardiography

Fetal echo is used to look at an unborn baby's heart. A doctor may recommend this test to check a baby for heart problems. Fetal echo is commonly done during pregnancy at about 18 to 22 weeks. For this test, the transducer is moved over the pregnant woman's belly.

Three-Dimensional Echocardiography

A three-dimensional (3D) echo creates 3D images of your heart. These images provide more information about how your heart looks and works.

During transthoracic echo or TEE, 3D images can be taken as part of the process used to do these types of echo.

3D echo may be used to diagnose heart problems in children. This method also may be used for planning and monitoring heart valve surgery.

Researchers continue to study new ways to use 3D echo.

Other Names for Echocardiography

- Echo
- Surface echo
- Ultrasound of the heart

What to Expect before Echocardiography

Echocardiography (echo) is done in a doctor's office or a hospital. No special preparations are needed for most types of echo. Usually you can eat, drink, and take any medicines as you normally would.

The exception is if you're having a transesophageal echo. This test usually requires that you don't eat or drink for 8 hours prior to the test.

If you're having a stress echo, there may be special preparations. Your doctor will let you know how to prepare for your echo test.

What to Expect during Echocardiography

Echocardiography (echo) is painless and usually takes less than an hour to do. For some types of echo, your doctor will need to inject saline or a special dye into one of your veins to make your heart show up more clearly on the test images. This special dye is different from the dye used during angiography (a test used to examine the body's blood vessels).

For most types of echo, you'll be asked to remove your clothing from the waist up. Women will be given a gown to wear during the test. You'll lay on your back or left side on an exam table or stretcher.

Soft, sticky patches called electrodes will be attached to your chest to allow an EKG (electrocardiogram) to be done. An EKG is a test that records the heart's electrical activity.

A doctor or sonographer (a person specially trained to do ultra-sounds) will apply gel to your chest. The gel helps the sound waves reach your heart. A wand-like device called a transducer will then be moved around on your chest.

The transducer transmits ultrasound waves into your chest. Echoes from the sound waves will be converted into pictures of your heart on a computer screen. During the test, the lights in the room will be dimmed so the computer screen is easier to see.

The sonographer will make several recordings of the pictures to show various locations in your heart. The recordings will be put on a computer disk or videotape for the cardiologist (heart specialist) to review.

During the test, you may be asked to change positions or hold your breath for a short time so that the sonographer can get good pictures of your heart.

At times, the sonographer may apply a bit of pressure to your chest with the transducer. This pressure can be a little uncomfortable, but it helps get the best picture of your heart. You should let the sonographer know if you feel too uncomfortable.

This process is similar for fetal echo. However, in that test the transducer is placed over the pregnant woman's belly at the location of the baby's heart.

Transesophageal Echocardiography

Transesophageal echo (TEE) is used when your doctor needs a more detailed view of your heart. For example, TEE may be used to look for blood clots in your heart. A doctor, not a sonographer, performs this type of echo.

The test uses the same technology as transthoracic echo, but the transducer is attached to the end of a flexible tube. The tube will be guided down your throat and into your esophagus (the passage leading from your mouth to your stomach). From this angle, your doctor can get a more detailed image of the heart and major blood vessels leading to and from the heart.

For TEE, you'll likely be given medicine to help you relax during the test. The medicine will be injected into one of your veins. Your blood pressure, the oxygen content of your blood, and other vital signs will be checked during the test. You'll be given oxygen through a tube in your nose. If you wear dentures or partials, you'll have to remove them.

The back of your mouth will be numbed with a gel or a spray so that you don't gag when the transducer is put down your throat. The tube with the transducer on the end will be gently placed in your throat and guided down until it's in place behind the heart.

The pictures of your heart are then recorded as your doctor moves the transducer around in your esophagus and stomach. You shouldn't feel any discomfort as this happens.

Although the imaging usually takes less than an hour, you may be watched for a few hours at the doctor's office or hospital after the test.

Stress Echocardiography

Stress echo is a transthoracic echo combined with either an exercise or pharmacological stress test.

For an exercise stress test, you'll walk or run on a treadmill or pedal a stationary bike to make your heart work hard and beat fast. For a pharmacological stress test, you'll be given medicine to make your heart work hard and beat fast.

A technician will take pictures of your heart using echo before you exercise and as soon as you finish.

What You May See and Hear during Echocardiography

As the doctor or sonographer moves the transducer around, different views of your heart can be seen on the screen of the echo machine. The structures of the heart will appear as white objects, while any fluid or blood will appear black on the screen.

Doppler ultrasound techniques often are used during echo tests. Doppler ultrasound is a special ultrasound that shows how blood is flowing through the blood vessels.

This test allows the sonographer to see blood flowing at different speeds and in different directions. The speeds and directions appear as different colors moving within the black and white images.

The human ear is unable to hear the sound waves used in echo. If Doppler ultrasound is used, you may be able to hear "whooshing" sounds. Your doctor can use these sounds to learn about blood flow through your heart.

What to Expect after Echocardiography

You usually can go back to your normal activities right after having echocardiography (echo).

If you have a transesophageal echo (TEE), you may be watched for a few hours at the doctor's office or hospital after the test. Your throat might be sore for a few hours after the test.

You also may not be able to drive right after a TEE. Your doctor will let you know whether you need to arrange for someone to take you home.

What Echocardiography Shows

Echocardiography (echo) shows the size, structure, and movement of the various parts of your heart. This includes the valves, the septum (the wall separating the right and left heart chambers), and the walls of the heart chambers. Doppler ultrasound shows the movement of blood through the heart.

Echo can be used to do the following:

- Diagnose heart problems

- Guide or determine next steps for treatment

- Monitor changes and improvement

- Determine the need for more tests

Echo can detect many heart problems. Some may be minor and pose no risk to you. Others can be signs of serious heart disease or other heart conditions. Your doctor may use echo to learn about:

- **The size of your heart:** An enlarged heart can be the result of high blood pressure, leaky heart valves, or heart failure.

- **Heart muscles that are weak and aren't moving (pumping) properly:** Weakened areas of heart muscle can be due to damage from a heart attack. Weakening also could mean that the area isn't getting enough blood supply, which may be due to coronary heart disease.

- **Problems with your heart's valves:** Echo can show whether any of the valves of your heart don't open normally or don't form a complete seal when closed.

- **Problems with your heart's structure:** Echo can detect many structural problems, such as a hole in the septum and other congenital heart defects. Congenital heart defects are structural problems present at birth.

- **Blood clots or tumors:** If you've had a stroke, echo might be done to check for blood clots or tumors that may have caused it.

Risks of Echocardiography

Transthoracic and fetal echocardiography (echo) have no risks. These tests are safe in adults, children, and infants.

If you have a transesophageal echo (TEE), some risks are associated with the medicine given to help you relax. These include a bad reaction to the medicine, problems breathing, or nausea (feeling sick to your stomach).

Your throat also might be sore for a few hours after the test. Rarely, the tube used during TEE can cause minor throat injuries.

Stress echo has some risks, but they're related to the exercise or medicine used to raise your heart rate, not to the echo. Serious complications from stress tests are very uncommon.

Chapter 40

Electrocardiogram

An electrocardiogram, or EKG, is a simple, painless test that records the heart's electrical activity. To understand this test, it helps to understand how the heart works.

With each heartbeat, an electrical signal spreads from the top of the heart to the bottom. As it travels, the signal causes the heart to contract and pump blood. The process repeats with each new heartbeat. The heart's electrical signals set the rhythm of the heartbeat.

An EKG shows the following:

- How fast your heart is beating

- Whether the rhythm of your heartbeat is steady or irregular

- The strength and timing of electrical signals as they pass through each part of your heart

This test is used to detect and evaluate many heart problems, such as heart attack, arrhythmia, and heart failure. EKG results also can suggest other disorders that affect heart function.

EKGs also are used to monitor how the heart is working. This text focuses on how EKGs are used for testing purposes.

Excerpted from text by the National Heart, Lung, and Blood Institute (NHLBI, www.nhlbi.nih.gov), part of the National Institutes of Health, November 2008.

Other Names for Electrocardiogram

An electrocardiogram also is called EKG or ECG. Sometimes the test is called a 12-lead EKG or 12-lead ECG because the electrical activity of the heart is most often recorded from 12 different places on the body at the same time.

Who Needs an Electrocardiogram?

Your doctor may recommend an electrocardiogram (EKG) if you have signs or symptoms that suggest a heart problem. Examples of such signs and symptoms include the following:

- Chest pain
- Heart pounding, racing, or fluttering, or the sense that your heart is beating unevenly
- Problems breathing
- Feeling tired and weak
- Unusual heart sounds when your doctor listens to your heartbeat

You may need to have more than one EKG so your doctor can diagnose certain heart conditions.

An EKG may be done as part of a routine health exam. The test can screen for early heart disease that has no symptoms. Your doctor is more likely to look for early heart disease if your mother, father, brother, or sister had heart disease—especially if it developed early.

You may have an EKG so your doctor can check how well heart medicine or a medical device, such as a pacemaker, is working. The test also may be used for routine screening before major surgery.

Your doctor may use EKG results to help plan your treatment for a heart condition.

What to Expect before an Electrocardiogram

No special preparation is needed for an electrocardiogram (EKG). Before the test, let your doctor or doctor's office know what medicines you're taking. Some medicines can affect EKG results.

What Happens during an Electrocardiogram?

An electrocardiogram (EKG) is painless and harmless. A technician attaches soft, sticky patches called electrodes to the skin of

362

your chest, arms, and legs. The patches are about the size of a quarter.

Typically, 12 patches are attached to detect your heart's electrical activity from many angles. To help the patches stick, the technician may have to shave areas of your skin.

After the patches are placed on your skin, you lie still on a table while the patches detect your heart's electrical signals. A machine records these signals on graph paper or displays them on a screen.

The entire test takes about 10 minutes.

Special Types of Electrocardiogram

The standard EKG described above, called a resting 12-lead EKG, records only seconds of heart activity at a time. It will show a heart problem only if the problem is present during the time that the test is run.

Many heart problems are present all the time, and a resting 12-lead EKG will detect them. But some heart problems, like those related to an irregular heartbeat, can come and go. They may occur for only a few minutes out of the day or only while you exercise.

Special EKGs, such as stress tests and Holter and event monitors, are used to help diagnose these kinds of problems.

Stress test: Some heart problems are easier to diagnose when your heart is working hard and beating fast. During stress testing, you exercise to make your heart work hard and beat fast while your heart's electrical activity is recorded. If you're not able to exercise, you're given medicine to make your heart work hard and beat fast.

Holter and event monitors: Holter and event monitors are small, portable devices. They record your heart's activity while you do your normal daily activities. A Holter monitor records the heart's electrical activity for a full 24-hour period or longer.

An event monitor only records your heart's electrical activity at certain times while you're wearing it. For many event monitors, you push a button to start the monitor when you feel symptoms. Other event monitors start automatically when they sense abnormal heart rhythms.

What to Expect after an Electrocardiogram

After an electrocardiogram (EKG), the electrodes (soft patches) are removed from your skin. You may get a rash or redness where the EKG patches were attached. This mild rash usually goes away without treatment.

You usually can go back to your normal daily routine after an EKG.

What an Electrocardiogram Shows

Many heart problems change the heart's electrical activity in distinct ways. An electrocardiogram (EKG) can help detect a number of heart problems.

EKG recordings can help doctors diagnose a heart attack that's happening now or has happened in the past. This is especially true if doctors can compare a current EKG recording to an older one.

An EKG also can show the following:

- Lack of blood flow to the heart muscle
- A heart that's beating too fast, too slow, or with an irregular rhythm (arrhythmia)
- A heart that doesn't pump forcefully enough (heart failure)
- Heart muscle that's too thick or parts of the heart that are too big
- Birth defects in the heart (congenital heart defects)
- Problems with the heart valves (heart valve disease)
- Inflammation of the sac that surrounds the heart (pericarditis)

An EKG also can reveal whether the heartbeat starts at the top right part of the heart like it should. The test shows how long it takes for the electrical signals to travel through the heart. Delays in signal travel time may suggest heart block or long QT syndrome.

Risks of an Electrocardiogram

An electrocardiogram (EKG) has no serious risks. It's a harmless, painless test that detects the heart's electrical activity. EKGs don't give off electrical charges, such as shocks.

You may have a mild rash where the electrodes (soft patches) were attached. This rash usually goes away without treatment.

Chapter 41

Exercise Stress Test (Treadmill Test)

Stress testing gives your doctor information about how your heart works during physical stress. Some heart problems are easier to diagnose when your heart is working hard and beating fast.

During a stress test, you exercise (walk or run on a treadmill or pedal a bicycle) to make your heart work hard and beat fast. Tests are done on your heart while you exercise.

You may have arthritis or another medical problem that prevents you from exercising during a stress test. If so, your doctor may give you medicine to make your heart work hard, as it would during exercise. This is called a pharmacological stress test.

Overview

Doctors usually use stress testing to help diagnose coronary heart disease (CHD), also called coronary artery disease. They also use stress testing to see how severe CHD is in people who have it.

CHD is a condition in which a fatty material called plaque builds up in the coronary arteries. These arteries supply oxygen-rich blood to your heart.

Plaque narrows the arteries and reduces blood flow to your heart muscle. It also makes it more likely that blood clots will form in your

Excerpted from "Stress Testing," by the National Heart, Lung, and Blood Institute (NHLBI, www.nhlbi.nih.gov), part of the National Institutes of Health, June 2009.

arteries. Blood clots can partly or completely block blood flow. This can lead to chest pain or a heart attack.

You may not have any signs or symptoms of CHD when your heart is at rest. But when your heart has to work harder during exercise, it needs more blood and oxygen. Narrowed arteries can't supply enough blood for your heart to work well. As a result, signs and symptoms of CHD may only occur during exercise.

A stress test can detect the following problems, which may suggest that your heart isn't getting enough blood during exercise.

- Abnormal changes in your heart rate or blood pressure

- Symptoms such as shortness of breath or chest pain, which are particularly important if they occur at low levels of exercise

- Abnormal changes in your heart's rhythm or electrical activity

During a stress test, if you can't exercise for as long as what's considered normal for someone your age, it may be a sign that not enough blood is flowing to your heart. However, other factors besides CHD can prevent you from exercising long enough (for example, lung disease, anemia, or poor general fitness).

A stress test also may be used to assess other problems, such as heart valve disease or heart failure.

Types of Stress Testing

There are two main types of stress testing: a standard exercise stress test and an imaging stress test.

Standard Exercise Stress Test

A standard exercise stress test uses an EKG (electrocardiogram) to detect and record the heart's electrical activity.

An EKG shows how fast your heart is beating and the heart's rhythm (steady or irregular). It also records the strength and timing of electrical signals as they pass through each part of your heart.

During a standard stress test, your blood pressure will be checked. You also may be asked to breathe into a special tube during the test. This allows your doctor to see how well you're breathing and measure the gases that you breathe out.

A standard stress test shows changes in your heart's electrical activity. It also may show signs that your heart isn't getting enough blood during exercise.

Imaging Stress Test

Some stress tests take pictures of the heart when you exercise and when you're at rest. These imaging stress tests can show how well blood is flowing in various parts of your heart and/or how well your heart squeezes out blood when it beats.

One type of imaging stress test involves echocardiography (echo). This test uses sound waves to create a moving picture of your heart. An exercise stress echo can show how well your heart's chambers and valves are working when your heart is under stress.

The test can identify areas of poor blood flow to your heart, dead heart muscle tissue, and areas of the heart muscle wall that aren't contracting normally. These areas may have been damaged during a heart attack, or they may not be getting enough blood.

Other imaging stress tests use radioactive dye to create pictures of the blood flow to your heart. The dye is injected into your bloodstream before the pictures of your heart are taken. The pictures show how much of the dye has reached various parts of your heart during exercise and while you're at rest.

Tests that use radioactive dye include a thallium or sestamibi stress test and a positron emission tomography (PET) stress test. The amount of radiation in the dye is thought to be safe and not a danger to you or those around you. However, if you're pregnant, you shouldn't have this test because of risks it might pose to your unborn child.

Imaging stress tests tend to be more accurate at detecting CHD than standard (nonimaging) stress tests. Imaging stress tests also can predict the risk of a future heart attack or premature death.

An imaging stress test may be done first (as opposed to a standard exercise stress test) if you have any of the following:

- Can't exercise for enough time to get your heart working at its hardest (Medical problems, such as arthritis or leg arteries clogged by plaque, may prevent you from exercising enough.)

- Have abnormal heartbeats or other problems that will cause a standard exercise stress test to be inaccurate

- Had a heart procedure in the past, such as coronary artery by-pass grafting or placement of a stent in a coronary artery

Other Names for Stress Testing

- Exercise echocardiogram or exercise stress echo
- Exercise test

- Myocardial perfusion imaging
- Nuclear stress test
- PET stress test
- Pharmacological stress test
- Sestamibi stress test
- Stress EKG
- Thallium stress test
- Treadmill test

Who Needs Stress Testing?

You may need stress testing if you've had chest pains, shortness of breath, or other symptoms of limited blood flow to your heart.

Imaging stress tests, particularly, can show whether you have coronary heart disease (CHD) or a heart valve problem. (Heart valves are like doors that let blood flow between the heart's chambers and into the heart's arteries. So, like CHD, faulty heart valves can limit the amount of blood reaching your heart.)

If you've been diagnosed with CHD or recently had a heart attack, a stress test can show whether you can tolerate an exercise program. If you've had angioplasty with or without stents or coronary artery bypass grafting, a stress test can show how well the treatment relieves your CHD symptoms.

You also may need a stress test if, during exercise, you feel faint, get a rapid heartbeat or a fluttering feeling in your chest, or have other symptoms of an arrhythmia (an abnormal heartbeat).

If you don't have chest pain when you exercise, but still get short of breath, you may need a stress test. The test can help show whether a heart problem, rather than a lung problem or being out of shape, is causing your breathing problems.

For such testing, you breathe into a special tube. This allows a technician to measure the gases you breathe out. Breathing into the special tube and checking the heart as part of a stress test also is done before a heart transplant to help assess whether you're a candidate for the surgery.

Stress testing isn't used as a routine screening test for CHD. Usually you have to have symptoms of CHD before a doctor will recommend stress testing.

However, your doctor may want to use a stress test to screen for CHD if you have diabetes. This disease increases your risk for CHD.

Currently, though, no evidence shows that having a stress test will improve your outcome if you have diabetes.

What to Expect before Stress Testing

Standard stress testing often is done in a doctor's office. Imaging stress testing usually is done at a hospital. Be sure to wear athletic or other shoes in which you can exercise comfortably. You may be asked to wear comfortable clothes, or you may be given a gown to wear during the test.

Your doctor may ask you not to eat or drink anything but water for a short time before the test. If you're diabetic, ask your doctor whether you need to adjust your medicines on the day of your test.

For some stress tests, you can't drink coffee or other caffeinated drinks for a day before the test. Certain over-the-counter or prescription medicines also may interfere with some stress tests. Discuss with your doctor whether you need to avoid certain drinks or food or change how you take your medicine before the test.

If you use an inhaler for asthma or other breathing problems, bring it to the test. Make sure you let the doctor know that you use it.

What to Expect during Stress Testing

During all types of stress testing, a technician or nurse will always be with you to closely check your health status.

Before you start the "stress" part of a stress test, the technician or nurse will put sticky patches called electrodes on the skin of your chest, arms, and legs. To help an electrode stick to the skin, the technician or nurse may have to shave a patch of hair where the electrode will be attached.

The electrodes are connected to an EKG (electrocardiogram) machine. This machine records your heart's electrical activity and shows how fast your heart is beating and the heart's rhythm (steady or irregular). An EKG also records the strength and timing of electrical signals as they pass through each part of your heart.

The technician or nurse will put a blood pressure cuff on your arm to check your blood pressure during the stress test. (The cuff will feel tight on your arm when it expands every few minutes.) Also, you may be asked to breathe into a special tube so the gases you breathe out can be measured.

After these preparations, you'll exercise on a treadmill or stationary bicycle. If such exercise poses a problem for you, you may instead turn a crank with your arms. During the test, the exercise level will get harder. You can stop whenever you feel the exercise is too much for you.

If you can't exercise, medicine may be injected into a vein in your arm or hand. This medicine will increase blood flow through your coronary arteries and/or make your heart beat fast, as would exercise. The stress test can then be done.

The medicine may make you flushed and anxious, but the effects go away as soon as the test is over. The medicine also may give you a headache.

While you're exercising or getting medicine to make your heart work harder, the technician will frequently ask you how you're feeling. You should tell him or her if you feel chest pain, short of breath, or dizzy.

The exercise or medicine infusion will continue until you reach a target heart rate, or until the following occur:

- You feel moderate to severe chest pain.
- You get too out of breath to continue.
- You develop abnormally high or low blood pressure or an arrhythmia (an abnormal heartbeat).
- You become dizzy.

The technician will continue to check your heart functions and blood pressure after the test until they return to your normal levels.

The "stress" part of a stress test (when you're exercising or given medicine that makes your heart work hard) usually lasts about 15 minutes or less.

However, there's prep time before the test and monitoring time afterward. Both extend the total test time to about an hour for a standard stress test, and up to 3 hours or more for some imaging stress tests.

Exercise Stress Echocardiogram Test

For an exercise stress echocardiogram (echo) test, the technician will take pictures of your heart using echocardiography before you exercise and as soon as you finish.

A sonographer (a person who specializes in using ultrasound techniques) will apply gel to your chest. Then, he or she will briefly put a transducer (a wand-like device) against your chest and move it around.

The transducer sends and receives high-pitched sounds that you usually can't hear. The echoes from the sound waves are converted into moving pictures of your heart on a screen.

You may be asked to lie on your side on an exam table for this test. Some stress echo tests also use a dye to improve imaging. This dye is injected into your bloodstream while the test occurs.

Sestamibi or Other Imaging Stress Tests Involving Radioactive Dye

For a sestamibi stress test, or other imaging stress tests that use radioactive dye, the technician will inject a small amount of dye (such as sestamibi) into your bloodstream. This is done through a needle placed in a vein in your arm or hand.

You're usually given the dye about a half-hour before you start exercising or take medicine to make your heart work hard. The amount of radiation in the dye is thought to be safe and not a danger to you or those around you. However, if you're pregnant, you shouldn't have this test because of risks it might pose to your unborn child.

Pictures will be taken of your heart at least two times: when it's at rest and when it's working its hardest. You'll lie down on a table, and a special camera or scanner that can see the dye in your bloodstream will take pictures of your heart.

Some pictures may not be taken until you lie quietly for a few hours after the stress test. Some patients may even be asked to return in a day or so for more pictures.

What to Expect after Stress Testing

After stress testing, you'll be able to return to your normal activities. If you had a test that involved radioactive dye, your doctor may ask you to drink plenty of fluids to flush it out of your body. You also shouldn't have certain other imaging tests until the dye is no longer in your body. Your doctor can advise you about this.

What Stress Testing Shows

Stress testing gives your doctor information about how your heart works during physical stress (exercise) and how healthy your heart is.

A standard exercise stress test uses an EKG (electrocardiogram) to monitor changes in your heart's electrical activity. Imaging stress tests take pictures of blood flow in various parts of your heart. They also show your heart valves and the movement of your heart muscle.

Both types of stress tests are used to look for signs that your heart isn't getting enough blood flow during exercise. Abnormal test results may be due to coronary heart disease (CHD) or other factors, such as a lack of physical fitness.

If you have a standard exercise stress test and the results are normal, no further testing or treatment may be needed. But if your test results are abnormal, or if you're physically unable to exercise, your doctor may want you to have an imaging stress test or other tests.

Even if your standard exercise stress test results are normal, your doctor may want you to have an imaging stress test if you continue having symptoms (such as shortness of breath or chest pain).

Imaging stress tests are more accurate than standard exercise stress tests, but they're much more expensive.

Imaging stress tests show how well blood is flowing in the heart muscle and reveal parts of the heart that aren't contracting strongly. They also can show the parts of the heart that aren't getting enough blood, as well as dead tissue in the heart, where no blood flows. (A heart attack can cause some tissue in the heart to die.)

If your imaging stress test suggests significant CHD, your doctor may want you to have more testing and/or treatment.

Risks of Stress Testing

There's little risk of serious harm from any type of stress testing. The chance of these tests causing a heart attack or death is about one in 5,000. More common, but less serious side effects linked to stress testing include:

- **Arrhythmia (an abnormal heartbeat):** Often, an arrhythmia will go away quickly once you're at rest. But if it persists, you may need monitoring or treatment in a hospital.

- **Low blood pressure, which can cause you to feel dizzy or faint:** This problem may go away once your heart stops working hard; it usually doesn't require treatment.

- **Jitteriness or discomfort while getting medicine to make your heart work harder (you may be given medicine if you can't exercise):** These side effects usually go away shortly after you stop getting the medicine. In some cases, the symptoms may last a few hours.

Also, some of the medicines used for pharmacological stress tests can cause wheezing, shortness of breath, and other asthma-like symptoms. In some cases, these symptoms may be severe and require treatment.

Chapter 42

Holter and Event Monitors

Holter and event monitors are medical devices that record the heart's electrical activity. Doctors most often use these monitors to diagnose arrhythmias. These are problems with the speed or rhythm of the heartbeat. During an arrhythmia, the heart can beat too fast, too slow, or irregularly.

Holter and event monitors also are used to detect silent myocardial ischemia. In this condition, not enough oxygen-rich blood reaches the heart muscle. "Silent" means that no symptoms occur.

These monitors also can check whether treatments for arrhythmia and silent myocardial ischemia are working.

This text focuses on using Holter and event monitors to diagnose problems with the heart's speed or rhythm.

Overview

Holter and event monitors are similar to an EKG (electrocardiogram). An EKG is a simple test that detects and records the heart's electrical activity. It's the most common test for diagnosing a heart rhythm problem.

However, a standard EKG only records the heartbeat for a few seconds. It won't detect heart rhythm problems that don't occur during the test.

Excerpted from text by the National Heart, Lung, and Blood Institute (NHLBI, www.nhlbi.nih.gov), part of the National Institutes of Health, December 2007.

Holter and event monitors are small, portable devices. You can wear one while you do your normal daily activities. This allows the monitor to record your heart for a longer time than an EKG.

Some people have heart rhythm problems that only occur during certain activities, such as sleep or physical exertion. Using a Holter or event monitor increases the chance of recording these problems.

Although similar, Holter and event monitors aren't the same. A Holter monitor records your heart's electrical activity the entire time you're wearing it. An event monitor only records your heart's electrical activity at certain times while you're wearing it.

Types of Holter and Event Monitors

Holter Monitors

Holter monitors are sometimes called continuous EKGs (electrocardiograms). This is because Holter monitors record the heart rhythm continuously for 24 to 48 hours.

A Holter monitor is about the size of a large deck of cards. You can clip it to a belt or carry it in a pocket. Wires connect the device to sensors (called electrodes) that are stuck to your chest using sticky patches. These sensors pick up your heart's electrical signals, and the monitor records your heart's rhythm.

Wireless Holter Monitors

Wireless Holter monitors have a longer recording time than standard Holter monitors. The wireless version records your heart's electrical activity for a preset amount of time.

These monitors are called wireless because they use a cell phone to send the data to your doctor's office. This happens automatically at certain times. These monitors still have wires that connect the device to the sensors stuck to your chest.

You can use a wireless Holter monitor for days or even weeks until signs or symptoms of a heart rhythm problem occur. These monitors usually are used to detect heart rhythm problems that don't occur often.

Although wireless Holter monitors work for longer periods, they have a down side. You must remember to write down the time of symptoms, so your doctor can match it to the heart rhythm recording. Also, the batteries in the wireless monitor must be changed every 1 to 2 days.

Event Monitors

Event monitors are similar to Holter monitors. You wear one while you do your normal daily activities. Most event monitors have wires that connect the device to sensors that are stuck to your chest using sticky patches.

Unlike Holter monitors though, event monitors don't continuously record the heart's electrical activity. They only record when symptoms occur. For many event monitors, you need to start the monitor when you feel symptoms.

Event monitors tend to be smaller than Holter monitors because they don't need to store as much data.

Different types of event monitors work in slightly different ways. Your doctor will explain how to use the monitor before you start wearing it.

Postevent recorders: Postevent recorders are among the smallest event monitors. You can wear a postevent recorder like a wristwatch or carry it in your pocket. The pocket version is about the size of a thick credit card. These recorders don't have wires that connect the device to chest sensors.

When you feel a symptom, you start the recorder. A postevent recorder only records what happens after you start it. It may miss a heart rhythm problem that occurs before and during the onset of symptoms. Also, it may be hard to start the monitor when a symptom is in progress.

In some cases, this missing data would have helped your doctor diagnose the heart rhythm problem.

Presymptom memory loop recorders: Presymptom memory loop recorders are the size of a small cell phone. They're also called continuous loop event recorders.

You can clip this event monitor to your belt or carry it in your pocket. Wires connect the device to sensors on your chest.

These recorders are always recording and erasing data. When you feel a symptom, you push a button on the device. The normal erase process stops. The recording will show a few minutes of the data from before, during, and after the symptom.

In some cases, this makes it possible for your doctor to see very brief changes in your heart's rhythm.

Autodetect recorders: Autodetect recorders are about the size of the palm of your hand. Wires connect the device to sensors on your chest.

You don't need to start an autodetect recorder during symptoms. These recorders detect abnormal heart rhythms and automatically record and send the data to your doctor's office.

Implantable loop recorders: You may need an implantable loop recorder if other event monitors can't provide enough data. Implantable loop recorders are about the size of a pack of gum. This type of event monitor is inserted under the skin on your chest. No wires or chest sensors are used.

The device records either when you activate it or automatically when symptoms occur. It depends on how your doctor programs it. Devices may differ, so your doctor will tell you how to use it. In some cases, a special card is held close to the recorder to start it.

Other Names for Holter and Event Monitors

- Ambulatory EKG (electrocardiogram)

- Continuous EKG

- EKG event monitors

- Episodic monitors

- Mobile cardiac outpatient telemetry systems (This is another name for autodetect recorders.)

- Thirty-day event recorders

- Transtelephonic event monitors (These are monitors that require the patient to send the collected data to a doctor's office. This is done using a telephone.)

Who Needs a Holter or Event Monitor?

You may need a Holter or event monitor if your doctor suspects you have an arrhythmia. This is a problem with the speed or rhythm of your heartbeat. Holter or event monitors are most often used to detect arrhythmias in people who have experienced the following:

- Fainting or sometimes feeling dizzy: A monitor may be used if causes other than a heart rhythm problem have been ruled out.

- Palpitations that recur with no known cause: Palpitations are the feeling that your heart is pounding, racing, fluttering, or beating unevenly.

People who are being treated for a heart rhythm problem also may need to use a Holter or event monitor. These monitors can show how treatment is working.

In some people, heart rhythm problems only occur during certain events, such as sleep or physical exertion. Holter and event monitors record the heart rhythm while a person does his or her normal daily routine. This allows the doctor to see how the heart responds to different daily activities, which helps diagnose the problem.

Holter and event monitors also are used for elderly people who may have trouble getting to and from clinics.

What to Expect before Using a Holter or Event Monitor

Your doctor will do a physical exam before giving you a Holter or event monitor. He or she will do the following:

- Check your pulse to find out how fast your heart is beating and measure your blood pressure.

- Listen to the rate and rhythm of your heart.

- Check for swelling in your legs or feet. This could be a sign of an enlarged heart or heart failure, which may cause arrhythmias (problems with the speed or rhythm of the heartbeat).

- Look for signs of other diseases (such as thyroid disease) that could be causing heart rhythm problems.

You may have an EKG (electrocardiogram) test before your doctor sends you home with a Holter or event monitor. An EKG detects and records the electrical activity of the heart for a few seconds. It shows how fast the heart is beating and its rhythm (steady or irregular). It also records the strength and timing of electrical signals as they pass through each part of the heart.

A standard EKG won't detect heart rhythm problems that don't happen during the test. For this reason, your doctor may give you a Holter or event monitor. These monitors are portable. You can wear one while doing your normal daily activities. This increases the chance of recording symptoms that only occur once in a while.

Your doctor will explain how to wear and use the Holter or event monitor. Usually, you will leave the office wearing it.

What to Expect When Using a Holter or Event Monitor

Your experience while using a Holter or event monitor depends on the type of monitor you have. However, most monitors have some factors in common.

Recording the Heart's Electrical Activity

All monitors record the heart's electrical activity. So, it's important to maintain a clear signal between the sensors (electrodes) and the recording device.

In most cases, the sensors are attached to your chest with sticky patches. Wires connect the sensors to the monitor. You usually can clip the monitor to your belt or carry it in your pocket. (Postevent and implantable loop recorders don't have chest sensors.)

A good stick between the patches and your skin helps provide a clear signal. Poor contact leads to a poor recording, which is hard for your doctor to read.

Oil, too much sweat, and hair can keep the patches from sticking to your skin. You may need to shave the area where your doctor will attach each patch. You will need to clean the area with a special prep pad that your doctor provides.

You may need to use a small amount of special paste or gel to make the patches stick to your skin better. Some patches come with paste or gel on them.

Too much movement can pull the patches away from the skin or create "noise" on the rhythm strip. A rhythm strip is a graph showing the pattern of the heartbeat. Noise looks like a lot of jagged lines and makes it hard for the doctor to see the real rhythm of the heart.

When you have a symptom, stop what you're doing. This way you can be sure that the recording shows the heart's activity rather than your movement.

Your doctor will tell you whether you need to adjust your activity level during the testing period. If you exercise, choose a cool location to avoid sweating too much. This will help the patches stay sticky.

Other everyday items also can disrupt the signal between the sensors and the monitor. These items include magnets, metal detectors, microwave ovens, and electric blankets, toothbrushes, and razors. Avoid using these items. Also avoid areas with high voltage.

Cell phones and iPods may interfere with the signal if they're too close to the monitor. When using any electronic device, try to keep it at least 6 inches away from the monitor.

Keeping a Diary

When using a Holter or event monitor, you need to keep a diary of your symptoms and activities. Write down when symptoms occur, what they are, and what you were doing at the time.

The most common symptoms of heart rhythm problems include the following:

- Palpitations
- Fainting or feeling dizzy

It's important to note the time symptoms occur, because your doctor matches the data with the information in your diary. This allows your doctor to see whether certain activities trigger changes in your heart rate and rhythm.

You also should include details in your diary about when you take any medicine or if you feel stress at certain times during the test.

What to Expect with Specific Monitors

Holter Monitor

The Holter monitor is about the size of a large deck of cards. You wear it for 24 to 48 hours. When the test is complete, you return the device to your doctor's office. The results are stored on the device.

You can't get the monitor wet, so you won't be able to bathe or shower. You can take a sponge bath if needed.

The recording period for a standard Holter monitor may be too short to capture a heart rhythm problem. If this is the case, you may need a wireless Holter monitor.

Wireless Holter Monitors

Wireless Holter monitors can record for a longer time than standard Holter monitors. A wireless monitor records for a preset amount of time. It then automatically sends data from the monitor to your doctor's office.

These monitors are called wireless because they use a cell phone to send the data to your doctor's office. They still have wires that connect the device to the sensors stuck to your chest.

You can use a wireless Holter monitor for days or even weeks until signs or symptoms of a heart rhythm problem occur.

The batteries in the wireless monitor must be changed every 1 to 2 days. You will need to detach the sensors to shower or bathe and then reattach them.

Event Monitors

Event monitors are slightly smaller than Holter monitors. Event monitors record heart rhythm problems when you activate them. They can be worn for weeks or until symptoms occur.

Most event monitors are worn like Holter monitors—clipped to a belt or carried in a pocket. When you have symptoms, you simply push a button to start recording.

Postevent Recorders

Postevent recorders may be worn like a wristwatch or carried in a pocket. The pocket version is about the size of a thick credit card. These recorders don't have wires that connect the device to chest sensors.

To start the recorder when you feel a symptom, you hold it to your chest. To start the wristwatch version, you touch a button on the side of the watch.

You send the stored data to your doctor's office using a telephone. Your doctor will explain how to use the monitor before you leave the office.

Autodetect Recorders

Autodetect recorders are about the size of the palm of your hand. Wires connect the device to sensors on your chest.

You don't need to start an autodetect recorder. This type of monitor automatically starts recording when it detects an abnormal heart rhythm. It then sends the data to your doctor's office.

Implantable Loop Recorders

Implantable loop recorders are about the size of a pack of gum. This type of event monitor is inserted under the skin on your chest. No chest sensors are used.

The device records either when you activate it or automatically when symptoms occur. It depends on how your doctor programs it. Devices may differ, so your doctor will tell you how to use it. In some cases, a special card is held close to the recorder to start it.

What to Expect after Using a Holter or Event Monitor

After you're finished using a Holter or event monitor, you return it to your doctor's office or the place you got it from.

If you were using an implantable loop recorder, you will need to have it removed. Your doctor will discuss the procedure with you.

Your doctor will tell you when to expect the results. Once your doctor has reviewed the recordings, he or she will discuss the results with you.

What a Holter or Event Monitor Shows

A Holter or event monitor may show what's causing symptoms of an arrhythmia. This is problem with the speed or rhythm of the heartbeat.

Holter and event monitors also can show whether a heart rhythm problem is harmless or whether it needs treatment. Treatment is needed if the problem causes serious symptoms or increases your chance for complications.

Serious symptoms may include dizziness, chest pain, and fainting. Complications may include heart failure, stroke, or sudden cardiac arrest.

If the symptoms of your heart rhythm problem occur often, a Holter or event monitor has a good chance of capturing them. You may not have symptoms while using a monitor. Even so, your doctor may learn more about your heart rhythm from the test results.

Sometimes, these monitors can't help doctors diagnose heart rhythm problems. If this happens, talk to your doctor about other steps you can take.

One option may be to try a different type of monitor. The wireless Holter monitor and the implantable loop recorder have longer recording periods. This may allow the monitor to get the data that your doctor needs to make a diagnosis.

Risks from Using a Holter or Event Monitor

The sticky patches used to attach the sensors (electrodes) to your chest have a small risk of skin irritation. You also may have an allergic reaction the paste or gel that's sometimes used to attach the patches. The irritation will go away once the patches are removed.

If you're using an implantable loop recorder, you may get an infection or have pain where the device is placed under the skin. You may be given medicine to treat these complications.

Chapter 43

Coronary Angiography

Coronary angiography is a test that uses dye and special x-rays to show the inside of your coronary arteries. The coronary arteries supply oxygen-rich blood to your heart.

A material called plaque can build up on the inside walls of the coronary arteries, causing them to narrow. When this happens, it's called coronary heart disease (CHD) or coronary artery disease.

CHD can prevent enough blood from flowing to your heart and can lead to angina and heart attack. (Angina is chest pain or discomfort.) Coronary angiography shows whether you have CHD.

Most of the time, the coronary arteries can't be seen on an x-ray. During coronary angiography, special dye is injected into the bloodstream to make the coronary arteries show up on an x-ray.

A procedure called cardiac catheterization is used to get the dye to your coronary arteries. A long, thin, flexible tube called a catheter is put into a blood vessel in your arm, groin (upper thigh), or neck.

The tube is then threaded into your coronary arteries, and the dye is injected into your bloodstream. Special x-rays are taken while the dye is flowing through the coronary arteries.

Cardiologists (heart specialists) usually do cardiac catheterization in a hospital. You're awake during the procedure. It usually causes little to no pain, although you may feel some soreness in the blood vessel where your doctor put the catheter.

Cardiac catheterization rarely causes serious complications.

From text by the National Heart, Lung, and Blood Institute (NHLBI, www .nhlbi.nih.gov), part of the National Institutes of Health, May 2009.

When Coronary Angiography Is Needed

Your doctor may recommend coronary angiography if you have signs or symptoms of coronary heart disease (CHD). Signs and symptoms include the following:

- **Angina:** This is unexplained pain or pressure in your chest. You also may feel it in your shoulders, arms, neck, jaw, or back. Angina may only happen when you're active. Emotional stress also can trigger the pain.

- **Sudden cardiac arrest:** This is a condition in which your heart suddenly and unexpectedly stops beating.

- **EKG results:** Results from an EKG (electrocardiogram), exercise stress test, or other test may suggest you have heart disease.

You also may need coronary angiography on an emergency basis if you're having a heart attack. This test, combined with a procedure called angioplasty, can open the blocked artery that's causing the heart attack and prevent further damage to your heart.

Coronary angiography also can help your doctor decide how to treat CHD after a heart attack. This is especially true if the heart attack caused major damage to your heart, or if you're still having chest pain.

What to Expect before Coronary Angiography

Before having coronary angiography, talk to your doctor about the following:

- How the test is done and how to prepare for it

- Any medicines you're taking, and whether you should stop taking them before the test

- Whether you have diabetes, kidney disease, or other conditions that may require taking extra steps during or after the test to avoid complications

Your doctor will tell you exactly which procedures will be done. For example, your doctor may recommend angioplasty if the angiography shows a blocked artery.

You will have the chance to ask questions about the procedure. Also, you'll be asked to provide written informed consent to have the procedures done.

It may not be safe to drive after having cardiac catheterization, which is part of coronary angiography, so you must arrange for a ride home.

What to Expect during Coronary Angiography

During coronary angiography, you're kept on your back and awake. That way, you can follow your doctor's instructions during the test. You'll be given medicine to help you relax. The medicine may make you sleepy.

Your doctor will numb the area where the catheter (a small plastic tube) will enter the blood vessel through a small cut in the arm, groin (upper thigh), or neck.

The doctor then threads the catheter through the vessel up to the opening of the coronary arteries. Special x-ray movies are taken of the catheter as it's moved up into the heart. The movies help your doctor see where to position the tip of the catheter.

Your doctor will put special dye in the catheter when it reaches the correct spot. This dye will flow through your coronary arteries and make them show up on an x-ray. This x-ray is called an angiogram. If the angiogram reveals blocked arteries, your doctor may use angioplasty to restore blood flow to your heart.

After your doctor completes the angiography, or the angiography and angioplasty, he or she will remove the catheter from your body. The opening left in the blood vessel will then be closed up and bandaged.

A small sandbag or other type of weight may be put on top of the bandage to apply pressure. This will help prevent major bleeding from the site.

What to Expect after Coronary Angiography

After coronary angiography, you'll be moved to a special care area, where you'll rest and be checked for several hours or overnight. During this time, you'll need to limit your movement to avoid bleeding from the site where the catheter was inserted.

While you recover in the special care area, nurses will check your heart rate and blood pressure regularly and see whether you're bleeding from the tube insertion site.

A small bruise may develop on your arm, groin (upper thigh), or neck at the site where the catheter was inserted. That area may feel sore or tender for about a week. Let your doctor know if you develop problems such as the following:

- A constant or large amount of blood at the catheter insertion site that can't be stopped with a small bandage
- Unusual pain, swelling, redness, or other signs of infection at or near the catheter insertion site

Talk to your doctor about whether you should avoid certain activities, such as heavy lifting, for a short time after the test.

Risks of Coronary Angiography

Coronary angiography is a common medical test that rarely causes serious problems. But complications can include the following:

- Bleeding, infection, and pain at the site where the catheter was inserted
- Damage to blood vessels
- An allergic reaction to the dye used

Damage to blood vessels is a very rare complication. It may occur if the catheter scrapes or pokes a hole in a blood vessel as it's threaded up to the heart.

Other less common complications of the test include:

- An arrhythmia (irregular heartbeat) that often goes away on its own, but may need treatment if it persists
- Damage to the kidneys caused by the dye used
- Blood clots that can trigger stroke, heart attack, or other serious problems
- Low blood pressure
- A buildup of blood or fluid in the sac that surrounds the heart

A buildup of fluid can prevent the heart from beating properly.

As with any procedure involving the heart, complications can sometimes be fatal. However, this is rare with coronary angiography.

The risk of complications from coronary angiography is higher if you have diabetes or kidney disease or if you're 75 years old or older. The risk of complications also is greater in women and in people having coronary angiography on an emergency basis.

Chapter 44

Cardiac Computed Tomography

Cardiac computed tomography, or cardiac CT, is a painless test that uses an x-ray machine to take clear, detailed pictures of your heart. It's a common test for showing problems of the heart. During a cardiac CT scan, the x-ray machine will move around your body in a circle and take a picture of each part of your heart.

Because an x-ray machine is used, cardiac CT scans involve radiation. However, the amount of radiation used is small. This test gives out a radiation dose similar to the amount of radiation you're naturally exposed to over 3 years. There is a very small chance that cardiac CT will cause cancer.

Each picture that the machine takes shows a small slice of the heart. A computer will put the pictures together to make a large picture of the whole heart. Sometimes an iodine-based dye is injected into one of your veins during the scan to help highlight blood vessels and arteries on the x-ray images.

Overview

Cardiac CT is a common test for finding and evaluating the following conditions:

- **Problems in the heart:** Iodine-based dye used with a cardiac CT scan can show pictures of the coronary arteries. The coronary

From "Cardiac CT," by the National Heart, Lung, and Blood Institute (NHLBI, www.nhlbi.nih.gov), part of the National Institutes of Health, July 2007.

arteries are blood vessels on the surface of the heart. If these blood vessels are narrowed or blocked, you may have chest pain or a heart attack. The CT scan also can find problems with heart function and heart valves.

- **Problems with the aorta:** The aorta is the main artery that carries oxygen-rich blood from the heart to the body. Cardiac CT can detect two serious problems in the aorta:

  - Aneurysms, diseased areas of a weak blood vessel wall that bulge out, can be life threatening because they can burst.

  - Dissections, which can occur when the layers of the aortic artery wall peel away from each other, can cause pain and also may be life threatening.

- **Blood clots in the lungs:** A cardiac CT scan also may be used to find a pulmonary embolism, a serious but treatable condition. A pulmonary embolism is a sudden blockage in a lung artery, usually due to a blood clot that traveled to the lung from the leg.

- **Pericardial disease:** This is a disease that occurs in the pericardium, a sac around your heart.

Because the heart is in motion, a fast type of CT scanner, called multidetector computed tomography (MDCT), is used to show high-quality pictures of the heart.

Another type of CT scanner, called electron-beam computed tomography (EBCT), is used to detect calcium in the coronary arteries. Calcium in the coronary arteries may be an early sign of coronary artery disease (CAD).

CAD occurs when the coronary arteries (the arteries that supply blood and oxygen to the heart muscle) harden and narrow due to the buildup of a material called plaque on their inner walls. CAD is the leading cause of death for both men and women in the United States.

Researchers also are studying new ways to use cardiac CT.

Other Names for Cardiac CT

- CAT scan
- Coronary CT angiography
- Coronary artery scan
- CT angiography (CTA)

What to Expect before Cardiac CT

Your doctor will give you instructions before the cardiac computed tomography (CT) scan. Usually he or she will ask you to avoid drinks that contain caffeine before the test. Normally you'll be able to drink water, but you won't be able to eat for 4 hours before the scan.

If you take medicines for diabetes, ask your doctor whether you will need to change how you take them on the day of your cardiac CT scan.

Tell your doctor if you are pregnant or may be pregnant. Even though cardiac CT uses a low radiation dose, you shouldn't have the scan if you're pregnant. The x-rays may harm the developing fetus.

Also, tell your doctor if you have asthma or kidney problems or are allergic to any medicines, iodine, and/or shellfish. These may increase your chance of having an allergic reaction to the contrast dye.

A technician will ask you to remove your clothes above the waist and wear a hospital gown. You also will be asked to remove any jewelry from around your neck or chest.

Taking pictures of the heart can be difficult because the heart is always beating (in motion). A slower heart rate will help produce better quality pictures. If you don't have asthma or heart failure, your doctor may give you a medicine called a beta-blocker to help slow your heart rate. The medicine will be given by mouth or injected into a vein.

What to Expect during Cardiac CT

The cardiac computed tomography (CT) scan will take place in a hospital or outpatient office.

Because an x-ray machine is used, cardiac CT scans involve radiation. However, the amount of radiation used is small. This test gives out a radiation dose similar to the amount of radiation you're naturally exposed to over 3 years. There's a very small chance that cardiac CT will cause cancer. A doctor who has experience with CT scanning will supervise the test.

If your doctor wants to use contrast dye during the cardiac CT scan, a small needle connected to an intravenous (IV) line will be put in a vein in your hand or arm.

The contrast dye will be injected through the IV during the scan. You may have a warm feeling during the injection. The dye will highlight your blood vessels on the x-ray pictures from the cardiac CT scan.

The technician who operates the cardiac CT scanner will clean areas of your chest and place small sticky patches on those areas. The patches are attached to an EKG (electrocardiogram) machine to record the electrical activity of your heart during the exam.

The CT scanner is a large, square machine that has a hollow, circular tube in the middle. You will lie on your back on a sliding table that can move up and down and goes inside the tunnel-like machine.

Inside the scanner, an x-ray tube moves around your body to take pictures of different parts of your heart. These pictures can be shown on a computer as one large, three-dimensional picture. The technician controls the machine from the next room. The technician can see you through a glass window and talk to you through an intercom system.

Moving your body can cause the pictures to blur. You will be asked to lie still and hold your breath for short periods, while each picture is taken.

A cardiac CT scan usually takes about 15 minutes to complete. However, it can take over an hour to get ready for the test and for the medicine to slow your heart rate enough.

What to Expect after Cardiac CT

Once the cardiac computed tomography (CT) scan is done, you're able to return to your normal activities.

A doctor who has experience with CT will provide your doctor with the results of your cardiac CT. Your doctor will discuss the findings with you.

What Cardiac CT Shows

Many x-rays are taken while you're in the computed tomography (CT) scanner. Each picture that the machine takes shows a small slice of the heart. A computer can put the pictures together to make a large picture of the whole heart. This picture shows the inside of the heart and the structures that surround the heart.

Because the heart is in motion, a fast type of CT scanner, called multidetector computed tomography (MDCT), is used to take high-quality pictures of the heart.

Another type of CT scanner, called electron-beam computed tomography (EBCT), is used to detect calcium in the coronary arteries. Calcium in the coronary arteries may be an early sign of coronary artery disease (CAD).

Risks of Cardiac CT

Cardiac computed tomography (CT) scans are safe, painless tests. Although cardiac CT uses radiation, the amount is small. This test gives out a radiation dose similar to the amount of radiation you're naturally exposed to over 3 years. There is a very small chance that cardiac CT will cause cancer.

Some people feel side effects from the contrast dye that's used during the cardiac CT scan, including an itchy feeling or a rash that may appear after the injection of the contrast dye. Neither one normally lasts for a long time, so medicine often isn't needed. If you do want medicine to relieve these symptoms, you can ask your doctor to prescribe you a medicine called an antihistamine, which is used to help stop allergic reactions.

Although rare, it's possible to have a serious allergic reaction that may lead to breathing difficulties. Medicines are used to treat serious reactions.

People who have asthma or emphysema may have breathing problems during cardiac CT if they're given beta-blockers to slow down their heart rates.

Chapter 45

Cardiac Magnetic Resonance Imaging

Magnetic resonance imaging (MRI) is a safe, noninvasive test that creates detailed pictures of your organs and tissues. Noninvasive means that no surgery is done and no instruments are inserted into your body.

MRI uses radio waves, magnets, and a computer to create pictures of your organs and tissues. Unlike computed tomography scans (also called CT scans) and standard x-rays, MRI doesn't use ionizing radiation or carry any risk of causing cancer.

Cardiac MRI creates pictures of your heart as it's beating, producing both still and moving pictures of your heart and major blood vessels. Doctors use cardiac MRI to get pictures of the beating heart and to look at its structure and function. These pictures can help them decide how to treat people who have heart problems.

Cardiac MRI is a common test. It's used to diagnose and evaluate a number of diseases and conditions, including the following:

- Coronary heart disease, also called coronary artery disease
- Damage caused by a heart attack
- Heart failure
- Heart valve problems
- Congenital heart defects

From "Cardiac MRI," by the National Heart, Lung, and Blood Institute (NHLBI, www.nhlbi.nih.gov), part of the National Institutes of Health, July 2009.

- Pericarditis (a condition in which the membrane, or sac, around your heart is inflamed)
- Cardiac tumors

Cardiac MRI can help explain results from other tests, such as x-rays and CT scans. Sometimes, cardiac MRI is used to avoid the need for invasive procedures or tests that use radiation (such as x-rays) or dyes containing iodine (these dyes may be harmful to people who have kidney problems).

Often during cardiac MRI, a contrast agent is injected into a vein to highlight portions of the heart or blood vessels. This contrast agent often is used for people who are allergic to the dyes used in CT scanning.

People who have severe kidney or liver problems may not be able to have the contrast agent. As a result, they may have an MRI that doesn't use the substance (a noncontrast MRI).

Other Names for Cardiac MRI

- Heart MRI
- Cardiovascular MRI
- Cardiac nuclear magnetic resonance (NMR)

What to Expect before Cardiac MRI

You'll be asked to fill out a screening form before having cardiac MRI. The form may ask whether you have had previous surgeries, have any metal objects in your body, or have any medical devices (like a cardiac pacemaker) surgically implanted in your body.

Most, but not all, implanted medical devices are allowed near the MRI machine. Talk to your doctor or the technician operating the machine if you have concerns about any implanted devices or conditions that may interfere with the MRI.

MRI can seriously affect some types of implanted medical devices.

- Implanted cardiac pacemakers and defibrillators can malfunction.
- Cochlear (inner-ear) implants can be damaged. Cochlear implants are small electronic devices that help people who are deaf or who can't hear well understand speech and the sounds around them.

- Brain aneurysm clips can move due to MRI's strong magnetic field. This can cause severe injury.

Your doctor will let you know if you shouldn't have a cardiac MRI because of a medical device. If this happens, consider wearing a medical ID [identification] bracelet or necklace or carrying a medical alert card that states that you shouldn't have an MRI.

Your doctor or technician will tell you whether you need to change into a hospital gown for the test. Don't bring hearing aids, credit cards, jewelry and watches, eyeglasses, pens, removable dental work, and anything that's magnetic near the MRI machine.

Tell your doctor if being in a fairly tight or confined space causes you anxiety or fear. This fear is called claustrophobia. If you have this condition, your doctor might give you medicine to help you relax. Your doctor may ask you to fast (not eat) for 6 hours before you take this medicine on the day of the test.

Some of the newer cardiac MRI machines are open on all sides. Ask your doctor to help you find a facility that has an open MRI machine if you're fearful in tight or confined spaces.

Your doctor will let you know whether you need to arrange for a ride home after the test.

What to Expect during Cardiac MRI

MRI machines usually are located at hospitals or special medical imaging facilities. A radiologist or other doctor who has special training in medical imaging oversees MRI testing.

Cardiac MRI usually takes 45 to 90 minutes, depending on how many pictures are needed. The test may take less time with some newer MRI machines.

The MRI machine will be located in a specially constructed room. This will prevent radio waves from disrupting the machine. It also will prevent the MRI machine's strong magnetic fields from interfering with other equipment.

Traditional MRI machines look like a long, narrow tunnel. Newer MRI machines, called short-bore systems, are shorter, wider, and don't completely surround you. Some of the newer machines are open on all sides. Your doctor will help decide which type of machine is best for you.

Cardiac MRI is painless and harmless. You'll lie on your back on a sliding table that goes inside the tunnel-like machine. The technician will control the machine from the next room. He or she will be able to see you through a glass window and talk to you through a speaker. Tell the technician if you have a hearing problem.

The MRI machine makes loud humming, tapping, and buzzing noises. Earplugs may help lessen the noises made by the MRI machine. Some facilities let you listen to music during the test.

You will need to remain very still during the test. Any movement may blur the pictures. If you're unable to lie still, you may be given medicine to help you relax.

You may be asked to hold your breath for 10 to 15 seconds at a time while the technician takes pictures of your heart.

Researchers are studying ways that will allow someone having a cardiac MRI to breathe freely during the exam, while achieving the same image quality.

A contrast agent, such as gadolinium, may be used to highlight your blood vessels or heart in the pictures. Contrast agent usually is injected into a vein in your arm with a needle.

You may feel a cool sensation during the injection and discomfort where the needle was inserted. Gadolinium doesn't contain iodine, so it won't cause problems for people who are allergic to iodine.

Your cardiac MRI may include a stress test to detect blockages in your coronary arteries. If so, you'll get other medicines to increase the blood flow in your heart or to increase your heart rate.

What to Expect after Cardiac MRI

If you didn't take medicine to help you relax, you'll be able to return to your normal routine once the cardiac MRI is done.

If you did take medicine to help you relax during the test, your doctor will tell you when you can return to your normal routine. You'll need someone to drive you home.

What Cardiac MRI Shows

The doctor supervising your scan will provide your doctor with the results of your cardiac MRI. Your doctor will discuss the findings with you.

Cardiac MRI can reveal various heart conditions and disorders, such as the following:

- Coronary heart disease
- Damage caused by a heart attack
- Heart failure

- Heart valve problems
- Congenital heart defects
- Pericarditis (a condition in which the membrane, or sac, around your heart is inflamed)
- Cardiac tumors

Cardiac MRI is a fast, accurate tool that can help diagnose a heart attack. The test does this by detecting areas of the heart that don't move normally, have poor blood supply, or are scarred.

Cardiac MRI can show whether any of the coronary arteries are blocked, causing reduced blood flow to your heart muscle.

Currently, coronary angiography is the most common procedure for looking at blockages in the coronary arteries. Coronary angiography is an invasive procedure that uses x-rays and iodine-based dyes.

Researchers have found that cardiac MRI can replace coronary angiography in some cases, avoiding the need to use x-ray radiation and iodine-based dyes. This use of MRI is called MRI angiography.

Researchers are finding new ways to use cardiac MRI. In the future, cardiac MRI may replace x-rays as the main way to guide invasive procedures such as cardiac catheterization. Also, improvements in cardiac MRI are likely to lead to better methods for detecting heart disease in the future.

Risks of Cardiac MRI

Cardiac MRI produces no side effects from the magnetic fields and radio waves. This method of taking pictures of organs and tissues doesn't carry a risk of causing cancer or birth defects.

Serious reactions to the contrast agent used for MRI are very rare. However, side effects are possible and include the following:

- Headache
- Nausea (feeling sick to your stomach)
- Dizziness
- Changes in taste
- Allergic reactions

Rarely, the contrast agent can be harmful in people who have severe kidney or liver disease.

If your cardiac MRI includes a stress test, more medicines will be used during the test. These medicines may have other side effects that aren't expected during a regular MRI scan, such as the following:

- Arrhythmias, or irregular heartbeats
- Chest pain
- Shortness of breath
- Palpitations (feelings that your heart is skipping a beat, fluttering, or beating too hard or fast)

Chapter 46

Coronary Calcium Scan

A coronary calcium scan is a test that can help show whether you have coronary artery disease (CAD). In CAD, a fatty material called plaque narrows your coronary (heart) arteries and limits blood flow to your heart. CAD is the most common type of heart disease in both men and women. It can lead to angina, heart attack, heart failure, and arrhythmia.

Coronary calcium scanning looks for specks of calcium (called calcifications) in the walls of the coronary arteries. Calcifications are an early sign of heart disease. The test can show, before other signs and symptoms occur, whether you're at increased risk for a heart attack or other heart problems.

A coronary calcium scan is most useful for people who are at moderate risk for a heart attack. You or your doctor can calculate your 10-year risk using the Risk Assessment Tool from the National Cholesterol Education Program. People at moderate risk have a 10 to 20 percent chance of having a heart attack within the next 10 years. The coronary calcium scan may help doctors decide who within this group needs treatment.

Two machines can show calcium in the coronary arteries—electron beam computed tomography (EBCT) and multidetector computed tomography (MDCT). Both use an x-ray machine to make detailed pictures of your heart. Doctors study the pictures to see whether you're at risk for heart problems in the next 2 to 10 years.

From text by the National Heart, Lung, and Blood Institute (NHLBI, www .nhlbi.nih.gov), part of the National Institutes of Health, April 2008.

A coronary calcium scan is simple and easy for the patient, who lies quietly in the scanner machine for about 10 minutes. Pictures of the heart are taken that show whether the coronary arteries have calcifications.

Other Names for Coronary Calcium Scans

- Calcium scan test
- Cardiac CT for calcium scoring

Sometimes people refer to a coronary calcium scan by the name of the machine used to take pictures of the heart:

- Electron-beam computed tomography (EBCT) or electron-beam tomography (EBT)
- Multidetector computed tomography (MDCT)

What to Expect before a Coronary Calcium Scan

No special preparation is needed. You may be asked to avoid caffeine and smoking for 4 hours before the test. For the scan, you will remove your clothes above the waist and wear a hospital gown. You also will remove any jewelry from around your neck or chest.

What to Expect during a Coronary Calcium Scan

Coronary calcium scans are done in a hospital or outpatient office. The x-ray machine that's used is called a computed tomography (CT) scanner.

The technician who operates the scanner will clean areas of your chest and apply small sticky patches called electrodes. The electrodes are attached to an EKG (electrocardiogram) monitor. The EKG measures the electrical activity of your heart during the scan. This makes it possible to take pictures of your heart when it's relaxed, between beats.

The CT scanner is a large machine that has a hollow, circular tube in the center. You will lie on your back on a sliding table. The table can move up and down and goes inside the tunnel-like machine.

The table will slowly slide into the opening in the machine. Inside the scanner, an x-ray tube moves around your body to take pictures of your heart. You may be asked to hold your breath for 10 to 20 seconds while the pictures are taken. This prevents movement in the image.

During the test, the technician will be in a nearby room with the computer that controls the CT scanner. The technician can see you through a window and talk to you through an intercom system.

You may be given medicine to slow down a fast heart rate. This helps the machine take better pictures of your heart. The medicine will be given by mouth or injected into a vein.

A coronary calcium scan takes about 5 to 10 minutes. During the test, the machine makes clicking and whirring sounds as it takes pictures. It causes no discomfort, but the exam room may be chilly to keep the machine working properly.

If you become nervous in enclosed spaces, you may need to take medicine to stay calm. This isn't a problem for most people, because your head will remain outside the opening in the machine.

What to Expect after a Coronary Calcium Scan

You're able to return to your normal activities after the coronary calcium scan is done. A doctor who is trained in reading these scans will discuss the results with you.

What the Coronary Calcium Scan Shows

After the coronary calcium scan, you will get a calcium score called an Agatston score. The score is based on the amount of calcium found in your coronary arteries. You may get an Agatston score for each major artery and a total score.

The test is negative if no sign of calcium deposits (calcifications) is found in your arteries. This means your chance of having a heart attack in the next 2 to 5 years is low.

The test is positive if calcifications are found in your arteries. Calcifications are a sign of atherosclerosis and coronary artery disease. (Atherosclerosis is when the arteries harden and narrow due to plaque buildup.) The higher your Agatston score, the greater the amount of atherosclerosis.

Risks of a Coronary Calcium Scan

Coronary calcium scanning has very few risks. The test isn't invasive, which means that no surgery is done and no instruments are inserted into your body. Coronary calcium scanning doesn't require an injection of contrast dye to make your heart or arteries visible on the x-ray images.

Because an x-ray machine is involved, you will be exposed to a small amount of radiation. Electron-beam computed tomography (EBCT) uses less radiation than multidetector computed tomography (MDCT). In either case, the amount of radiation is less than or equal to the amount of radiation you're naturally exposed to in a single year.

Chapter 47

Carotid Ultrasound

Carotid ultrasound is a painless and harmless test that uses high-frequency sound waves to create pictures of the insides of the two large arteries in your neck.

These arteries, called carotid arteries, supply your brain with oxygen-rich blood. You have one carotid artery on each side of your neck.

Carotid ultrasound shows whether a substance called plaque has narrowed your carotid arteries. Plaque is made up of fat, cholesterol, calcium, and other substances found in the blood. Plaque builds up on the insides of your arteries as you age. This condition is called carotid artery disease.

Too much plaque in a carotid artery can cause a stroke. The plaque can slow down or block the flow of blood through the artery, allowing a blood clot to form. A piece of the blood clot can break off and get stuck in the artery, blocking blood flow to the brain. This is what causes a stroke.

A standard carotid ultrasound shows the structure of your carotid arteries. Your carotid ultrasound test may include a Doppler ultrasound. Doppler ultrasound is a special test that shows the movement of blood through your blood vessels.

Your doctor often will need results from both types of ultrasound to fully assess whether there's a problem with blood flow through your carotid arteries.

From text by the National Heart, Lung, and Blood Institute (NHLBI, www.nhlbi.nih.gov), part of the National Institutes of Health, May 2009.

Other Names for Carotid Ultrasound

- Doppler ultrasound
- Carotid duplex ultrasound

Who Needs Carotid Ultrasound?

Carotid ultrasound checks for plaque buildup in the carotid arteries. Plaque can narrow or block your carotid arteries, preventing oxygen-rich blood from reaching your brain.

Your doctor may recommend a carotid ultrasound if you had a stroke or mini-stroke recently. During a mini-stroke, you may have some or all of the symptoms of a stroke. However, the symptoms usually go away on their own within 24 hours.

Your doctor may also recommend a carotid ultrasound if you have an abnormal sound in your carotid artery called a carotid bruit. Your doctor can hear a carotid bruit with the help of a stethoscope put on your neck over the carotid artery. A bruit may suggest a partial blockage in your carotid artery that could lead to a stroke.

Your doctor also may recommend a carotid ultrasound if he or she suspects you may have the following:

- Blood clots that can slow blood flow in your carotid artery
- A split between the layers of your carotid artery wall that weakens the wall or reduces blood flow to your brain

A carotid ultrasound also may be done to see whether carotid artery surgery, also called carotid endarterectomy, has restored normal blood flow through your carotid artery.

If you had a procedure called carotid stenting, you may have carotid ultrasound afterward to check the position of the stent put in your carotid artery. (The stent, a small mesh tube, helps prevent the artery from becoming narrowed or blocked again.)

Sometimes carotid ultrasound is used as a preventive screening test in people who have medical conditions that increase their risk of stroke, including high blood pressure and diabetes.

People who have these conditions may benefit from having their carotid arteries checked regularly, even if they show no signs of plaque buildup.

What to Expect before Carotid Ultrasound

Carotid ultrasound is a painless test, and typically there is little to do in advance. Your doctor will tell you how to prepare for your carotid ultrasound.

What to Expect during Carotid Ultrasound

Carotid ultrasound usually is done in a doctor's office or hospital. The test is painless and often doesn't take more than 30 minutes.

The ultrasound machine includes a computer, a video screen, and a transducer. A transducer is a handheld device that sends and receives ultrasound waves into and from the body.

You will lie on your back on an exam table for the test. Your technician or doctor will put a gel on your neck where your carotid arteries are located. This gel helps the ultrasound waves reach the arteries better.

Your technician or doctor will put the transducer against different spots on your neck and move it back and forth. The transducer gives off ultrasound waves and detects their echoes after they bounce off the artery walls and blood cells. Ultrasound waves can't be heard by the human ear.

A computer uses the echoes to create and record pictures of the insides of the arteries (usually in black and white) and your blood flowing through them (usually in color; this is the Doppler ultrasound). A video screen displays these live images for your doctor to review.

What to Expect after Carotid Ultrasound

You usually don't have to take any special steps after a carotid ultrasound. You should be able to return to normal activities right away.

Often, your doctor will be able to tell you the results of the carotid ultrasound when it occurs or soon afterward.

What a Carotid Ultrasound Shows

A carotid ultrasound can show whether plaque buildup has narrowed one or both of your carotid arteries and reduced blood flow to your brain.

If plaque has narrowed your carotid arteries, you may be at risk of having a stroke. That risk depends on how much of your artery is blocked and how much blood flow is restricted.

To reduce your risk for stroke, your doctor may recommend medical or surgical treatments to reduce or remove the plaque buildup in your carotid arteries.

Risks of Carotid Ultrasound

There are no risks linked to having a carotid ultrasound, because the test uses harmless sound waves. These are the same type of sound waves that doctors use to record pictures of fetuses in pregnant women.

Chapter 48

Nuclear Heart Scan

A nuclear heart scan is a type of medical test that allows your doctor to get important information about the health of your heart. During a nuclear heart scan, a safe, radioactive material called a tracer is injected through a vein into your bloodstream. The tracer then travels to your heart. The tracer releases energy, which special cameras outside of your body detect. The cameras use the energy to create pictures of different parts of your heart.

Nuclear heart scans are used for three main purposes:

- **It provides information about the flow of blood throughout the heart muscle.** If the scan shows that one part of the heart muscle isn't receiving blood, it's a sign of a possible narrowing or blockage in the coronary arteries (the arteries that supply blood and oxygen to your heart). Decreased blood flow through the coronary arteries may mean you have coronary artery disease (CAD). CAD can lead to angina, heart attack, and other heart problems. When a nuclear heart scan is performed for this purpose, it's called myocardial perfusion scanning.

- **It looks for damaged heart muscle.** Damage may be due to a previous heart attack, injury, infection, or medicine. When a nuclear heart scan is performed for this purpose, it's called myocardial viability testing.

From text by the National Heart, Lung, and Blood Institute (NHLBI, www .nhlbi.nih.gov), part of the National Institutes of Health, July 2007.

- **It sees how well your heart pumps blood out to your body.** When a nuclear heart scan is performed for this purpose, it's called ventricular function scanning.

Usually, two sets of pictures are taken during a nuclear heart scan. The first set is taken when the heart is beating fast due to you exercising. This is called a cardiac stress test. If you can't exercise, your heart rate can be increased using medicines such as adenosine, dipyridamole, or dobutamine.

The second set of pictures is taken later, when the heart is at rest and beating at a normal rate.

Types of Nuclear Heart Scanning

There are two main types of nuclear heart scanning:

- Single positron emission computed tomography (SPECT)
- Cardiac positron emission tomography (PET)

SPECT is the most well-established and widely used type, while PET is newer. There are specific reasons for using each, which are discussed in the following paragraphs.

Single Positron Emission Computed Tomography

Cardiac SPECT is the most commonly used nuclear scanning test for diagnosing coronary artery disease (CAD). Combining SPECT with a cardiac stress test can show problems with blood flow to the heart that can be detected only when the heart is working hard and beating fast.

SPECT also is used to look for areas of damaged or dead heart muscle tissue, which may be due to a previous heart attack or other cause of injury.

SPECT also can show how well the heart's left ventricle pumps blood to the body. Weak pumping ability may be the result of heart attack, heart failure, and other causes.

The most commonly used tracers in SPECT are called thallium-201, technetium-99m sestamibi (Cardiolite®), and technetium-99m tetrofosmin (Myoview™).

Positron Emission Tomography

PET uses different kinds of tracers than SPECT. PET can provide more detailed pictures of the heart. However, PET is newer and has some technical limits that make it less available than SPECT. Research into advances in both SPECT and PET is ongoing. Right now, there is no clear cut advantage of using one over the other in all situations.

PET can be used for the same purposes as SPECT—to diagnose CAD, check for damaged or dead heart muscle, and evaluate the heart's pumping strength.

PET takes a clearer picture through thick layers of tissue (such as abdominal or breast tissue). PET also is better than SPECT at showing whether CAD is affecting more than one of your heart's blood vessels. A PET scan also may be used if a SPECT scan wasn't able to produce good enough pictures.

Other Names for a Nuclear Heart Scan

Names used for nuclear heart scans include the following:

- Nuclear stress test
- SPECT scan
- PET scan

What to Expect before a Nuclear Heart Scan

Talk to your doctor about how the nuclear heart scan is done. Discussing your overall health, including health problems such as asthma, chronic obstructive pulmonary disease (COPD), diabetes, and kidney disease, is important. If you have lung disease or diabetes, your doctor will give you special instructions before the nuclear heart scan.

Also, let your doctor know about any medicines you take, including prescription and over-the-counter medicines, vitamins, minerals, and other supplements. Some medicines and supplements can cause problems when used with adenosine, dipyridamole, or dobutamine (medicines used to increase your heart rate during a stress test).

If you are having a stress test as part of your nuclear heart scan, wear comfortable walking shoes and loose-fitting clothes for the test. You may be asked to wear a hospital gown during the test.

A nuclear heart scan can take a lot of time. Most take between 2 to 5 hours, especially if two sets of pictures are needed.

What to Expect during a Nuclear Heart Scan

Many, but not all, nuclear medicine centers are located in hospitals. A doctor who has special training in nuclear heart scans—a cardiologist or radiologist—will oversee the test. (Cardiologists are doctors who specialize in diagnosing and treating heart problems. Radiologists are doctors who specialize in diagnostic techniques such as nuclear scans.)

Before the test begins, the doctor or a technician will use a needle to insert an intravenous (IV) line into a vein in your arm. Through this IV line, he or she will put the radioactive tracers into your bloodstream at the right time. You also will have EKG (electrocardiogram) patches attached to your body to check your heart rate during the test.

If you're having an exercise stress test as part of your nuclear scan, you will walk on a treadmill or pedal a stationary bicycle, while attached to EKG and blood pressure monitors.

You will be asked to exercise until you're too tired to continue, short of breath, or having chest or leg pain. You can expect that your heart will beat faster, you will breathe faster, your blood pressure will increase, and you will sweat. Report any chest, arm, or jaw pain or discomfort; dizziness; lightheadedness; or any other unusual symptoms.

If you're unable to exercise, your doctor can give you medicine to make your heart beat faster. This is called a chemical stress test. The medicine used may make you feel anxious, sick, dizzy, or shaky for a short time. If the side effects are severe, other medicine can be given for relief.

Before the exercise or the chemical stress test stops, the tracer is injected through the IV line.

The nuclear heart scan will start shortly after the exercise or chemical stress test. You will be asked to lie very still on a padded table.

The nuclear heart scan camera, called a gamma camera, is enclosed in a metal housing. The part of the camera that detects the radioactivity from the tracer can be put in several positions around your body as you lie on the padded table. For some nuclear heart scans, the metal housing is shaped like a doughnut and you lie on a table that goes slowly through the doughnut hole. The computer used to collect the pictures of your heart is nearby or in another room.

Two sets of pictures will be taken. One will be taken right after your exercise or chemical stress test and the other will be taken after a period of rest. The pictures may be taken all in 1 day or over 2 days. Each set of pictures takes about 15 to 30 minutes to do.

Some people find it hard to stay in one position for some time. Others may feel anxious while lying in the doughnut-shaped scanner. The table may feel hard. Sometimes, the room feels chilly because of the air conditioning needed to maintain the machines.

Let the person performing the test know how you're feeling during the test so he or she can respond as needed.

What to Expect after a Nuclear Heart Scan

You may be asked to return to the nuclear medicine center the next day for more pictures. Outpatients will be allowed to go home after the scan or leave the nuclear medicine center between the two scans.

Most people can go back to daily activities after a nuclear heart scan. The radioactivity will naturally leave the body in the urine or stool. It's helpful to drink plenty of fluids after the test.

The cardiologist or radiologist will read and interpret the results of the test within 1 to 3 days. Results will be reported to your doctor, who will contact you to discuss the results. Or, the cardiologist may discuss the results directly with you.

What a Nuclear Heart Scan Shows

The results from a nuclear heart scan can help doctors do the following:

- Diagnose heart conditions, such as coronary artery disease (CAD), and decide on a course of treatment

- Manage certain heart diseases, such as CAD and heart failure, and predict short-term or long-term survival

- Determine your risk for a heart attack

- Decide whether you will be helped by other heart tests, such as coronary angiography or cardiac catheterization

- Decide whether procedures that can increase blood flow to the coronary arteries, such as angioplasty or coronary artery bypass grafting (CABG), can help you

- Monitor procedures or surgeries that have been done, such as CABG or a heart transplant

Risks of a Nuclear Heart Scan

The radioactive tracers used during a nuclear heart scan expose the body to a very small amount of radiation. No long-term effects have been reported from these doses.

If you have coronary artery disease, you may have chest pain during exercise or when you take medicine to increase your heart rate. Medicine can be given to relieve this symptom.

411

Some people may be allergic to the radioactive tracers, but this is very rare.

Women who are pregnant should tell their doctor and technician before the scan is done. It may be postponed until after the pregnancy.

Part Six

Managing Cardiovascular Disorders

Chapter 49

Cardiovascular Specialists and Your Health Care

Cardiology, or the discipline of medicine that specializes in heart disease, is a complex and sophisticated field. Generally, three types of cardiology specialists care for your heart.

A cardiologist has special training and skill in finding, treating, and preventing diseases of the heart and blood vessels in adults.

A pediatric cardiologist has special training and skill in finding, treating, and preventing heart and blood vessel disease in infants, children, and teenagers. In some cases, the pediatric cardiologist begins diagnosis and treatment in the fetus and continues into adulthood.

A cardiac surgeon has special training and skills to perform delicate operations on the heart, blood vessels, and lungs.

Training

After 4 years of medical school, these highly trained doctors spend from 6 to 8 more years in specialized training. A cardiologist receives 3 years of training in internal medicine and 3 or more years in specialized cardiology training. A pediatric cardiologist receives 3 years of training in pediatrics, and 3 or more years in specialized pediatric cardiology training. A cardiac surgeon must complete 5 years of training in general surgery before starting a 2-or 3-year cardiothoracic

"Cardiovascular Specialists and Your Heart," © 2003 American College of Cardiology (www.acc.org). Reprinted with permission. Reviewed by David A. Cooke, MD, FACP, October 1, 2009.

training program. Some cardiac surgeons have additional training to perform pediatric or transplant surgery.

Qualifications

At each stage of their training, these specialists must pass rigorous exams that test their knowledge and judgment, as well as their ability to provide superior care.

Cardiologists, pediatric cardiologists, and cardiac surgeons must first become board-certified in their primary specialty (internal medicine, pediatrics, and surgery respectively), and then certified in their subspecialty (cardiology, pediatric cardiology, and cardiothoracic surgery respectively).

Membership in the American College of Cardiology

If your cardiology specialist adds F.A.C.C.—Fellow of the American College of Cardiology—to his or her name, it is a sign of significant accomplishment and commitment to a profession, to a specialty, and to the provision of the best health care for the patient.

Election to ACC membership is based on training, specialty board certification, scientific and professional accomplishments, length of active participation in a cardiovascular-related field, and peer recognition. Members are expected to conform to high moral and ethical standards.

Cardiologists

Referral to a Cardiologist

Any time you have a significant heart or related condition, you may require the attention of a cardiologist. Symptoms like shortness of breath, chest pains, or dizzy spells often require special testing. Heart murmurs or ECG [electrocardiogram] changes are best evaluated by a cardiologist. Most importantly, cardiologists treat heart attacks, heart failure, and serious heart rhythm disturbances. Their skills and training are required for decisions about heart catheterization, balloon angioplasty, heart surgery, and other procedures.

Diagnostic Tests Which May Be Necessary

Your cardiologist will review your medical history and perform a physical examination which may include checking your blood pressure, weight, heart, lungs, and blood vessels. While some problems may be diagnosed from this examination, your cardiologist may order an ECG, x-ray, or blood tests. In addition, an ambulatory ECG, echocardiogram, exercise test, heart catheterization, and/or nuclear imaging may be required.

The Cardiologist and Your Primary Care Physician

The cardiologist usually serves as a consultant to other doctors, although many provide general medical care for their patients. Your primary care physician may recommend a cardiologist or you may choose one yourself. As your cardiac care proceeds, your cardiologist will guide your care and plan tests and treatment with the doctors and nurses who are looking after you.

Pediatric Cardiologists

Referral to a Pediatric Cardiologist

Children who have heart murmurs are often referred for evaluation. Many of these turn out to be normal and no follow-up by the pediatric cardiologist is necessary. About one in every 100 babies is born with heart disease (congenital heart disease) which requires a pediatric cardiologist's care.

Referrals are also made for cyanosis ("blue-baby" condition), rapid breathing, heart enlargement, high blood pressure, infections involving the heart and blood vessels, chest pain, heart rhythm disturbances, fainting episodes, and questions about participation in sports. Some pediatric cardiologists see and advise congenital heart patients into adulthood.

The skills of a pediatric cardiologist are required whenever decisions are made about procedures such as heart catheterization and heart surgery. The pediatric cardiologist may also advise about the prevention of heart attacks in later life and screen for high cholesterol levels.

The Pediatric Cardiologist and Your Pediatrician

A pediatric cardiologist usually serves as a consultant to other doctors. Your pediatrician may recommend a pediatric cardiologist, or you may choose one for your child. As your child's cardiac care proceeds, your pediatric cardiologist will guide the care and plan tests and treatments with the doctors and nurses who are looking after your child. If heart surgery is indicated, your child's pediatric cardiologist and cardiac surgeon work as a team. In follow-up, the pediatric cardiologist keeps you, your pediatrician, and/or surgeon informed.

Cardiac Surgeons

Cardiac surgeons perform many operations—coronary artery bypass, pacemaker insertion, heart rhythm surgery, valve replacement or repairs, heart transplants, and repairs of complex heart problems present from birth (congenital heart disease). They are also qualified to operate on organs other than the heart, such as the lungs, esophagus, and blood vessels.

Referral to a Cardiac Surgeon

If your general medical doctor, pediatrician, or cardiologist feels that surgery may be the best treatment for your heart condition and that medication alone will not be enough, then you will be referred to a cardiac surgeon for further evaluation. The surgeon will review your medical records and test, especially the heart catheterization results, if bypass, cardiac valve, or heart surgery for a congenital defect is being considered. The cardiac surgeon will then discuss your case with you and your doctors, to give further advice about the risks and benefits of surgery.

The Cardiac Surgeon and Your Cardiologist

The cardiac surgeon leads a team of doctors and nurses responsible for the immediate evaluation prior to surgery, final decision for surgery, as well as the recovery period after the operation until you are discharged. After leaving the hospital, you will usually be seen by both the cardiac surgeon and the cardiologist to assure that your recovery period is progressing smoothly.

Chapter 50

Medications for Cardiovascular Disease

Chapter Contents

Section 50.1

Anticoagulant Therapy Helps Blood Flow More Easily

Excerpted from "Blood Thinner Pills: Using Them Safely," by the Agency for Healthcare Research and Quality (AHRQ, www.ahrq.gov), September 2009.

Your doctor has prescribed a medicine called a blood thinner to prevent blood clots. Blood clots can put you at risk for heart attack, stroke, and other serious medical problems. A blood thinner is a kind of drug called an anticoagulant. "Anti" means against and "coagulant" means to thicken into a gel or solid.

Blood thinner drugs work well when they are used correctly. You and your doctor will work together as a team to make sure that taking your blood thinner does not stop you from living well and safely. The information in this text will help you understand why you are taking a blood thinner and how to keep yourself healthy.

How to Take Your Blood Thinner

Always take your blood thinner as directed. For example, some blood thinners need to be taken at the same time of day, every day.

Never skip a dose, and never take a double dose.

If you miss a dose, take it as soon as you remember. If you don't remember until the next day, call your doctor for instructions. If this happens when your doctor is not available, skip the missed dose and start again the next day. Mark the missed dose in a diary or on a calendar.

A pillbox with a slot for each day may help you keep track of your medicines.

Check Your Medicine

Check your medicine when you get it from the pharmacy.

- Does the medicine seem different from what your doctor prescribed or look different from what you expected?

- Does your pill look different from what you used before?

- Are the color, shape, and markings on the pill the same as what you were previously given?

If something seems different, ask the pharmacist to double check it. Many medication errors are found by patients.

Using Other Medicines

Tell your doctor about every medicine you take. The doctor needs to know about all your medicines, including medicines you were taking before you started taking a blood thinner.

Other medicines can change the way your blood thinner works. Your blood thinner can also change the way your other medicines work.

It is very important to talk with your doctor about all the medicines that you take, including other prescription medicines, over-the-counter medicines, vitamins, and herbal products.

Products that contain aspirin may lessen the blood's ability to form clots and may increase your risk of bleeding when you also are taking a blood thinner. Talk with your doctor about whether or not you should take aspirin and which dose is right for you.

Medicines you get over the counter may also interact with your blood thinner. Following is a list of some common medicines that you should talk with your doctor or pharmacist about before using.

Pain relievers, cold medicines, or stomach remedies, such as the following:

- Advil®
- Aleve®
- Alka-Seltzer®
- Excedrin®
- Ex-Lax®
- Midol®
- Motrin®
- Nuprin®
- Pamprin HB®
- Pepto Bismol®
- Sine-Off®

- Tagamet HB®
- Tylenol®

Vitamins and herbal products, such as the following:

- Centrum®, One a Day®, or other multivitamins
- Garlic
- Ginkgo biloba
- Green tea

Always tell your doctor about all the medicines you are taking. Tell your doctor when you start taking new medicine, when you stop taking a medicine, and if the amount of medicine you are taking changes. When you visit your doctor, bring a list of current medicines, over-the-counter drugs—such as aspirin—and any vitamins and herbal products you take.

Possible Side Effects

When taking a blood thinner it is important to be aware of its possible side effects. Bleeding is the most common side effect.

Call your doctor immediately if you have any of the following signs of serious bleeding:

- Menstrual bleeding that is much heavier than normal
- Red or brown urine
- Bowel movements that are red or look like tar
- Bleeding from the gums or nose that does not stop quickly
- Vomit that is brown or bright red
- Anything red in color that you cough up
- Severe pain, such as a headache or stomachache
- Unusual bruising
- A cut that does not stop bleeding
- A serious fall or bump on the head
- Dizziness or weakness

Some people who take a blood thinner may experience hair loss or skin rashes, but this is rare.

Stay Safe while Taking Your Blood Thinner

Call your doctor and go to the hospital immediately if you have had a bad fall or a hard bump, even if you are not bleeding. You can be bleeding but not see any blood. For example, if you fall and hit your head, bleeding can occur inside your skull. Or, if you hurt your arm during a fall and then notice a large purple bruise, this means you are bleeding under your skin.

Because you are taking a blood thinner, you should try not to hurt yourself and cause bleeding. You need to be careful when you use knives, scissors, razors, or any sharp object that can make you bleed.

You also need to avoid activities and sports that could cause injury. Swimming and walking are safe activities. If you would like to start a new activity that will increase the amount of exercise you get every day, talk to your doctor.

You can still do many things that you enjoy. If you like to work in the yard, you still can. Just be sure to wear sturdy shoes and gloves to protect yourself. Or, if you like to ride your bike, be sure you wear a helmet.

To prevent injury indoors, take the following precautions:

- Be very careful using knives and scissors.
- Use an electric razor.
- Use a soft toothbrush.
- Use waxed dental floss.
- Do not use toothpicks.
- Wear shoes or non-skid slippers in the house.
- Be careful when you trim your toenails.
- Do not trim corns or calluses yourself.

To prevent injury outdoors, take the following precautions:

- Always wear shoes.
- Wear gloves when using sharp tools.
- Avoid activities and sports that can easily hurt you.
- Wear gardening gloves when doing yard work.

Ask your doctor about whether you should wear a medical alert bracelet or necklace. If you are badly injured and unable to speak, the bracelet lets health care workers know that you are taking a blood thinner.

Food and Your Blood Thinner

The foods you eat can affect how well your blood thinner works for you. High amounts of vitamin K might work against some blood thinners, like warfarin (Coumadin®). Other blood thinners are not affected by vitamin K. Ask your doctor if you need to pay attention to the amount of vitamin K you eat.

Examples of some foods that contain medium to high levels of vitamin K and can affect how your blood thinner work include the following:

- Asparagus
- Avocado
- Broccoli
- Brussels sprouts
- Cabbage
- Canola oil
- Cranberries
- Endive
- Green onions
- Kale
- Lettuce
- Liver
- Margarine
- Mayonnaise
- Parsley
- Soybean oil
- Soybeans
- Spinach
- Turnip, collard, and mustard greens

You should also avoid drinking alcohol if you are taking a blood thinner.

Call your doctor if you are unable to eat for several days, for whatever reason. Also call if you have stomach problems, vomiting, or diarrhea that lasts more than 1 day. These problems could affect your blood thinner dose.

Keep your diet the same. Do not make any major changes in your diet or start a weight loss plan before calling your doctor first.

Talk to Your Other Doctors

Because you take a blood thinner, you will be seen regularly by the doctor who prescribed the medicine. You may also see other doctors for different problems. When you see other doctors, it is very important that you tell them you are taking a blood thinner. You should also tell your dentist and the person who cleans your teeth.

If you use different pharmacies, make sure each pharmacist knows that you take a blood thinner.

Blood thinners can interact with medicines and treatments that other doctors might prescribe for you. If another doctor orders a new medicine for you, tell the doctor who ordered your blood thinner because dose changes for your blood thinner may be needed.

Blood Tests

You might have to have your blood tested often if you are taking a blood thinner. The blood test helps your doctor decide how much medicine you need.

The International Normalized Ratio (INR) blood test measures how fast your blood clots and lets the doctor know if your dose needs to be changed. Testing your blood helps your doctor keep you in a safe range. If there is too much blood thinner in your body, you could bleed too much. If there is not enough, you could get a blood clot.

Once the blood test is in the target range and the correct dose is reached, this test is done less often. Because your dose is based on the INR blood test, it is very important that you get your blood tested on the date and at the time that you are told.

Illness can affect your INR blood test and your blood thinner dose. If you become sick with a fever, the flu, or an infection, call your doctor. Also call if you have diarrhea or vomiting lasting more than 1 day.

Section 50.2

Aspirin for Reducing the Risk of Heart Attack or Stroke

From text by the U.S. Food and Drug Administration
(FDA, www.fda.gov), April 30, 2009.

You can walk into any pharmacy, grocery, or convenience store and buy aspirin without a prescription. The Drug Facts label on medication products will help you choose aspirin for relieving headache, pain, swelling, or fever. The Drug Facts label also gives directions that will help you use the aspirin so that it is safe and effective.

But what about using aspirin for a different use, time period, or in a manner that is not listed on the label? For example, using aspirin to lower the risk of heart attack and clot-related strokes. In these cases, the labeling information is not there to help you with how to choose and how to use the medicine safely. Since you don't have the labeling directions to help you, you need the medical knowledge of your doctor, nurse practitioner or other health professional.

You can increase the chance of getting the good effects and decrease the chance of getting the bad effects of any medicine by choosing and using it wisely.

Fact: Daily use of aspirin is not right for everyone.

Aspirin has been shown to be helpful when used daily to lower the risk of heart attack, clot-related strokes, and other blood flow problems. Many medical professionals prescribe aspirin for these uses. There may be a benefit to daily aspirin use for you if you have some kind of heart or blood vessel disease or if you have evidence of poor blood flow to the brain. However, the risks of long-term aspirin use may be greater than the benefits if there are no signs of or risk factors for heart or blood vessel disease.

Every prescription and over-the-counter medicine has benefits and risks—even such a common and familiar medicine as aspirin. Aspirin use can result in serious side effects, such as stomach bleeding, bleeding in the brain, kidney failure, and some kinds of strokes. No medicine is completely safe. By carefully reviewing many different factors, your health professional can help you make the best choice for you.

When you don't have the labeling directions to guide you, you need the medical knowledge of your doctor, nurse practitioner, or other health professional.

Fact: Daily aspirin can be safest when prescribed by a medical health professional.

Before deciding if daily aspirin use is right for you, your health professional will need to consider the following factors:

- Your medical history and the history of your family members
- Your use of other medicines, including prescription and over-the-counter
- Your use of other products, such as dietary supplements, including vitamins and herbals
- Your allergies or sensitivities and anything that affects your ability to use the medicine
- What you have to gain, or the benefits, from the use of the medicine
- Other options and their risks and benefits
- What side effects you may experience
- What dose and what directions for use are best for you
- How to know when the medicine is working or not working for this use

Make sure to tell your health professional all the medicines (prescription and over-the-counter) and dietary supplements, including vitamins and herbals, that you use—even if only occasionally.

Fact: Aspirin is a drug.

If you are at risk for heart attack or stroke your doctor may prescribe aspirin to increase blood flow to the heart and brain. But any drug—including aspirin—can have harmful side effects, especially when mixed with other products. In fact, the chance of side effects increases with each new product you use.

New products includes prescription and other over-the-counter medicines, dietary supplements, (including vitamins and herbals), and sometimes foods and beverages. For instance, people who already use a prescribed medication to thin the blood should not use aspirin unless recommended by a health professional. There are also dietary supplements known to thin the blood. Using aspirin with alcohol or with another product that also contains aspirin, such as a cough-sinus drug, can increase the chance of side effects.

Your health professional will consider your current state of health. Some medical conditions, such as pregnancy, uncontrolled high blood pressure, bleeding disorders, asthma, peptic (stomach) ulcers, liver and kidney disease, could make aspirin a bad choice for you.

Make sure that all your health professionals are aware that you are using aspirin to reduce your risk of heart attack and clot-related strokes.

Fact: Once your doctor decides that daily use of aspirin is for you, safe use depends on following your doctor's directions.

There are no directions on the label for using aspirin to reduce the risk of heart attack or clot-related stroke. You may rely on your health professional to provide the correct information on dose and directions for use. Using aspirin correctly gives you the best chance of getting the greatest benefits with the fewest unwanted side effects. Discuss with your health professional the different forms of aspirin products that might be best suited for you.

Aspirin has been shown to lower the risk of heart attack and stroke, but not all over-the-counter pain and fever reducers do that. Even though the directions on the aspirin label do not apply to this use of aspirin, you still need to read the label to confirm that the product you buy and use contains aspirin at the correct dose. Check the Drug Facts label for "active ingredients: aspirin" or "acetylsalicylic acid" at the dose that your health professional has prescribed.

Remember, if you are using aspirin everyday for weeks, months, or years to prevent a heart attack, stroke, or for any use not listed on the label—without the guidance from your health professional—you could be doing your body more harm than good.

Section 50.3

Blood Pressure Medications

Excerpted from "High Blood Pressure—Medicines to Help You,"
by the U.S. Food and Drug Administration (FDA, www.fda.gov),
October 8, 2009.

It is important to take your blood pressure medicines every day.
Take your medicines even when your blood pressure comes down—
even when you do not feel bad. Do not stop taking your medicine until your doctor says that it is OK.

Most people who take high blood pressure medicines do not get any
side effects. Like all medicines, high blood pressure medicines can
sometimes cause side effects. Some people have common problems like
headaches, dizziness, or an upset stomach. These problems are small
compared to what could happen if you do not take your medicine.

High Blood Pressure Medicines

Use this information to help you talk to your doctor about your
blood pressure medicines. Ask your doctor about the risks of taking
your medicine. This information only talks about some of the risks.

Tell your doctor about any problems you are having. Also, tell your
doctor if you are pregnant, nursing, or planning to get pregnant. Your
doctor will help you find the medicine that is best for you.

The different kinds of blood pressure medicines are listed in the
following text. The drugs are listed in groups. The brand names and
generic names are given for the drugs in each group.

Find your drug. Then read some basic information about your kind
of drug.

Types of High Blood Pressure Medicines

- ACE [angiotensin-converting enzyme] inhibitors
- Beta-blockers
- Calcium channel blockers

- Peripherally acting alpha-adrenergic blockers
- Angiotensin II antagonists
- Vasodilators
- Centrally-acting alpha adrenergics
- Combination medicines
- Diuretics (sometimes called water pills)
- Renin inhibitors

ACE Inhibitors: What You Should Know

For brand and generic names of ACE inhibitors see Table 50.1.

Warnings

- Women who are pregnant should talk to their doctor about the risks of using these drugs late in pregnancy.
- People who have kidney or liver problems, diabetes, or heart problems should talk to their doctor about the risks of using ACE drugs.
- People taking diuretics (water pills) should talk to their doctor about the risks of using ACE drugs.

Common Side Effects

- Cough
- Dizziness

Table 50.1. Angiotensin-Converting Enzyme (ACE) Inhibitors

Brand Name	Generic Name
Aceon	Perindopril
Accupril	Quinapril
Altace	Ramipril
Capoten	Captopril
Lotensin	Benazepril
Mavik	Trandolapril
Monopril	Fosinopril
Prinivil	Lisinopril
Univasc	Moexipril
Vasotec	Enalapril
Zestril	Lisinopril

- Feeling tired
- Headache
- Problems sleeping
- Fast heartbeat

Warning Signs

Call your doctor if you have any of these signs:

- Chest pain
- Problems breathing or swallowing
- Swelling in the face, eyes, lips, tongue, or legs

Beta-Blockers: What You Should Know

For brand and generic names of beta-blockers, see Table 50.2.

Warnings

- Do not use these drugs if you have slow heart rate, heart block, or shock.
- Women who are pregnant or nursing should talk to their doctor before they start using beta-blockers.
- The elderly and people who have kidney or liver problems, asthma, diabetes, or overactive thyroid should talk to their doctor about the specific risks of using any of these beta-blockers.

Common Side Effects

- Feeling tired
- Upset stomach
- Headache
- Dizziness
- Constipation/diarrhea
- Feeling lightheaded

Warning Signs

Call your doctor if you have any of these signs:

- Chest pain
- Problems breathing

- Slow or irregular heartbeat
- Swelling in the hands, feet, or legs

Table 50.2. Beta-Blockers

Brand Name	Generic Name
Bystolic	Nebivolol
	Timolol
Coreg	Carvedilol
Corgard	Nadolol
Inderal	Propranolol
Inderal LA	Propranolol
Kerlone	Betaxolol
Levatol	Penbutolol
Lopressor	Metoprolol
Sectral	Acebutolol
Tenormin	Atenolol
Toprol XL	Metoprolol
Trandate	Labetalol
Visken	Pindolol
Zebeta	Bisoprolol

Table 50.3. Calcium Channel Blockers

Brand Name	Generic Name
Norvasc	Amlodipine
Cleviprex	Clevidipine
Cardizem	Diltiazem
Dilacor XR	Diltiazem
Tiazac	Diltiazem
Plendil	Felodipine
DynaCirc CR	Isradipine
Cardene	Nicardipine
Adalat CC	Nifedipine
Procardia	Nifedipine
	Nimodipine
Sular	Nisoldipine
Calan	Verapamil
Covera HS	Verapamil
Isoptin	Verapamil
Verelan	Verapamil

Calcium Channel Blockers: What You Should Know

For brand and generic names of calcium channel blockers, see Table 50.3.

Warnings

- Do not use calcium channel blockers if you have a heart condition or if you are taking nitrates, quinidine, or fentanyl.
- People who have liver or kidney problems should talk to their doctor about the specific risks of using any calcium channel blocker.
- Women who are pregnant or nursing should talk to their doctor before they start using these drugs.

Common Side Effects

- Feeling drowsy
- Headache
- Upset stomach
- Ankle swelling
- Feeling flushed (warm)

Warning Signs

Call your doctor if you have any of these signs:

- Chest pain
- Serious rashes
- Swelling of the face, eyes, lips, tongue, arms, or legs
- Fainting
- Irregular heartbeat

Peripherally Acting Alpha-Adrenergic Blockers: What You Should Know

For brand and generic names of peripherally acting alpha-adrenergic blockers, see Table 50.4.

Warnings

The elderly and people who have liver problems should talk to their doctor about the risks of using these drugs.

Common Side Effects

- Dizziness
- Feeling tired
- Feeling lightheaded
- Vision problems
- Swelling of the hands, feet, ankles, or legs
- Decreased sexual ability

Warning Signs

Call your doctor if you have any of these signs:

- Chest pain
- Irregular heartbeat
- Painful erection in men

Table 50.4. Peripherally Acting Alpha-Adrenergic Blockers

Brand Name	Generic Name
Cardura	Doxazosin
Dibenzyline	Phenoxybenzamine
Minipress	Prazosin
Hytrin	Terazosin

Vasodilators: What You Should Know

For generic names of vasodilators, see Table 50.5.

Warnings

- Do not use these drugs if you are also taking bisulfates.
- Women who are pregnant or nursing should talk to their doctor before they start using these drugs.
- People who have diabetes, heart disease, or uremia (buildup of waste in your blood) should talk to their doctor about the risks of using any of these drugs.
- People taking diuretics (water pills), insulin, phenytoin, corticosteroids, estrogen, warfarin, or progesterone should talk to their doctor about the risks of using any of these drugs.

Common Side Effects

- Headache
- Upset stomach
- Dizziness
- Growth in body hair

Warning Signs

Call your doctor if you have any of these signs:

- Fever
- Fast heartbeat
- Fainting
- Chest pain
- Problems breathing
- Sudden weight gain

Table 50.5. Vasodilators

Brand Name	Generic Name
	Hydralazine
	Minoxidil

Angiotensin II Antagonists: What You Should Know

For brand and generic names of angiotensin II antagonists, see Table 50.6.

Warnings

- Do not use these drugs if you are pregnant or nursing.
- People who have kidney disease, liver disease, low blood volume, or low salt in their blood should talk to their doctor about the risks of taking these drugs.
- People taking diuretics (water pills) should talk to their doctor about the risks of taking these drugs.

Common Side Effects

- Sore throat

Table 50.6. Angiotensin II Antagonists

Brand Name	Generic Name
Atacand	Candesartan
Avapro	Irbesartan
Benicar	Olmesartan
Cozaar	Losartan
Diovan	Valsartan
Micardis	Telmisartan
Teveten	Eprosartan

- Sinus problems
- Heartburn
- Dizziness
- Diarrhea
- Back pain

Warning Signs

Call your doctor if you have any of these signs:

- Problems breathing
- Fainting
- Swelling of the face, throat, lips, eyes, hands, feet, ankles, or legs

Centrally-Acting Alpha Adrenergics: What You Should Know

For brand and generic names of centrally-acting alpha adrenergics, see Table 50.7.

Table 50.7. Centrally-Acting Alpha Adrenergics

Brand Name	Generic Name
Catapres	Clonidine
Tenex	Guanfacine

Warnings

- Women who are pregnant or nursing should talk to their doctor before using these drugs.
- People with heart disease, recent heart attack, or kidney disease should talk to their doctor before using these drugs.
- Drinking alcohol may make side effects worse.

Common Side Effects

- Dizziness
- Dry mouth
- Upset stomach
- Feeling drowsy or tired

Warning Signs

Call your doctor if you have any of these signs:

- Fainting
- Slow or irregular heartbeat
- Fever
- Swollen ankles or feet

Combination Drugs: What You Should Know

For brand and generic names of combination drugs, see Table 50.8.

- These medicines are made up of two different kinds of blood pressure medicines.
- The warnings and side effects for brand-name drugs vary depending on the generic drugs they contain.

Caduet

Caduet is used to treat people who have both high blood pressure and high cholesterol.

- Do not take Caduet if you are pregnant or planning to become pregnant.
- Do not take Caduet if you are breastfeeding.
- Do not take Caduet if you have liver problems.

Common side effects of Caduet include the following:

- Swelling of the legs or ankles (edema)
- Muscle or joint pain
- Headache
- Diarrhea or constipation
- Feeling dizzy
- Feeling tired or sleepy
- Gas
- Rash
- Nausea
- Stomach pain
- Fast or irregular heartbeat
- Face feels hot or warm (flushing)

Call your doctor if you have any of these signs:

- Muscle problems like weakness, tenderness, or pain that happens without a good reason (like exercise or injury)
- Brown or dark-colored urine
- Skin or eyes look yellow (jaundice)
- Feel more tired than usual

Table 50.8. Combination Medicines

Brand Name	Generic Name
Diovan HCT	Hydrochlorothiazide and Valsartan
Exforge	Amlodipine and Valsartan
Hyzaar	Hydrochlorothiazide and Losartan
Lexxel	Enalapril and Felodipine
Lotrel	Benazepril and Amlodipine
Tarka	Verapamil and Trandolapril
Caduet	Amlodipine and Atorvastatin

Diuretics: What You Should Know

For brand and generic names of diuretics, see Table 50.9.

Warnings

- Tell you doctor if you are breastfeeding. These medicines may pass into your breast milk.
- Do not use these medicines if you have problems making urine.
- People with kidney or liver problems, pregnant women, and the elderly should talk to their doctor about the risks of using diuretics.

Common Side Effects

- Dizziness
- Frequent urination
- Headache
- Feeling thirsty
- Muscle cramps
- Upset stomach

Table 50.9. Diuretics

Brand Name	Generic Name
Aldactazide; Aldactone	Spironolactone
Demadex	Torsemide
Diuril	Chlorothiazide
Enduron	Methyclothiazide
Microzide; Oretic	Hydrochlorothiazide
Lasix	Furosemide
	Indapamide
Saluron	Hydroflumethiazide
Thalitone	Chlorthalidone
Zaroxolyn	Metolazone

Warning Signs

Call your doctor if you have any of these signs:

- Severe rash
- Problems breathing or swallowing
- Hyperuricemia (Gout)

Renin Inhibitors: What You Should Know

For brand and generic names of renin inhibitors, see Table 50.10.

Warnings

- Women who are pregnant or planning to become pregnant should talk to their doctor before using this drug.
- People with kidney problems should talk to their doctor before using this drug.
- Tell your doctor if you are taking water pills (diuretics), high blood pressure medicines, heart medicines, or medicines to treat a fungus.

Common Side Effects

- Diarrhea

Warning Signs

Call your doctor if you have any of these signs:

- Low blood pressure
- Swelling of the face, throat, lips, eyes, or tongue

Table 50.10. Renin Inhibitors

Brand Name	Generic Name
Tekturna	Aliskiren

Section 50.4

Digoxin

Dosage forms

- Oral tablets: 0.125 mg, 0.250 mg
- Oral capsules: 0.05 mg, 0.1 mg, 0.2 mg

About This Drug

Digoxin (dye-JOX-in) is used to improve the strength (contraction) of the heart. It is also commonly used to control heart rate and prevent irregular heartbeats.

Side Effects

Common side effects are:

- loss of appetite;
- nausea;
- diarrhea; and
- tiredness.

Rare side effects include:

- rash;
- confusion or hallucinations;
- blurred vision; and
- irregular or decreased heart beat.

If any of these side effects become severe or bother you, call your doctor. Do not take over-the-counter medicines for your symptoms.

Drug Interactions

Tell your doctor or pharmacist about any prescription medicine, over-the-counter medicine, or herbal products that you are taking. He or she will check for interactions.

If You Miss a Dose

If you miss a medicine dose, take it as soon as you remember—if it is within 12 hours of when you were supposed to take it. If it has been more than 12 hours since your scheduled dose time, skip that dose. Take your next dose at its scheduled time, and continue your usual dosing schedule. Do not "double up" on doses to catch up.

Don't Stop Taking This Medicine

Do not stop taking this medicine unless your doctor tells you to.

How to Take This Medicine

Take this medicine every morning (once a day), unless your doctor tells you otherwise. You may take it with or without food.

Section 50.5

Nitroglycerin for Chest Pain

Why is this medication prescribed?

Nitroglycerin is used to prevent chest pain (angina). It works by relaxing the blood vessels to the heart, so the blood flow and oxygen supply to the heart is increased.

This medication is sometimes prescribed for other uses; ask your doctor or pharmacist for more information.

How should this medicine be used?

Nitroglycerin comes as a sublingual tablet, buccal tablet, extended-release (long-acting) capsule, or spray to be used orally. The buccal extended-release tablets and the extended-release tablets and capsules are usually taken three to six times a day. Do not crush, chew, or divide the extended-release tablets or capsules. The sublingual tablet and spray are used as needed to relieve chest pain that has already started or to prevent pain before activities known to provoke attacks (e.g., climbing stairs, sexual activity, heavy exercise, or cold weather). The buccal extended-release tablets also may be used during an attack and just before situations known to provoke attacks. Follow the directions on your prescription label carefully, and ask your doctor or pharmacist to explain any part you do not understand. Take nitroglycerin exactly as directed. Do not take more or less of it or take it more often than prescribed by your doctor.

Nitroglycerin controls chest pain but does not cure it. Continue to use nitroglycerin even if you feel well. Do not stop taking nitroglycerin without talking to your doctor. Stopping the drug abruptly may cause chest pain.

Nitroglycerin can lose its effectiveness when used for a long time. This effect is called tolerance. If your angina attacks happen more often, last longer, or are more severe, call your doctor.

443

If you are using the buccal extended-release tablet, place the tablet between your cheek and gum and allow it to dissolve. Do not chew or swallow it. If you feel dizzy, sit down after placing the tablet in your mouth. Try not to swallow saliva until the tablet dissolves. Buccal extended-release tablets start to work within 2 to 3 minutes. To make the tablet dissolve faster, touch it with your tongue before placing it in your mouth or drink a hot liquid. If an attack occurs while you have a buccal extended-release tablet in place, place a second tablet on the opposite side of your mouth. If chest pain persists, use sublingual tablets, call for emergency assistance, or go to a hospital emergency department immediately.

If you are taking nitroglycerin sublingual tablets or spray for acute chest pain, you should carry the tablets and spray with you at all times. Sit down when an acute attack occurs. The drug starts to work within 2 minutes and goes on working for up to 30 minutes. If you are taking nitroglycerin tablets and your chest pain is not relieved within 5 minutes, take another dose. If you are using nitroglycerin spray and your chest pain is not relieved in 3 to 5 minutes, repeat the process. Call for emergency assistance or go to a hospital emergency department if pain persists after you have taken three tablets (at 5-minute intervals) or have used three sprays (at 3- to 5-minute intervals) and 15 minutes have passed.

To use the tablets, place a tablet under your tongue or between your cheek and gum and allow it to dissolve. Do not swallow the tablet. Try not to swallow saliva too often until the tablet dissolves.

To use the spray, follow these steps:

- Do not shake the drug container. Hold it upright with the opening of the spray mechanism as close as possible to your opened mouth.

- Press the spray mechanism with your forefinger to release the spray. Spray the drug onto or under your tongue and close your mouth immediately. Do not inhale or swallow the spray.

Other uses for this medicine: Nitroglycerin tablets also are used with other drugs to treat congestive heart failure and heart attacks. Talk to your doctor about the possible risks of using this drug for your condition.

What special precautions should I follow?

Before taking nitroglycerin:

- Tell your doctor and pharmacist if you are allergic to nitroglycerin, isosorbide (Imdur, Isordil, Sorbitrate), or any other drugs.

- Tell your doctor and pharmacist what prescription and nonprescription medications you are taking, especially aspirin; beta-blockers such as atenolol (Tenormin), carteolol (Cartrol), labetalol (Normodyne, Trandate), metoprolol (Lopressor), nadolol (Corgard), propranolol (Inderal), sotalol (Betapace), and timolol (Blocadren); calcium channel blockers such as amlodipine (Norvasc), diltiazem (Cardizem), felodipine (Plendil), isradipine (DynaCirc), nifedipine (Procardia), and verapamil (Calan, Isoptin); dihydroergotamine (D.H.E. 45); sildenafil (Viagra); and vitamins.

- Tell your doctor if you have low red blood cell counts (anemia), glaucoma, or recent head trauma.

- Tell your doctor if you are pregnant, plan to become pregnant, or are breastfeeding. If you become pregnant while taking nitroglycerin, call your doctor.

- If you are having surgery, including dental surgery, tell the doctor or dentist that you are taking nitroglycerin.

- You should know that this drug may make you drowsy or dizzy. Do not drive a car or operate machinery until you know how it affects you.

- Ask your doctor about the safe use of alcoholic beverages while you are taking nitroglycerin. Alcohol can make the side effects from nitroglycerin worse.

What special dietary instructions should I follow?

Take nitroglycerin extended-release tablets and capsules on an empty stomach with a full glass of water.

What should I do if I forget a dose?

Take the missed dose as soon as you remember it. However, if it is almost time for the next dose, skip the missed dose and continue your regular dosing schedule. Do not take a double dose to make up for a missed one.

What side effects can this medication cause?

Side effects from nitroglycerin are common. Tell your doctor if any of these symptoms are severe or do not go away:

- Headache
- Rash
- Dizziness
- Upset stomach
- Flushing (feeling of warmth)

If you experience any of the following symptoms, call your doctor immediately:

- Blurred vision
- Dry mouth
- Chest pain
- Fainting

If you experience a serious side effect, you or your doctor may send a report to the Food and Drug Administration's (FDA) MedWatch Adverse Event Reporting program online [at http://www.fda.gov/Med Watch/index.html] or by phone [800-332-1088].

What storage conditions are needed for this medicine?

Keep this medication in the container it came in, tightly closed, and out of reach of children. Store it at room temperature and away from excess heat and moisture (not in the bathroom). Avoid puncturing the spray container and keep it away from excess heat. Do not open a container of sublingual nitroglycerin until you need a dose. Do not use tablets that are more than 12 months old. Throw away any medication that is outdated or no longer needed. Talk to your pharmacist about the proper disposal of your medication.

In case of emergency/overdose: In case of overdose, call your local poison control center at 800-222-1222. If the victim has collapsed or is not breathing, call local emergency services at 911.

What other information should I know?

Keep all appointments with your doctor and the laboratory. Nitroglycerin extended-release capsules should not be used for acute angina attacks. Continue to use nitroglycerin tablets or spray to relieve chest pain that has already started.

If headache continues, ask your doctor if you may take acetaminophen. Your nitroglycerin dose may need to be adjusted. Do not take aspirin or any other medication for headache while taking nitroglycerin unless your doctor tells you to.

The tablets may cause a sweet, tingling sensation when placed under your tongue. This sensation is not an accurate indicator of drug strength; the absence of a tingling sensation does not mean that the drug is not working.

Do not let anyone else take your medication. Ask your pharmacist any questions you have about refilling your prescription.

It is important for you to keep a written list of all of the prescription and nonprescription (over-the-counter) medicines you are taking, as well as any products such as vitamins, minerals, or other dietary supplements. You should bring this list with you each time you visit a doctor or if you are admitted to a hospital. It is also important information to carry with you in case of emergencies.

Brand Names

- Nitro-Bid®
- Nitrogard®
- Nitroglycerin Slocaps®
- Nitrolingual® Pumpspray
- NitroQuick®
- Nitrostat®
- NitroTab®
- Nitro-Time®

Section 50.6

Statins to Control Cholesterol

From "Controlling Cholesterol with Statins," by the U.S. Food and Drug Administration (FDA, www.fda.gov), October 27, 2009.

When it comes to keeping your heart healthy, what foods you eat and the genes you inherit matter. Good heart health also may depend on the drugs you take. Several medicines are effective at lowering blood cholesterol levels—a key factor in good heart health. Chief among them are the statins.

Statins (HMG-CoA reductase inhibitors) are one class of many drugs used to lower the level of cholesterol in the blood by reducing the production of cholesterol by the liver. Statins block the enzyme in the liver that is responsible for making cholesterol. Too much cholesterol can increase a person's chance of getting heart disease. According to the Centers for Disease Control and Prevention, heart disease is the leading cause of death for both women and men in the United States.

Understanding Cholesterol

Cholesterol is a waxy substance found in all parts of the body. It is critical to the normal function of all cells. The body needs cholesterol for making hormones, digesting dietary fats, building cell walls, and other important processes. Your body makes all the cholesterol it needs, but cholesterol is also in some of the foods you eat.

When there is too much cholesterol in your blood, it can build up on the walls of the arteries (blood vessels that carry blood from the heart to other parts of the body). This buildup is called plaque. Over time, plaques can cause narrowing or hardening of the arteries—a condition called atherosclerosis. In short, too much cholesterol can clog your arteries and keep your heart from getting the blood it needs.

Cholesterol Numbers That Matter

There are no warning symptoms of high cholesterol. But a simple blood test by your doctor will measure the different kinds of cholesterol.

Low-density lipoprotein (LDL) or "bad" cholesterol can clog the arteries. Lower numbers of LDL are best. The higher the LDL level, the greater the risk for heart disease.

High-density lipoprotein (HDL) or "good" cholesterol carries bad cholesterol out of your blood, back to the liver, where it can be eliminated, to keep it from building up in the arteries. The higher the HDL level, the lower the risk for heart disease.

What Affects Cholesterol?

The following factors affect blood cholesterol levels:

- **Certain foods**—Eating too much saturated fat, found mostly in animal products, and too much cholesterol, found only in animal products, can raise cholesterol.

- **Heredity**—Genes play a role in influencing the levels.

- **Weight**—Excess weight tends to increase the levels.

- **Exercise**—Regular physical activity may not only lower LDL cholesterol, but it may increase the level of desirable HDL cholesterol.

- **Smoking**—Cigarette smoking lowers HDL cholesterol.

- **Age and gender**—Cholesterol levels naturally rise as men and women age. Menopause is often associated with increased LDL cholesterol in women.

State of the Statins

The main goal of cholesterol treatment is to lower LDL to levels that will not lead to or worsen heart disease. When a patient without heart disease is first diagnosed with elevated blood cholesterol, the National Cholesterol Education Program guidelines advise a 6-month program of reduced dietary saturated fat and cholesterol, together with physical activity and weight control, as the primary treatment to bring levels down.

When diet and exercise alone are not enough to reduce cholesterol to goal levels, doctors often prescribe medication—the most prominent being the statins. By interfering with the production of cholesterol, statin medications can slow the formation of plaques in the arteries.

Statins are relatively safe for most people, but some can respond differently to the drugs. Certain people may have fewer side effects with one statin drug than another. Some statins, in particular Lovastatin and Simvastatin, also are known to interact adversely with other drugs. This information, coupled with the degree of cholesterol-lowering desired, will help guide the decision about which statin to use, or whether another type of drug should be used.

Statin medications (HMG-CoA reductase inhibitors) are prescribed keeping the following in mind:

- Statins work in the liver to prevent formation of cholesterol.
- Statins are effective in lowering bad cholesterol levels and raising good cholesterol.
- Statins are not recommended for pregnant patients or those with active or chronic liver disease.
- Statins can cause serious muscle problems.

Currently available statins including the following:

- Lovastatin (Mevacor, Altoprev)
- Pravastatin (Pravachol)
- Simvastatin (Zocor)
- Fluvastatin (Lescol)
- Atorvastatin (Lipitor)
- Rosuvastatin (Crestor)

Tips for Consumers

- Have your blood cholesterol levels checked at least once every 5 years if you are an adult 20 years or older.
- Check with your doctor. You may be able to lower your cholesterol levels by eating better and exercising more.
- Maintain a healthy weight. Being overweight increases your risk for heart disease.
- Stay active every day.
- Use the food label to choose foods lower in saturated fat, including trans fats, and calories.
- Eat more fruits and vegetables.
- Don't stop taking any cholesterol-lowering medications you may be on without first talking to your doctor.

Section 50.7

Stroke Medications

Excerpted from "Stroke: Hope Through Research," by the
National Institute of Neurological Disorders and Stroke (NINDS,
www.ninds.nih.gov), May 15, 2009.

Medication or drug therapy is the most common treatment for stroke. The most popular classes of drugs used to prevent or treat stroke are antithrombotics (antiplatelet agents and anticoagulants) and thrombolytics.

Antithrombotics prevent the formation of blood clots that can become lodged in a cerebral artery and cause strokes. Antiplatelet drugs prevent clotting by decreasing the activity of platelets, blood cells that contribute to the clotting property of blood. These drugs reduce the risk of blood-clot formation, thus reducing the risk of ischemic stroke. In the context of stroke, physicians prescribe antiplatelet drugs mainly for prevention. The most widely known and used antiplatelet drug is aspirin. Other antiplatelet drugs include clopidogrel, ticlopidine, and dipyridamole.

Anticoagulants reduce stroke risk by reducing the clotting property of the blood. The most commonly used anticoagulants include warfarin (also known as Coumadin®), heparin, and enoxaparin (also known as Lovenox).

Thrombolytic agents are used to treat an ongoing, acute ischemic stroke caused by an artery blockage. These drugs halt the stroke by dissolving the blood clot that is blocking blood flow to the brain. Recombinant tissue plasminogen activator (rt-PA) is a genetically engineered form of t-PA, a thrombolytic substance made naturally by the body. It can be effective if given intravenously within 3 hours of stroke symptom onset, but it should be used only after a physician has confirmed that the patient has suffered an ischemic stroke. Thrombolytic agents can increase bleeding and therefore must be used only after careful patient screening. The NINDS rt-PA Stroke Study showed the efficacy of t-PA and in 1996 led to the first FDA [U.S. Food and Drug Administration]-approved treatment for acute ischemic stroke. Other thrombolytics are currently being tested in clinical trials.

Neuroprotectants are medications that protect the brain from secondary injury caused by stroke. Although no neuroprotectants are FDA-approved for use in stroke at this time, many are in clinical trials. There are several different classes of neuroprotectants that show promise for future therapy, including glutamate antagonists, antioxidants, apoptosis inhibitors, and many others.

Chapter 51

Cardiac Catheterization

Cardiac catheterization is a medical procedure used to diagnose and treat certain heart conditions.

A long, thin, flexible tube called a catheter is put into a blood vessel in your arm, groin (upper thigh), or neck and threaded to your heart. Through the catheter, doctors can do diagnostic tests and treatments on your heart.

For example, your doctor may put a special dye in the catheter. This dye will flow through your bloodstream to your heart. Once the dye reaches your heart, it will make the inside of your coronary (heart) arteries show up on an x-ray. This test is called coronary angiography.

The dye can show whether a substance called plaque has narrowed or blocked any of your coronary arteries. Plaque is made up of fat, cholesterol, calcium, and other substances found in your blood.

Plaque narrows the inside of the arteries and, in time, may restrict blood flow to your heart. When plaque builds up in the coronary arteries, the condition is called coronary heart disease (CHD) or coronary artery disease.

Blockages in the coronary arteries also can be seen using ultrasound during cardiac catheterization. Ultrasound uses sound waves to create detailed pictures of the heart's blood vessels.

Doctors may take samples of blood and heart muscle during cardiac catheterization and do minor heart surgery.

Excerpted from text by the National Heart, Lung, and Blood Institute (NHLBI, www.nhlbi.nih.gov), part of the National Institutes of Health, May 2009.

Cardiologists (heart specialists) usually do cardiac catheterization in a hospital. You're awake during the procedure, and it causes little to no pain. However, you may feel some soreness in the blood vessel where the catheter was inserted. Cardiac catheterization rarely causes serious complications.

When Cardiac Catheterization Is Needed

Cardiac catheterization is used to diagnose and/or treat many heart conditions. Doctors may recommend this procedure for various reasons. The most common reason is to evaluate chest pain.

Chest pain may be a symptom of coronary heart disease (CHD). Cardiac catheterization can show whether plaque is narrowing or blocking your heart's arteries.

Doctors can treat CHD during cardiac catheterization with a procedure called angioplasty. During angioplasty, a tiny balloon is put through the catheter and into the blocked artery. When the balloon is inflated, it pushes the plaque against the artery wall. This creates a wider pathway for blood to flow to the heart.

Sometimes a stent is placed in the artery during angioplasty. A stent is a small mesh tube that's used to treat narrowed or weakened arteries in the body.

Most people who have heart attacks have partly or completely blocked coronary arteries. Thus, cardiac catheterization may be done on an emergency basis while you're having a heart attack. When used with angioplasty, the procedure allows your doctor to open up blocked arteries and prevent more damage to your heart.

Cardiac catheterization also can help your doctor figure out the best treatment for your CHD if you have experienced the following:

- Recently recovered from a heart attack, but are having chest pain
- Had a heart attack that caused major damage to your heart
- Had an EKG (electrocardiogram), stress test, or other test with results that suggested heart disease

You also may need cardiac catheterization if your doctor suspects you have a heart defect or if you're about to have heart surgery. The procedure shows the overall shape of your heart and the four large spaces (heart chambers) inside it. This inside view of the heart will show certain heart defects and help your doctor plan your heart surgery.

Sometimes doctors do cardiac catheterization to see how well the valves at the openings and exits of the heart chambers are working. Valves control the flow of blood in the heart.

To check your valves, your doctor will measure blood flow and oxygen levels in different parts of your heart. Cardiac catheterization also can check how well a man-made heart valve is working and how well your heart is pumping blood.

If your doctor thinks you have a heart infection or tumor, he or she may take samples of your heart muscle through the catheter. With the help of cardiac catheterization, doctors can even do minor heart surgery, such as repair certain heart defects.

What to Expect before Cardiac Catheterization

Before having cardiac catheterization, discuss the following with your doctor:

- How to prepare for the procedure

- Any medicines you're taking, and whether you should stop taking them before the procedure

- Whether you have diabetes, kidney disease, or other conditions that may require taking extra steps during or after the procedure to avoid complications

It may not be safe to drive after having cardiac catheterization, so you must arrange for a ride home.

What to Expect during Cardiac Catheterization

Cardiac catheterization is done in a hospital. During the procedure, you'll be kept on your back and awake. This allows you to follow your doctor's instructions during the procedure. You'll be given medicine to help you relax, which may make you sleepy.

Your doctor will numb the area on the arm, groin (upper thigh), or neck where the catheter will enter your blood vessel. A needle is used to make a small hole in the blood vessel. Through this hole your doctor will put a tapered tube called a sheath.

Next, your doctor will put a thin, flexible wire through the sheath and into your blood vessel. This guide wire is then threaded through your blood vessel to your heart. The wire helps your doctor position the catheter correctly. Your doctor then puts a catheter through the sheath and slides it over the guide wire and into the coronary arteries.

Special x-ray movies are taken of the guide wire and the catheter as they're moved into the heart. The movies help your doctor see where to position the tip of the catheter.

When the catheter reaches the right spot, your doctor will use it to do tests or treatments on your heart. For example, your doctor may do angioplasty and stenting.

During the procedure, your doctor may put a special dye in the catheter. This dye will flow through your bloodstream to your heart. Once the dye reaches your heart, it will make the inside of your heart's arteries show up on an x-ray called an angiogram. This test is called coronary angiography.

Coronary angiography can show how well blood is being pumped out of the heart's main pumping chambers, which are called ventricles. When the catheter is inside your heart, your doctor may use it to take blood samples from different parts of the heart or to do minor heart surgery.

To get a more detailed view of a blocked coronary artery, your doctor may do intracoronary ultrasound. For this test, your doctor will thread a tiny ultrasound device through the catheter and into the artery. This device gives off sound waves that bounce off the artery wall (and its blockage) to make an image of the inside of the artery.

If the angiogram or intracoronary ultrasound shows blockages or other possible problems in the heart's arteries, your doctor may use angioplasty to open the blocked arteries.

After your doctor does all of the needed tests or treatments, he or she will pull back the catheter and take it out along with the sheath. The opening left in the blood vessel will then be closed up and bandaged. A small weight may be put on top of the bandage for a few hours to apply more pressure. This will help prevent major bleeding from the site.

What to Expect after Cardiac Catheterization

After cardiac catheterization, you will be moved to a special care area. You will rest there for several hours or overnight. During that time, your movement will be limited to avoid bleeding from the site where the catheter was inserted.

While you recover in this area, nurses will check your heart rate and blood pressure regularly. They also will check for bleeding from the catheter insertion site.

A small bruise may develop on your arm, groin (upper thigh), or neck at the site where the catheter was inserted. That area may feel sore or tender for about a week. Let your doctor know if you develop problems such as the following:

- A constant or large amount of bleeding at the insertion site that can't be stopped with a small bandage
- Unusual pain, swelling, redness, or other signs of infection at or near the insertion site

Talk to your doctor about whether you should avoid certain activities, such as heavy lifting, for a short time after the procedure.

Risks of Cardiac Catheterization

Cardiac catheterization is a common medical procedure that rarely causes serious problems. However, complications can include the following:

- Bleeding, infection, and pain where the catheter was inserted
- An allergic reaction to the dye used
- Damage to blood vessels

Rarely, the catheter may scrape or poke a hole in a blood vessel as it's threaded to the heart.

Other, less common complications of the procedure include the following:

- Arrhythmias (irregular heartbeats) can occur. These often go away on their own, but may need treatment if they persist.
- Damage to the kidneys caused by the dye used may occur.
- Blood clots that can trigger stroke, heart attack, or other serious problems can develop as a complication.
- Low blood pressure may occur.
- A buildup of blood or fluid in the sac that surrounds the heart may develop. This fluid can prevent the heart from beating properly.

As with any procedure involving the heart, complications can sometimes be fatal. However, this is rare with cardiac catheterization.

The risk of complications with cardiac catheterization is higher if you have diabetes or kidney disease or if you're aged 75 or older. The risk of complications also is greater in women and in people having cardiac catheterization on an emergency basis.

Chapter 52

Catheter Ablation

Catheter ablation is a medical procedure used to treat some arrhythmias. An arrhythmia is a problem with the speed or rhythm of the heartbeat.

During catheter ablation, a long, thin, flexible tube is put into a blood vessel in your arm, groin (upper thigh), or neck. This tube is called an ablation catheter. It's then guided to your heart through the blood vessel. A special machine sends energy through the catheter to your heart. This energy finds and destroys small areas of heart tissue where abnormal heartbeats may cause an arrhythmia to start.

Overview

The heart's electrical system controls the speed and rhythm of your heartbeat. With each heartbeat, an electrical signal spreads from the top of the heart to the bottom. As it travels, the electrical signal causes the heart to contract and pump blood.

The process repeats with each new heartbeat. A problem with any part of this process can cause an arrhythmia.

Catheter ablation is one of several treatments for arrhythmia. Your doctor may recommend it if the following apply to you:

- The medicines you take don't control your arrhythmia.

Excerpted from text by the National Heart, Lung, and Blood Institute (NHLBI, www.nhlbi.nih.gov), part of the National Institutes of Health, November 2007.

- You can't tolerate the medicines your doctor has prescribed for your arrhythmia.
- You have certain types of arrhythmia, such as Wolff-Parkinson-White syndrome.

Though few, catheter ablation has risks. These include bleeding, infection, and pain where the catheter is inserted. More serious problems include blood clots and puncture of the heart. Your doctor will explain the risks to you.

Cardiologists (doctors who specialize in treating people with heart problems) sometimes perform ablation through open-heart surgery. But this method isn't as common as catheter ablation, which doesn't require surgery to open the chest cavity.

Outlook

Catheter ablation alone doesn't always restore a normal heart rate and rhythm. Other treatments may need to be used as well.

Also, some people who have the procedure may need to have it done again. This can happen when the first procedure doesn't fully correct the problem.

Other Names for Catheter Ablation

- Ablation
- Cardiac ablation
- Cardiac catheter ablation
- Radiofrequency ablation
- Catheter cryoblation

When Catheter Ablation Is Needed

Your doctor may recommend catheter ablation if the following apply to you:

- You have an arrhythmia that medicine can't control.
- You can't tolerate the medicines your doctor has prescribed for your arrhythmia.
- You have certain types of arrhythmia, such as Wolff-Parkinson-White syndrome or some forms of atrial fibrillation.

- You have abnormal electrical activity in your heart that raises your risk for ventricular fibrillation (a life-threatening arrhythmia) and sudden cardiac arrest.

What to Expect before Catheter Ablation

Before having catheter ablation, discuss the following with your doctor:

- Discuss how to prepare for the procedure, including limits on eating and drinking. You will likely need to stop eating and drinking by midnight before the procedure. Your doctor will give you specific instructions.

- Talk about any medicines you're taking, and whether you should stop taking them before the procedure.

- Mention whether you have diabetes, kidney disease, or other conditions that may require taking extra steps during or after the procedure to avoid complications.

Some people go home the same day as the procedure. Others need to stay overnight for 1 or more days. Driving after the procedure may not be safe. Your doctor will let you know if you need to arrange for someone to drive you home.

What to Expect during Catheter Ablation

Catheter ablation is done in a hospital. Doctors who do this procedure have special training in cardiac electrophysiology (the electrical system of the heart) and ablation (destruction) of diseased heart tissue.

At the Start

Before the procedure, you're given medicine through an intravenous (IV) line inserted in a vein in your arm. The medicine will help you relax. It may make you sleepy. You're also connected to several machines that check your heart's activity during the procedure.

Once you're drowsy, your doctor numbs an area on your arm, groin (upper thigh), or neck. A needle is used to make a small hole through the skin into a blood vessel. Your doctor puts a tapered tube called a sheath through this hole.

461

Your doctor then puts a thin, flexible wire and an ablation catheter (a long, thin, flexible tube) through the sheath and into your blood vessel. The guide wire is threaded through your blood vessel to your heart. The wire helps your doctor place the catheter correctly.

Then, your doctor puts a special dye into the catheter. The dye makes the inside of your heart show up on special x-ray images called angiograms. The images help your doctor place the tip of the catheter in the correct spot in the heart.

During the Procedure

Electrodes at the end of the catheter are used to stimulate the heart and record its electrical activity. This helps your doctor learn where abnormal heartbeats are starting in your heart.

Your doctor aims the tip of the catheter at the small area of heart tissue where the abnormal heartbeats are starting. A special machine sends energy through the catheter to create a scar line, also called an ablation line. The types of energy used include radiofrequency (heat generated by electrodes), laser, or cryoablation, which uses very cold temperatures.

The scar line creates a barrier between the damaged heart tissue and the surrounding healthy heart tissue. This stops abnormal electrical signals from traveling to the rest of the heart and causing arrhythmias.

What You May Feel

You may sleep on and off during the procedure. You generally will not feel anything except for the following:

- A burning sensation when the doctor injects medicine into the area where the catheter will be inserted

- Discomfort or burning in your chest when the energy is applied

- A faster heartbeat during studies of your heart's electrical system

The procedure lasts 3 to 6 hours. When the procedure is done, your doctor will pull back the ablation catheter and take it out along with the sheath and guide wire.

The opening left in the blood vessel is closed and bandaged. Nurses apply pressure to this site to help prevent major bleeding and to help the site begin to heal.

What to Expect after Catheter Ablation

After the procedure, you're moved to a special care unit where you lie still for 4 to 6 hours of recovery. Lying still prevents bleeding at the site where the catheter was inserted.

While you're in the special care unit, you're connected to special devices that measure your heart's electrical activity and blood pressure. The nurses check these monitors continuously. Nurses also check to make sure that there's no bleeding at the catheter insertion site.

Going Home

Your doctor determines whether you need to stay overnight in the hospital. Some people go home the same day. Others need to stay overnight for 1 or more days.

Before you go home, your doctor will tell you the following:

• Which medicines you need to take

• How much physical activity you can do

• How to care for the area where the catheter was inserted

• When to see the doctor again

Driving after the procedure may not be safe. Your doctor will let you know if you need to arrange for someone to drive you home.

Recovery and Recuperation

Recovery from catheter ablation is usually quick. You may feel stiff and achy from lying still for 4 to 6 hours after the procedure. In addition, a small bruise may form at the site where the ablation catheter was inserted. The area may feel sore or tender for about a week. Most people are able to return to normal activity in a few days.

Talk to your doctor about signs and symptoms to watch for. Let your doctor know if you have problems such as the following:

• A constant or large amount of bleeding at the catheter insertion site that you can't stop with a small bandage

• Unusual pain, swelling, redness, or other signs of infection at or near the catheter insertion site

• Strong, rapid, or other irregular heartbeats

• Fainting

Risks of Catheter Ablation

Though few, catheter ablation does have risks. Possible problems include the following:

- Bleeding, infection, and pain where the catheter was inserted are risks of catheter ablation.

- Damage to blood vessels is another risk of catheter ablation. This complication is very rare. It's caused by the catheter scraping or poking a hole in a blood vessel as it's guided to the heart.

- Puncture of the heart may occur.

- Damage to the heart's electrical system may lead to the need for a permanent pacemaker. A pacemaker is a small device that's placed under the skin of your chest or abdomen to help control abnormal heart rhythms.

- Blood clots, which could lead to stroke or other damage, may occur.

- Narrowing of the veins that carry blood from the lungs to the heart, called stenosis, is a risk of catheter ablation.

As with any heart procedure, complications can sometimes, although rarely, be fatal. The risk of complications is higher if you have diabetes or kidney disease. It also is higher if you're 75 years old or older.

Chapter 53

Cardioversion

What Is Cardioversion?

Cardioversion is a procedure used to restore a fast or irregular heartbeat to a normal rhythm. A fast or irregular heartbeat is called an arrhythmia.

Arrhythmias can prevent your heart from pumping enough blood to your body. They also can raise your risk for stroke, heart attack, or sudden cardiac arrest.

Overview

To understand arrhythmias, it helps to understand how the heart works. Your heart has an internal electrical system that controls the rate and rhythm of your heartbeat. With each heartbeat, an electrical signal spreads from the top of your heart to the bottom.

As it travels, the signal causes your heart to contract and pump blood. The process repeats with each new heartbeat.

A problem with any part of this process can cause an arrhythmia. During an arrhythmia, the heart can beat too fast, too slow, or with an irregular rhythm. Cardioversion is used to correct fast or irregular heartbeats.

Cardioversion is done two ways: using an electrical procedure or using medicines.

From text by the National Heart, Lung, and Blood Institute (NHLBI, www .nhlbi.nih.gov), part of the National Institutes of Health, July 2008.

For the electrical procedure, low-energy shocks are given to your heart to trigger a normal rhythm. You're temporarily put to sleep before the shocks are given. This type of cardioversion is done in a hospital as an outpatient procedure. This means you can go home after the procedure is done.

Cardioversion also can be done by taking medicines that correct arrhythmias. This type of cardioversion usually is done in the hospital. It also can be done at home or in a doctor's office.

This text only discusses the electrical procedure.

Many doctors prefer to do electrical cardioversions because they work better and are more predictable. It's also easier to find out right away if the procedure worked.

Cardioversion isn't the same as defibrillation, although they both involve shocking the heart. Defibrillation gives high-energy shocks to the heart to treat very irregular and severe arrhythmias. Defibrillation is used to restore normal heartbeats during life-threatening situations, such as cardiac arrest.

Outlook

Cardioversion successfully restores normal heart rhythms in more than 75 percent of people who have the procedure. However, fast or irregular heartbeats can occur again. For this reason, you may need to have more than one cardioversion over time.

The procedure has some risks. For example, it may worsen arrhythmias. However, serious complications are rare.

Who Needs Cardioversion?

You may need cardioversion if you have an arrhythmia that's causing troublesome symptoms. These symptoms may include dizziness, shortness of breath, extreme fatigue (tiredness), and chest discomfort.

Atrial fibrillation, or AF, is the most common type of arrhythmia treated with cardioversion. In AF, the electrical signals travel through the upper chambers of your heart (the atria) in a fast and disorganized way. This causes the atria to quiver instead of contract.

Atrial flutter, which is similar to AF, also may be treated with cardioversion. In atrial flutter, the electrical signals travel through the atria in a fast, but regular, rhythm.

Less commonly, you may have cardioversion to treat a rapid heart rhythm in the lower chambers of your heart.

You may need cardioversion on an emergency basis if your symptoms are severe. However, you usually schedule this procedure in advance.

Cardioversion may not be right for you if you have other heart conditions as well as an arrhythmia. Talk to your doctor about whether cardioversion is an option for you.

What to Expect before Cardioversion

You usually can't have any food or drinks for about 12 hours before the cardioversion (as your doctor advises).

You're at increased risk for dangerous blood clots during and after a cardioversion. This is because the procedure can dislodge blood clots that may have formed due to an arrhythmia. Your doctor may prescribe anticlotting medicine to prevent these clots. People often take this medicine for several weeks before the procedure and for several weeks to months after the procedure.

To find out whether you need anticlotting medicine, your doctor may have you undergo a transesophageal echocardiogram (TEE) before the cardioversion. A TEE is a special type of ultrasound. An ultrasound is a test that uses sound waves to look at the organs and structures in the body.

You will be given medicine to make you sleep during the TEE. A special wand that transmits sound waves is put on the end of a tube. The tube is put down your throat into your esophagus (the passage from your mouth to your stomach). The tube is placed close to your heart, and the sound waves create pictures of your heart. Your doctor will look at these pictures to see whether you have any blood clots.

The TEE will be scheduled for the same time as the cardioversion or just before the procedure. If blood clots are found, your cardioversion may be put off for a few weeks. During this time, you will take anticlotting medicine.

Even if no blood clots are found, you will be given anticlotting medicine through a vein during the cardioversion. You also will take medicine after the procedure to prevent blood clots.

Before a cardioversion, you're given medicine to make you sleep through the procedure. This medicine can affect your awareness when you wake up. You will need to arrange for someone to drive you home after the procedure.

What to Expect during Cardioversion

A nurse or technician will stick soft patches, called electrodes, on your chest and possibly on your back. Some shaving may be needed to get the patches to stick to your skin.

These patches are attached to a cardioversion machine. This machine records your heart's electrical activity. The machine also sends low-energy shocks through the patches to restore a normal heart rhythm.

Your nurse will use a needle to insert an intravenous (IV) line into a vein in your arm. Through this line, the doctor or nurse will give you medicine to make you fall asleep. While you're asleep, a cardiologist (heart specialist) will give one or more low-energy electrical shocks to your heart. You won't feel any pain from the shocks because of the medicine used to make you sleep.

Your heart rhythm and blood pressure will be closely watched during the procedure for any signs of complications.

Cardioversion takes just a few minutes. However, you will likely be in the hospital for a few hours due to the prep time and monitoring after the procedure.

What to Expect after Cardioversion

You will be closely watched for an hour or so after the procedure for any signs of complications. Your doctor or nurse will let you know when you can go home.

You may feel drowsy for several hours after the cardioversion because of the medicine used to make you sleep. You shouldn't drive or operate heavy machinery the day of the procedure. You will need to arrange for someone to drive you home from the hospital. Until the medicine wears off, it also may affect your awareness and ability to make decisions.

You may have some redness or soreness on your chest where the electrodes were placed. This may last for a few days after the procedure. You also may have slight bruising or soreness at the site where the intravenous (IV) line was inserted.

You will take medicine for several weeks to months after the procedure to prevent blood clots. During this time, you also may take medicine to prevent repeat arrhythmias.

What Are the Risks of Cardioversion?

Cardioversion can sometimes worsen arrhythmias. Rarely, it can cause life-threatening arrhythmias. These irregular heartbeats will occur within minutes of the procedure. They're treated right away with electrical shocks or medicines, so they usually don't cause serious problems.

Rarely, cardioversion can cause stroke or other complications due to blood clots in the heart traveling to other organs or tissues. The risk of this happening is less than 5 percent if you take anticlotting drugs before and after the procedure.

Chapter 54

Implantable Cardioverter Defibrillators

An implantable cardioverter defibrillator (ICD) is a small device that's placed in your chest or abdomen. The device uses electrical pulses or shocks to help control life-threatening, irregular heartbeats, especially those that could cause sudden cardiac arrest (SCA).

SCA is a condition in which the heart suddenly and unexpectedly stops beating. If the heart stops beating, blood stops flowing to the brain and other vital organs. This usually causes death if it's not treated in minutes.

Overview

A problem with any part of the heart's electrical system can cause irregular heartbeats called arrhythmias. During an arrhythmia, the heart can beat too fast, too slow, or with an irregular rhythm. Faulty electrical signaling in the heart causes arrhythmias.

ICDs use electrical pulses or shocks to treat life-threatening arrhythmias that occur in the ventricles (the heart's lower chambers).

When ventricular arrhythmias occur, the heart can't effectively pump blood. You can pass out within seconds and die within minutes if not treated. To prevent death, the condition must be treated right away with an electric shock to the heart. This treatment is called defibrillation.

Excerpted from "Implantable Cardioverter Defibrillator," by the National Heart, Lung, and Blood Institute (NHLBI, www.nhlbi.nih.gov), part of the National Institutes of Health, August 2009.

An ICD has wires with electrodes on the ends that connect to your heart chambers. The ICD will continually monitor your heart rhythm. If the device detects an irregular rhythm in your ventricles, it will use low-energy electrical pulses to restore a normal rhythm.

If the low-energy pulses don't restore your normal heart rhythm, or if your ventricles start to quiver rather than contract strongly, the ICD will switch to high-energy electrical pulses for defibrillation. These pulses last only a fraction of a second, but they can be painful.

Doctors also treat arrhythmias with another device called a pacemaker. An ICD is similar to a pacemaker, but there are some differences.

Pacemakers can only give off low-energy electrical pulses. They're often used to treat less dangerous heart rhythms, such as those that occur in the upper chambers of your heart. Most new ICDs can act as both pacemakers and defibrillators.

Patients who have heart failure may need a special device called a cardiac resynchronization therapy (CRT) device. The CRT device is able to pace both ventricles at the same time. This allows them to work together and do a better job pumping blood out of the heart. CRT devices that have a defibrillator are called CRT-D.

Who Needs an Implantable Cardioverter Defibrillator?

Implantable cardioverter defibrillators (ICDs) are used in children, adolescents, and adults. Your doctor may recommend an ICD if you're at risk for certain types of arrhythmia.

ICDs are used to treat life-threatening ventricular arrhythmias, such as those that cause the ventricles to beat too fast or quiver. You may be considered at high risk for a ventricular arrhythmia if you have had the following:

- A ventricular arrhythmia before
- A heart attack that has damaged your heart's electrical system

ICDs often are recommended for people who have survived sudden cardiac arrest (SCA). People who have certain heart conditions that put them at high risk for SCA also may need ICDs.

For example, some people who have long QT syndrome, Brugada syndrome, or congenital heart disease may benefit from an ICD, even if they've never had ventricular arrhythmias before.

Some people who have heart failure may need a CRT-D device. This device combines a type of pacemaker called a cardiac resynchronization therapy (CRT) device with a defibrillator. CRT-D devices help both ventricles work together. This allows them to do a better job of pumping blood out of the heart.

How an Implantable Cardioverter Defibrillator Works

An implantable cardioverter defibrillator (ICD) has wires with electrodes on the ends that connect to one or more of your heart's chambers. These wires carry the electrical signals from your heart to a computer in the ICD. The computer monitors your heart rhythm.

If the ICD detects an irregular rhythm, it sends low-energy electrical pulses to prompt your heart to beat at a normal rate. If the low-energy pulses restore your heart's normal rhythm, you may avoid the high-energy pulses or shocks of the defibrillator (which can be painful).

Single-chamber ICDs have a wire that connects to either the right atrium or right ventricle. The wire senses electrical activity and corrects faulty electrical signaling within that chamber.

Dual-chamber ICDs have wires that connect to both an atrium and a ventricle. These ICDs provide low-energy pulses to either or both chambers. Some dual-chamber ICDs have three wires. They connect to an atrium and both ventricles.

The wires on an ICD connect to a small metal box implanted in your chest or abdomen. The box contains a battery, pulse generator, and computer. When the computer detects irregular heartbeats, it triggers the ICD's pulse generator to send electrical pulses. Wires carry these pulses to the heart.

The ICD also can record the heart's electrical activity and heart rhythms. The recordings can help your doctor fine-tune the programming of your ICD so it works better to correct irregular heartbeats.

The type of ICD you get is based on your heart's pumping abilities, structural defects, and the type of irregular heartbeats you've had. Whichever type of ICD you get, it will be programmed to respond to the type of irregular heartbeat you're most likely to have.

What to Expect during Implantable Cardioverter Defibrillator Surgery

Placing an implantable cardioverter defibrillator (ICD) requires minor surgery, which usually is done in a hospital. You'll be given medicine right before the surgery that will help you relax and may make you fall asleep.

471

Your doctor will give you medicine to numb the area where he or she will put the ICD so you don't feel any pain. Your doctor also may give you antibiotics to prevent infection.

First, your doctor will thread the ICD wires through a vein to the correct location in your heart. An x-ray "movie" of the wires as they pass through your vein and into your heart will help your doctor place them.

Once the wires are in place, your doctor will make a small cut into the skin of your chest or abdomen. He or she will then slip the ICD's small metal box through the cut and just under your skin. The box contains the battery, pulse generator, and computer.

Once the ICD is in place, your doctor will test it. You'll be given medicine to help you sleep during this testing so you don't feel any electrical pulses. Then your doctor will sew up the cut. The entire surgery takes a few hours.

What to Expect after Implantable Cardioverter Defibrillator Surgery

Expect to stay in the hospital 1 to 2 days so your health care team can check your heartbeat and make sure your implantable cardioverter defibrillator (ICD) is working properly.

You'll need to arrange for a ride home from the hospital because you won't be able to drive for at least a week while you recover from the surgery.

For a few days to weeks after the surgery, you may have pain, swelling, or tenderness in the area where your ICD was placed. The pain usually is mild, and over-the-counter medicines can help relieve it. Talk to your doctor before taking any pain medicines.

Your doctor may ask you to avoid vigorous activities and heavy lifting for about a month after ICD surgery. Most people return to their normal activities within a few days of having the surgery.

Risks of Having an Implantable Cardioverter Defibrillator

Unnecessary Electrical Pulses

The most common problem with implantable cardioverter defibrillators (ICDs) is that they can sometimes give electrical pulses or shocks that aren't needed.

A damaged wire or a very fast heart rate due to extreme physical activity may trigger unnecessary pulses. Unnecessary pulses also may occur if you forget to take your medicines.

Children tend to be more physically active than adults, and younger people who have ICDs are more likely to receive unnecessary pulses than older people.

Pulses delivered too often or at the wrong time can damage the heart or trigger an irregular, sometimes dangerous heartbeat. They also can be painful and emotionally upsetting. If this occurs, your doctor can reprogram your ICD or prescribe medicines so the unnecessary pulses occur less often.

Risks Related to Surgery

Although rare, some ICD risks are linked to the surgery used to place the device. These risks include the following:

- Swelling, bruising, or infection at the area where the ICD was placed
- Bleeding from the site where the ICD was placed
- Blood vessel, heart, or nerve damage
- A collapsed lung
- A bad reaction to the medicine used to make you sleep during the surgery

Other Risks

People who have ICDs may be at increased risk for heart failure. Heart failure is when your heart can't pump enough blood to meet your body's needs. It's not known for sure whether an ICD increases the risk of heart failure or whether heart failure is just more common in people who need ICDs.

Although rare, an ICD may not work properly. This will prevent the device from correcting irregular heartbeats. If this happens, your doctor may be able to reprogram the device. If that doesn't work, the ICD may need to be replaced.

The longer you have an ICD, the more likely it may be that you'll experience some of the related risks.

How an Implantable Cardioverter Defibrillator Affects Lifestyle

The low-energy electrical pulses your implantable cardioverter defibrillator (ICD) gives aren't painful. You may not notice them, or you may feel a fluttering in your chest.

The high-energy pulses or shocks your ICD gives last only a fraction of a second and feel like a thumping or painful kick in the chest, depending on their strength.

Your doctor may give you medicine to decrease the number of irregular heartbeats you have. This will reduce the number of high-energy pulses sent to your heart. Such medicines include amiodarone or sotalol and beta-blockers.

Your doctor may want you to call his or her office or come in within 24 hours of getting a strong shock from your ICD. See your doctor or go to an emergency room right away if you get many strong shocks within a short time.

Devices That Can Disrupt Implantable Cardioverter Defibrillator Functions

Once you have an ICD, you have to avoid close or prolonged contact with electrical devices or devices that have strong magnetic fields. Devices that can interfere with an ICD include the following:

- Cell phones and MP3 players (for example, iPods)
- Household appliances, such as microwave ovens
- High-tension wires
- Metal detectors
- Industrial welders
- Electrical generators

These devices can disrupt the electrical signaling of your ICD and prevent it from working properly. You may not be able to tell whether your ICD has been affected.

How likely a device is to disrupt your ICD depends on how long you're exposed to it and how close it is to your ICD.

To be on the safe side, some experts recommend not putting your cell phone or MP3 player in a shirt pocket over your ICD (if they're turned on). You may want to hold your cell phone up to the ear that's opposite the site where your ICD was implanted. If you strap your MP3 player to your arm while listening to it, put it on the arm that's farther from your ICD.

You can still use household appliances, but avoid close and prolonged exposure, as it may interfere with your ICD.

You can walk through security system metal detectors at your normal pace. Someone can check you with a metal detector wand as long as it isn't held for too long over your ICD site. You should avoid sitting or standing close to a security system metal detector. Notify airport screeners if you have an ICD.

Stay at least 2 feet away from industrial welders or electrical generators. Rarely, ICDs have caused inappropriate shocks during long, high-altitude flights.

Procedures That Can Disrupt Implantable Cardioverter Defibrillator Functions

Some medical procedures can disrupt your ICD. These procedures include the following:

- Magnetic resonance imaging, or MRI
- Shock-wave lithotripsy to treat kidney stones
- Electrocauterization to stop bleeding during surgery

Let all of your doctors, dentists, and medical technicians know that you have an ICD. Your doctor can give you a card that states what kind of ICD you have. Carry this card in your wallet. You may want to consider wearing a medical identification bracelet or necklace that explains that you have an ICD.

Chapter 55

Pacemakers

A pacemaker is a small device that's placed under the skin of your chest or abdomen to help control abnormal heart rhythms. This device uses electrical pulses to prompt the heart to beat at a normal rate.

Pacemakers are used to treat heart rhythms that are too slow, fast, or irregular. These abnormal heart rhythms are called arrhythmias. Pacemakers can relieve some symptoms related to arrhythmias, such as fatigue (tiredness) and fainting. A pacemaker can help a person who has an abnormal heart rhythm resume a more active lifestyle.

Overview

Faulty electrical signaling in the heart causes arrhythmias. A pacemaker uses low-energy electrical pulses to correct faulty electrical signaling. Pacemakers can do the following:

- Speed up a slow heartbeat

- Help end an abnormal and fast rhythm (only in implantable cardioverter defibrillator/pacemaker combination devices)

- Make sure the ventricles contract normally if the atria are quivering instead of beating in a normal rhythm (a condition called atrial fibrillation)

Excerpted from "Pacemaker," by the National Heart, Lung, and Blood Institute (NHLBI, www.nhlbi.nih.gov), May 2008.

- Coordinate the electrical signaling between the upper and lower chambers of the heart

- Coordinate the electrical signaling between the ventricles (cardiac resynchronization therapy used in heart failure)

Pacemakers also can monitor and record your heart's electrical activity and the rhythm of your heartbeat. Newer pacemakers can monitor your blood temperature, breathing rate, and other factors and adjust your heart rate to changes in your activity.

Pacemakers can be temporary or permanent. Temporary pacemakers are used to treat temporary heartbeat problems, such as a slow heartbeat due to heart attack, heart surgery, or an overdose of medicine. Temporary pacemakers are used in emergencies until a permanent pacemaker can be implanted or until the temporary condition goes away. A person with a temporary pacemaker will stay in the hospital as long as the pacemaker is in place.

In this text, "pacemakers" refers to permanent devices, unless stated otherwise.

Doctors also treat arrhythmias with another device called an implantable cardioverter defibrillator (ICD). An ICD is like a pacemaker in some ways, but it can use higher energy electrical pulses to treat certain dangerous types of arrhythmia.

When a Pacemaker Is Needed

Doctors recommend pacemakers to patients for a number of reasons. The most common reason is when a patient's heart is beating too slow or there are long pauses between heartbeats.

A pacemaker may be helpful if any of the following are true:

- Aging or heart disease damages your sinus node's ability to set the correct pace for your heartbeat. Such damage can make your heart beat too slow, or it can cause long pauses between heartbeats. The damage also can cause your heart rhythm to alternate between slow and fast.

- You need to take certain heart medicines (such as beta-blockers), but these medicines slow down your heartbeat too much.

- The electrical signals between your heart's upper and lower chambers are partially or completely blocked or slowed down (this is called heart block). Aging, damage to the heart from a heart attack, or other heart conditions can prevent electrical signals from reaching all the heart's chambers.

• You often faint due to a slow heartbeat. For example, this may happen if the main artery in your neck that supplies your brain with blood is sensitive to pressure. In you have this condition, just quickly turning your neck can cause your heart to beat slower than normal. When that happens, not enough blood may flow to your brain, causing you to faint.

• You have had a medical procedure to treat an arrhythmia called atrial fibrillation. A pacemaker can help regulate your heartbeat after the procedure.

• You have heart muscle problems that cause electrical signals to travel through your heart muscle too slow. (Your pacemaker will provide cardiac resynchronization therapy for this problem.)

To decide whether a pacemaker will benefit you, your doctor will consider any symptoms you have of an irregular heartbeat, such as dizziness, unexplained fainting, or shortness of breath. He or she also will consider whether you have a history of heart disease, what medicines you're currently taking, and the results of heart tests.

A pacemaker won't be recommended unless your heart tests show that you have irregular heartbeats.

How a Pacemaker Works

A pacemaker consists of a battery, a computerized generator, and wires with electrodes on one end. The battery powers the generator, and a thin metal box surrounds both it and the generator. The wires connect the generator to the heart.

The pacemaker's generator sends the electrical pulses that correct or set your heart rhythm. A computer chip figures out what types of electrical pulses to send to the heart and when those pulses are needed. To do this, the computer chip uses the information it receives from the wires connected to the heart. It also may use information from sensors in the wires that detect your movement, blood temperature, breathing, or other factors that indicate your level of physical activity. That way, it can make your heart beat faster when you exercise.

The computer chip also records your heart's electrical activity and heart rhythms. Your doctor will use these recordings to set your pacemaker so it works better at making sure you have a normal heart rhythm. Your doctor can program the computer in the pacemaker without having to use needles or directly contacting the pacemaker.

The wires in your pacemaker send electrical pulses to and from your heart and the generator. Pacemakers have one to three wires that are each placed in different chambers of the heart.

- The wires in a single-chamber pacemaker usually carry pulses between the right ventricle (the lower right chamber of your heart) and the generator.

- The wires in a dual-chamber pacemaker carry pulses between the right atrium and the right ventricle and the generator. The pulses help coordinate the timing of these two chambers' contractions.

- The wires in a triple-chamber pacemaker are used for heart muscle weakness and carry pulses between an atrium and both ventricles and the generator. The pulses help coordinate the timing of the two ventricles with each other.

Types of Pacemaker Programming

There are two main types of programming for pacemakers—demand pacing and rate-responsive pacing.

A demand pacemaker monitors your heart rhythm. It only electrically stimulates your heart if it's beating too slow or if it misses a beat.

A rate-responsive pacemaker will speed up or slow down your heart rate depending on how active you are. To do this, the rate-responsive pacemaker monitors your sinus node rate, breathing, blood temperature, or other factors to determine your activity level. Most people who need a pacemaker to continually set the pace of their heartbeat have rate-responsive pacemakers.

What to Expect during Pacemaker Surgery

Placement of a pacemaker requires minor surgery, which is usually done in a hospital or special heart treatment laboratory. You will be given medicine right before the surgery that will help you relax and may make you fall nearly asleep. Your doctor will give you a local anesthetic so you won't feel anything in the area where he or she puts the pacemaker.

First, your doctor will place a needle in a large vein, usually near the shoulder opposite your dominant hand. The doctor will then use the needle to thread the pacemaker wires into a vein and to the correct location in your heart.

An x-ray "movie" of the wires as they pass through your vein and into your heart will help your doctor place the wires. Once the wires are in place, your doctor will make a small cut into the skin of your chest or abdomen. He or she will then slip the pacemaker generator/ battery box through the cut, place it just under your skin, and connect it to the wires that lead to your heart.

Once the pacemaker is in place, your doctor will sew up the cut. The entire surgery takes a few hours.

What to Expect after Pacemaker Surgery

Expect to stay in the hospital overnight so your heartbeat can be monitored and your doctor can make sure your pacemaker is working properly. You probably will have to arrange for a ride to and from the hospital because your doctor may not want you to drive yourself.

For a few days to weeks after surgery, you may have pain, swelling, or tenderness in the area where your pacemaker was placed. The pain is usually mild and often relieved by over-the-counter medicines. Consult with your doctor before taking any pain medicines.

Your doctor also may ask you to avoid any vigorous activities and heavy lifting for about a month. Most people return to normal activities within a few days of having pacemaker surgery.

Risks of Pacemaker Surgery

Your chance of having any problems from pacemaker surgery is less than 5 percent. These problems may include the following:

- Swelling, bleeding, bruising, or infection in the area where the pacemaker was placed

- Blood vessel or nerve damage

- A collapsed lung

- A bad reaction to the medicine used to make you sleep during the procedure

- Infections that can become difficult to treat

Chapter 56

Stents

Chapter Contents

Section 56.1

What Are Stents?

Excerpted from "Stents," by the National Heart, Lung, and
Blood Institute (NHLBI, www.nhlbi.nih.gov), part of the National
Institutes of Health, July 2009.

A stent is a small mesh tube that's used to treat narrowed or weakened arteries in the body. Arteries are blood vessels that carry blood away from your heart to other parts of your body.

You may have a stent placed in an artery as part of a procedure called angioplasty. Angioplasty restores blood flow through narrowed or blocked arteries. Stents help prevent the arteries from becoming narrowed or blocked again in the months or years after angioplasty.

You also may have a stent placed in a weakened artery to improve blood flow and to help prevent the artery from bursting.

Stents usually are made of metal mesh, but sometimes they're made of fabric. Fabric stents, also called stent grafts, are used in larger arteries.

Some stents are coated with medicines that are slowly and continuously released into the artery. These stents are called drug-eluting stents. The medicines help prevent the artery from becoming blocked again.

How Stents Are Used

For the Coronary Arteries

In a condition called coronary heart disease (CHD), or coronary artery disease, a fatty substance called plaque can build up inside the coronary (heart) arteries. Plaque narrows the coronary arteries, reducing the flow of oxygen-rich blood to the heart muscle.

High blood cholesterol, high blood pressure, diabetes, and smoking may lead to CHD. When your coronary arteries are narrowed or blocked, oxygen-rich blood can't reach your heart muscle. This can cause angina (chest pain) or a heart attack.

During angioplasty, doctors use an expanding balloon inside the artery to compress plaque and widen the passage. Angioplasty improves blood flow to the heart, which reduces angina and other CHD symptoms.

Unless an artery is too small, doctors usually place a stent in the treated portion of the artery during angioplasty. The stent supports the inner artery wall and reduces the chance of the artery becoming narrowed or blocked again. A stent also can support an artery that was torn or injured during angioplasty.

When stents are used in coronary arteries, there's about a 10 to 20 percent chance that the arteries will renarrow or close in the first year after angioplasty. When stents aren't used, the risk of the arteries closing can be twice as high.

For the Carotid Arteries

Both the right and left sides of your neck have blood vessels called carotid arteries. These arteries carry blood from the heart to the brain. Plaque also can narrow the carotid arteries. When this happens, the condition is called carotid artery disease.

Plaque deposits in the carotid arteries limit blood flow to the brain and put you at risk for stroke. The same factors that raise your risk for CHD also increase your risk for carotid artery disease.

Stents are used to help keep the carotid arteries fully open after they're widened with angioplasty. How well this treatment works long term still isn't known. Research is ongoing to explore the risks and benefits of carotid artery stenting.

For Other Arteries

The arteries in the kidneys may become narrowed. This reduces blood flow to the kidneys, which can affect their function and ability to control blood pressure. This can cause severe high blood pressure.

Plaque can narrow the arteries in the arms and legs over time. When this happens, the condition is called peripheral arterial disease, or P.A.D.

This narrowing can cause pain and cramping in the affected limbs. If the narrowing is severe, it can completely cut off blood flow to a limb, which could require surgery.

To relieve these problems, doctors may do angioplasty on a narrowed kidney, arm, or leg artery. This procedure often is followed by placing a stent in the treated artery. The stent helps keep the artery fully open.

For the Aorta in the Abdomen or Chest

The major artery coming out of the heart that supplies blood to the body is called the aorta. The aorta travels through the chest and down into the abdomen. Over time, some areas of the aorta's walls can become weak. These weakened areas can cause a bulge in the artery called an aneurysm.

An aorta with an aneurysm can burst, leading to potentially deadly internal bleeding. When aneurysms occur, they're usually in the part of the aorta in the abdomen.

To help avoid a burst, doctors may place a fabric stent in the weakened area of the abdominal aorta. The stent creates a stronger inner lining for the artery.

Aneurysms also can develop in the part of the aorta in the chest. These aneurysms also can be treated with stents. How well these stents work over the long term still isn't known.

To Close off Aortic Tears

Another problem that can develop in the aorta is a tear in its inner wall. Blood can be forced into this tear, causing it to widen.

The tear can reduce blood flow to the tissues that the aorta serves. Over time, the tear can block blood flow through the artery or burst. When this occurs, it's usually in the part of the aorta that's in the chest.

Fabric stents are being developed and used experimentally to prevent aortic tears by stopping blood from flowing into the tear. A fabric stent placed within the torn area of the aorta can help restore normal blood flow and reduce the risk of a burst aorta. Researchers are still studying stents to treat aortic tears.

Placing Stents

To place a stent, your doctor will make a small opening in a blood vessel in your groin (upper thigh), arm, or neck. Through this opening, your doctor will thread a thin, flexible tube called a catheter with a deflated balloon on its end.

A stent may be placed around the deflated balloon. The tip of the catheter is threaded up to the narrowed section of the artery or to the aneurysm or aortic tear site.

Special x-ray movies are taken of the tube as it's threaded up into your blood vessel. These movies help your doctor position the catheter.

For Arteries Narrowed by Plaque

Once the tube is in the area of the artery that needs treatment, the doctor will take the following steps:

- Your doctor uses a special dye to help see narrowed areas of the blood vessel.

- Your doctor inflates the balloon. It pushes against the plaque and compresses it against the artery wall. The fully extended balloon also expands the surrounding stent, pushing it into place in the artery.

- The balloon is deflated and taken out along with the catheter. The stent remains in your artery. Cells in your artery eventually grow to cover the mesh of the stent and create an inner layer that looks like the inside of a normal blood vessel.

A very narrow artery, or one that's hard to reach with a catheter, may require more steps to place a stent. This type of artery usually is first expanded by inflating a small balloon. The balloon is then removed and replaced by another larger balloon with the collapsed stent around it. At this point, your doctor can follow the standard practice of compressing the plaque and placing the stent.

When angioplasty and stent placement are done on carotid arteries, a special filter device is used. The filter helps keep blood clots and loose pieces of plaque from passing into the bloodstream and traveling up to the brain during the procedure.

For Aortic Aneurysms

The procedure to place a stent in an artery with an aneurysm is very similar to the one used for an artery narrowed by plaque. The stent used to treat an aneurysm is different, though. It's made out of pleated fabric, often with one or more tiny hooks.

Once the stent has been placed and expanded to fit tight against the artery wall, the hooks on the stent latch on to the artery wall. This anchors the stent.

The stent creates a new inner lining for that portion of the artery. Cells in the artery eventually grow to cover the fabric and create an inner layer that looks like the inside of a normal blood vessel.

What to Expect before a Stent Procedure

Most stent procedures require an overnight stay in the hospital and someone to take you home. Discuss with your doctor the following issues:

- When to stop eating and drinking before coming to the hospital

- What medicines you should or shouldn't take on the day of the procedure

- When to come to the hospital and where to go

If you have diabetes, kidney disease, or other conditions, talk with your doctor about whether you need to take any extra steps during or after the procedure to avoid complications.

Before the procedure, your doctor may talk with you about medicines you'll probably need to take after the stent is placed. These medicines help prevent blood clots from forming.

It's important that you know how long you should take these medicines and why they're important.

What to Expect during a Stent Procedure

For Arteries Narrowed by Plaque

This procedure usually takes about an hour. It could take longer if stents are inserted into more than one artery during the procedure.

Before the procedure starts, you'll get medicine to help you relax. You'll be on your back and awake during the procedure so you can follow the doctor's instructions.

The area where the catheter is inserted will be numbed, and you won't feel the doctor threading the catheter, balloon, or stent inside the artery. You may feel some pain when the balloon is expanded to push the stent into place.

For Aortic Aneurysms

This procedure takes a few hours. It usually requires a 2- to 3-day stay in the hospital.

Before the procedure, you'll be given medicine to help you relax. If a stent is placed in the abdominal aorta, your doctor may give medicine to numb the area, but you'll be awake during the procedure.

If a stent is placed in the chest portion of the aorta, your doctor will likely give you medicine to make you sleep through the procedure.

Once you're numbed or asleep, your doctor will make a small cut in your groin (upper thigh). He or she will insert a catheter into the blood vessel through this cut.

Sometimes, two cuts (one in the groin area of each leg) are needed to place fabric stents that come in two parts. You will not feel the doctor threading the catheter, balloon, or stent into the artery.

What to Expect after a Stent Procedure

Recovery

After either type of stent procedure (for arteries narrowed by plaque or aortic aneurysms), the catheter will be removed and the tube insertion site will be bandaged.

A small sandbag or other type of weight may be put on top of the bandage to apply pressure and help prevent bleeding. You'll recover in a special care area where your movement will be limited.

While you're in recovery, a nurse will check your heart rate and blood pressure regularly. The nurse also will see whether there's any bleeding from the insertion site. Eventually, a small bruise and sometimes a small, hard "knot" will appear at the insertion site. This area may feel sore or tender for about a week.

You should let your doctor know if any of the following occur:

- You have a constant or large amount of bleeding at the site that can't be stopped with a small bandage.

- You have any unusual pain, swelling, redness, or other signs of infection at or near the insertion site.

Common Precautions after a Stent Procedure

Blood Clotting Precautions

After a stent procedure, your doctor will likely recommend that you take aspirin and another anticlotting medicine. These medicines help prevent blood clots from forming in the stent. A blood clot can lead to heart attack, stroke, or other serious problems.

If you have a metal stent, your doctor will likely recommend aspirin and another anticlotting medicine for at least 1 month. If your stent is coated with medicine, your doctor may recommend aspirin and another anticlotting medicine for 12 months or more. Your doctor will work with you to determine the best course of treatment.

The risk of developing a blood clot significantly increases if you stop taking the anticlotting medicine too early. It's important to take these medicines for as long as your doctor recommends. He or she may recommend lifelong treatment with aspirin.

If you're considering surgery for some other reason while you're on these medicines, talk to your doctor about whether it can wait until after you've stopped the medicine. Anticlotting medicines may increase the risk of bleeding.

In addition to an increased risk of bleeding, anticlotting medicines can cause other side effects, such as an allergic rash. Talk to your doctor about how to reduce the risk of these side effects.

Other Precautions

You should avoid vigorous exercise and heavy lifting for a short time after the stent procedure. Your doctor will let you know when you can go back to your normal activities.

If you have a metal stent, you shouldn't have a magnetic resonance imaging (MRI) test within the first couple of months after the procedure. Metal detectors used in airports and other screening areas don't affect stents. Your stent shouldn't cause metal detectors to go off.

If you have an aortic fabric stent, your doctor will probably recommend that you have followup imaging tests (for example, chest x-ray) within the first year of having the procedure. After the first year, he or she may recommend yearly imaging tests.

Risks of Having a Stent

Risks Related to Angioplasty

Angioplasty, the procedure used to place stents, is a common medical procedure. Angioplasty carries a small risk of the following serious complications:

- Bleeding from the site where the catheter was inserted into the skin

- Damage to the blood vessel from the catheter

- Arrhythmias (irregular heartbeats)

- Damage to the kidneys caused by the dye used during the procedure

- An allergic reaction to the dye used during the procedure
- Infection

Another problem after angioplasty is too much tissue growth within the treated portion of the artery. This can cause the artery to narrow or close again, which is called restenosis.

This problem often is avoided with the use of drug-eluting stents. These stents are coated with medicines that help prevent too much tissue growth.

Treating the tissue around the stent with radiation also can prevent tissue growth. For this procedure, the doctor puts a wire through a catheter to where the stent is placed. The wire releases radiation and stops cells around the stent from growing and blocking the artery.

Risks Related to Stents

About 1 to 2 percent of people who have a stented artery develop a blood clot at the stent site. Blood clots can cause heart attack, stroke, or other serious problems.

The risk of blood clots is greatest during the first few months after the stent is placed in the artery. Your doctor will likely recommend that you take aspirin and another anticlotting medicine, such as clopidogrel, for at least 1 month or up to a year or more after having a stent procedure. These medicines help prevent blood clots.

The length of time you need to take anticlotting medicines depends on the type of stent you get. Your doctor may recommend lifelong treatment with aspirin.

Stents coated with medicine, which often are used to keep clogged heart arteries open, may increase your risk for potentially dangerous blood clots. However, no conclusive evidence shows that these stents increase the chances of having a heart attack or dying, if used as recommended.

Risks Related to Aortic Stents in the Abdomen

Although rare, a few serious complications can occur when surgery or a fabric stent is used to repair an aneurysm in the abdominal region of the aorta. These complications include the following:

- A burst artery (aneurysm rupture)
- Blocked blood flow to the stomach or lower body

- Paralysis in the legs due to interruption of blood flow to the spinal cord (this complication is very rare)

Another possible complication is the fabric stent moving further down the aorta. This sometimes happens years after the stent is first placed. Such stent movement may require a doctor to place another fabric stent in the area of the aneurysm.

Section 56.2

Patients Who Receive Medicine-Coated Stents Have Lower Risk of Death

Excerpted from "AHRQ-Funded Study Finds Lower Risk of Death and Heart Attack in Patients with Drug-Coated Stent Implants Compared to Those with Bare Metal Stents." Press Release, March 28, 2009. Agency for Healthcare Research and Quality (AHRQ, www.ahrq.gov), Rockville, MD.

Heart disease patients 65 and older who receive stents coated with medicine to prevent blockages are more likely to survive and less likely to suffer a heart attack than people fitted with stents not coated with medication, according to a new study supported by Health and Human Services' (HHS) Agency for Healthcare Research and Quality (AHRQ) and the American College of Cardiology's National Cardiovascular Data Registry.

The comparative effectiveness study of 262,700 Medicare patients who received stents—spring-like tubes to keep heart vessels open—is the largest ever to compare drug-coated stents with bare metal ones.

A team of researchers from Duke University, AHRQ, and Kaiser Permanente found that, compared with patients who received bare metal stents, those fitted with stents coated with medication, called drug-eluting stents, had an 18 percent better survival rate over the 30-month study period and were 16 percent less likely to suffer a heart attack.

"The findings provide important new evidence for decision making by heart disease patients and their physicians," said AHRQ Director

Carolyn M. Clancy, MD. "These results should help resolve many lingering questions regarding the safety of drug-eluting stents in recent years."

HHS' Food and Drug Administration approved two stents coated with drugs in 2003 and 2004, but then issued precautionary advisories in 2006 after receiving scattered reports of blood clot formation, or thrombosis, and deaths. Subsequent clinical trials and other studies produced conflicting results.

The researchers in the AHRQ-funded study found that 16.5 percent of the patients implanted with bare metal stents died within 30 months of implantation, compared with 13.5 percent of those with drug-eluting stents, after adjusting for population differences. They also found that 8.9 percent of the patients with bare metal stents suffered heart attacks during the period, compared with 7.5 percent of those with drug-eluting stents—a 16 percent higher rate.

The researchers further found that patients fitted with drug-eluting stents in 2005 and 2006 had a lower risk of death than those given the stents in 2004.

"Some previous studies have suggested that drug-eluting stents are associated with an excess long-term death rate, whereas others have not," said the study's lead author, Pamela S. Douglas, MD, Geller professor of medicine at Duke University.

The researchers found no significant differences in the percentages of drug-eluting and bare metal stent in patients who required a repeat angioplasty or coronary artery bypass graft surgery (roughly 23 percent) and in the percentages of patients who suffered strokes or major bleeding (about 3 percent and 3.5 percent, respectively). The results were not affected by age, gender, race, ethnicity, or other factors.

According to AHRQ's Art Sedrakyan, MD, PhD, a co-author of the study, the better outcomes found for patients with drug-eluting stents may be at least partially explained because those patients are required to take blood-thinning drugs, such as clopidogrel, for a long time after their procedure. Patients who receive bare metal stents are usually prescribed blood-thinner medications for a shorter period of time and may take them less often. In addition, patients with drug-eluting stents may visit their doctors more often after hospital discharge and may receive prescriptions for drugs and therapies to lower their cholesterol levels and manage other heart conditions more often than patients who received bare metal stents.

The researchers based their study on data from the American College of Cardiology's National Cardiovascular Data Registry on patients who underwent angioplasty with drug-eluting or bare metal stent implantation at 650 hospitals, together with Medicare national claims data to capture post-hospital discharge information. The authors call for longer follow-up studies to further support the study's results and to confirm the possible effects of postimplantation treatment with blood-thinning drugs such as clopidogrel.

Chapter 57

Heart Surgery

Chapter Contents

Section 57.1

Overview of Heart Surgery

Excerpted from "Heart Surgery," by the National Heart,
Lung, and Blood Institute (NHLBI, www.nhlbi.nih.gov), part
of the National Institutes of Health, September 2007.

Heart surgery is done to correct problems with the heart. More
than half a million heart surgeries are done each year in the United
States for a variety of heart problems.

Heart surgery is used to correct heart problems in children and
adults. This text discusses heart surgeries for adults.

Overview

The most common type of heart surgery for adults is coronary artery bypass grafting (CABG). During CABG, surgeons use healthy
arteries or veins taken from another part of the body to bypass (that
is, go around) blocked arteries. CABG relieves chest pain and reduces
the risk of heart attack.

Heart surgery also is done to perform the following:

- Repair or replace valves that control blood flow through the
  heart

- Repair abnormal or damaged structures in the heart

- Implant medical devices that regulate heart rhythms or blood
  flow

- Replace a damaged heart with a healthy heart from a donor
  (heart transplant)

Traditional heart surgery, often called "open heart surgery," is done
by opening the chest wall to operate on the heart. Almost always, the
chest is opened by cutting through a patient's breastbone. Once the
heart is exposed, the patient is connected to a heart-lung bypass machine. The machine takes over the pumping action of the heart. This
allows surgeons to operate on a still heart.

In recent years, new ways of doing heart surgery have been developed. One new way is called off-pump, or beating heart, surgery. It's like traditional open-heart surgery, but it doesn't use a heart-lung bypass machine.

Minimally invasive heart surgery uses smaller incisions (cuts) than traditional open-heart surgery. Some types of minimally invasive heart surgery use a heart-lung bypass machine and others don't.

These new methods may reduce risks and speed up recovery time. Studies are under way to compare these new types of heart surgery to traditional open-heart surgery. The results of these studies will help doctors decide the best procedure to use for each patient.

Outlook

The results of heart surgery in adults are often excellent. For very ill people with severe heart problems, heart surgery can reduce symptoms, improve quality of life, and increase lifespan.

Types of Heart Surgery

Different types of heart surgery are used to fix different heart problems.

Coronary Artery Bypass Grafting

Coronary artery bypass grafting (CABG) is the most common type of heart surgery. More than 500,000 of these surgeries are done each year in the United States. CABG improves blood flow to the heart. It's used for people with severe coronary artery disease (CAD).

In CAD, a fatty material called plaque builds up inside your coronary (heart) arteries. It narrows the arteries and limits blood flow to your heart muscle. CAD can cause angina (chest pain or discomfort), shortness of breath, and can even lead to a heart attack.

During CABG, a surgeon takes a vein or an artery from your chest, your leg, or another part of your body and connects, or grafts, it to the blocked artery. The grafted artery bypasses (that is, goes around) the blockage. This allows oxygen-rich blood to reach the heart muscle. Surgeons can bypass as many as four blocked coronary arteries during one surgery.

Sometimes you can choose between CABG and angioplasty to treat CAD. Talk to your doctor about these different treatments.

Transmyocardial Laser Revascularization

Transmyocardial laser revascularization, or TLR, is a surgery used to treat angina when no other treatments work. For example, if you've already had one CABG procedure and can't have another one, TLR may be an option. This type of heart surgery isn't common.

During TLR, the surgeon uses lasers to make channels in the heart muscle. These channels allow oxygen-rich blood to flow from a heart chamber directly into the heart muscle.

Valve Repair or Replacement

For the heart to work right, blood must flow in only one direction. The heart's valves make this possible. Healthy valves open and close in a precise way as the heart pumps blood.

Each valve has a set of flaps called leaflets. The leaflets open to allow blood to pass from the heart chambers into the arteries. Then the leaflets close tightly to stop blood from flowing back into the chambers.

Heart surgery is done to fix leaflets that don't open as wide as they should. This can happen when they become thick or stiff or fuse together. As a result, not enough blood flows through the valve into the artery.

Heart surgery also is done to fix leaflets that don't close tightly. This means blood can leak backward into the chambers, rather than only moving forward into the artery as it should.

To fix these problems, surgeons either repair the valve or replace it. Replacement valves are taken from animals, made from human tissue, or made from man-made substances.

Arrhythmia Treatment

An arrhythmia is a problem with the speed or rhythm of the heartbeat. During an arrhythmia, the heart can beat too fast, too slow, or with an irregular rhythm.

Most arrhythmias are harmless, but some can be serious or even life threatening. When the heart rate is abnormal, the heart may not be able to pump enough blood to the body. Lack of blood flow can damage the brain, heart, and other organs.

Arrhythmias are usually treated with medicine first. If medicines don't work well enough, you may need surgery. For example, your doctor may use surgery to give you a pacemaker or an implantable cardioverter defibrillator (ICD).

A pacemaker is a small device that's placed under the skin of your chest or abdomen. Wires lead from the pacemaker to the heart's chambers. The pacemaker sends electrical signals through the wires to control the speed of the heartbeat. Most pacemakers have a sensor that activates the device only when the heartbeat is abnormal.

An ICD is another small device that's placed in your chest or abdomen. This device also is connected to the heart with wires. It checks your heartbeat for dangerous arrhythmias. If it senses one, it sends an electric shock to the heart to restore a normal heartbeat.

Another type of surgery for arrhythmia is called Maze surgery. In this operation, the surgeon makes new paths (a maze) for the heart's electrical signals to travel through. This type of surgery is used to treat atrial fibrillation, the most common type of serious arrhythmia.

Aneurysm Repair

An aneurysm is an abnormal bulge or "ballooning" in the wall of an artery or the heart muscle. This bulge happens when the wall weakens. Pressure from blood moving through the artery or heart causes the weak area to bulge out. Over time an aneurysm can grow and can burst, causing dangerous, often fatal bleeding inside the body.

Aneurysms in the heart most often occur in the heart's lower left chamber. They can develop after a heart attack.

Repairing an aneurysm involves surgery to replace the weak section of the artery or heart wall with a patch or graft.

Ventricular Assist Devices

Ventricular assist devices (VADs) are mechanical pumps that support your heart or take over your heart's pumping action. VADs are used when your heart can't pump enough blood to support your body.

You may need a VAD if you have heart failure or if you're waiting for a heart transplant. You can use a VAD for a short time or for months or years, depending on your situation.

Heart Transplant

A heart transplant is surgery in which a diseased heart is replaced with a healthy heart from a deceased donor. Heart transplants are done on patients whose hearts are so damaged or weak that they can't pump enough blood to meet the body's needs.

This type of surgery is a life-saving measure that's used when medical treatment and less drastic surgery have failed.

Because donor hearts are in short supply, patients who need a heart transplant go through a careful selection process. They need to be sick enough to need a new heart, yet healthy enough to receive it.

Patients on the waiting list for a donor heart receive ongoing treatment for heart failure and other medical conditions. VADs may be used to treat these patients.

Surgical Approaches

In recent years, new ways of doing heart surgery have been developed. Depending on a patient's heart problem, general health, and other factors, he or she can now have open-heart surgery or minimally invasive heart surgery.

Open-heart surgery: Open-heart surgery is any kind of surgery where the chest wall is opened and surgeons operate on the heart. "Open" refers to the chest, not the heart. Depending on the type of surgery, the heart may be opened, too.

Open-heart surgery is used to bypass blocked arteries in the heart, repair or replace heart valves, fix atrial fibrillation, and transplant hearts.

In recent years, more surgeons have started to use off-pump, or beating heart, surgery to do CABG. This approach is like traditional open-heart surgery, but surgeons don't use a heart-lung bypass machine.

Off-pump heart surgery may reduce complications that can occur when a heart-lung bypass machine is used. It also may speed up recovery time.

Off-pump heart surgery isn't right for all patients. Your doctor will decide whether you should have this type of surgery. He or she will carefully consider your heart problem, age, overall health, and other factors that may affect the surgery.

Minimally invasive heart surgery: For minimally invasive heart surgery, a surgeon doesn't make a large incision (cut) down the center of the chest to open the rib cage. Instead, he or she makes small incisions in the side of the chest between the ribs.

A heart-lung bypass machine is used in some types of minimally invasive heart surgery, but not others.

This newer heart surgery is used for some CABG and Maze procedures. It's also used to repair or replace heart valves and insert pacemakers.

One type of minimally invasive heart surgery that's still being developed is robotic-assisted surgery. For this surgery, a surgeon uses a computer to control surgical tools on thin robotic arms. The tools are inserted through small incisions in the chest. This allows surgeons to perform complex and highly precise surgery. The surgeon is always in total control of the robotic arms; they don't move on their own.

Benefits of minimally invasive heart surgery compared to open-heart surgery include smaller incisions and scars, lower risk of infection, less pain, a shorter hospital stay, and a faster recovery.

What to Expect before Heart Surgery

There are many types of heart surgery. The type you need depends on your situation. One person's experience before an operation can be very different from another's.

Some people carefully plan their surgeries with their doctors. They know exactly when and how it will happen. Other people need emergency heart surgery. Others are diagnosed with blocked coronary arteries and are admitted to the hospital right away for surgery as soon as possible.

If you're having a planned surgery, you may be admitted to the hospital the afternoon or morning before your surgery. Your doctors and others on your health care team will meet with you to explain what will happen. They will give you instructions on how to prepare for the surgery.

You also may need to have some tests, such as an EKG (electrocardiogram), chest x-ray, or blood tests. An intravenous (IV) line will be placed in your arm to give you fluids and medicines. Hair near the incision site may be shaved. Your skin may be washed with special soap to reduce the risk of infection.

Just before the surgery, you will be moved to the operating room. You will be given medicine so that you fall asleep and feel no pain during the surgery.

What to Expect during Heart Surgery

Heart surgery is done in a hospital. A team of experts is involved. Cardiothoracic surgeons perform the surgery with a team of other doctors and nurses who assist.

The length of time for the surgery depends on the type of surgery. CABG, the most common type of heart surgery, usually takes 3 to 5 hours.

Traditional Open-Heart Surgery

For this type of surgery, you're given medicine to make you fall asleep. A doctor checks your heartbeat, blood pressure, oxygen levels, and breathing during the surgery. A breathing tube is placed in your lungs through your throat and connected to a ventilator (breathing machine).

A surgeon makes a 6- to 8-inch incision (cut) down the center of your chest wall. Your chest bone is cut and your rib cage is opened so that the surgeon can get to your heart.

You're given medicine to thin your blood and keep it from clotting. A heart-lung bypass machine is connected to your heart. This machine takes over for your heart by replacing the heart's pumping action. A specialist oversees the machine. The bypass machine allows the surgeon to operate on a heart that isn't moving and full of blood.

You're given medicines to stop your heartbeat once you're connected to the heart-lung bypass machine. A pipe is placed in your heart to drain blood to the machine. The machine removes carbon dioxide (a waste product) from your blood, adds oxygen, and then pumps the blood back into your body. Tubes are inserted into your chest to drain fluid.

Once the bypass machine begins to work, the surgeon performs the surgery to repair your heart problem.

At the end of the surgery, your heart is restarted using mild electric shocks. The pipes and tubes are removed from your heart, and the heart-lung bypass machine is stopped. You're given medicine to allow your blood to clot again.

Your chest bone is closed with wires. Stitches or staples are used to close the incision. The breathing tube is removed.

An advantage of traditional open-heart surgery is that it's easier for the surgeon to operate. This is very important for long and complex surgeries.

Off-Pump Heart Surgery

This type of surgery is the same as traditional open-heart surgery, except you aren't connected to a heart-lung bypass machine. Instead, your heart is steadied with a mechanical device while the surgeon works on it. Your heart continues to pump blood to your body.

The advantages of off-pump heart surgery are that there are no complications related to using a heart-lung bypass machine and there is faster recovery from the surgery.

Minimally Invasive Heart Surgery

For this type of heart surgery, the surgeon makes small incisions in the side of your chest between the ribs. These incisions can be as small as 2 to 3 inches. Then the surgeon inserts surgical tools through these small incisions. A tool with a small video camera at the tip also is inserted through an incision. This allows the surgeon to see inside the body.

Some types of minimally invasive heart surgery use a heart-lung bypass machine; other types don't.

The advantages of minimally invasive heart surgery are the following:

- Less bleeding during surgery and a lower chance of needing a blood transfusion
- Lower risk of infection
- Less pain
- Smaller incisions and scars
- A shorter hospital stay and faster recovery

Patients who don't need the heart-lung bypass machine aren't at risk for the complications that the machine may cause.

What to Expect after Heart Surgery

Recovery in the Hospital

Depending on the type of heart surgery, you may spend 1 day or more in the hospital's intensive care unit. Then you will be moved to another part of hospital for several days before you go home.

While you're in the hospital, doctors and nurses will closely watch your heart rate, blood pressure, breathing, vital signs, and incision site(s). You may have an intravenous (IV) needle inserted in your arm to give you fluids until you're ready to drink on your own.

You also may be given extra oxygen through a face mask or nasal prongs that fit just inside your nose. These pieces of equipment are removed when you don't need them any more.

Recovery at Home

Each person responds differently to heart surgery. Your recovery at home also will depend on what kind of heart problem and surgery you had. Your doctor will give you specific instructions about how to care for your healing incisions, recognize signs of infection or other complications, and cope with after-effects of surgery.

You also will get information about followup appointments, medicines, and situations when you should call the doctor right away.

After-effects of heart surgery are normal. They may include the following:

- Muscle pain

- Chest pain
- Swelling (especially if you have an incision in your leg from coronary artery bypass grafting, or CABG)

Other after-effects may include loss of appetite, difficulty sleeping, constipation, and mood swings and depression. After-effects gradually go away.

Recovery time varies with type of heart surgery. Full recovery from traditional open-heart CABG may take 6 to 12 weeks or more. Less recovery time is needed for off-pump heart surgery and minimally invasive heart surgery.

Your doctor will let you know when you can go back to your daily activities, such as working, driving, and physical activity.

Section 57.2

Heart Valve Surgery

"Heart valve surgery," © 2009 A.D.A.M., Inc.
Reprinted with permission.

Heart valve surgery is used to repair or replace diseased heart valves.

Description

There are four valves in your heart:

1. Aortic valve
2. Mitral valve
3. Tricuspid valve
4. Pulmonary valve

The valves control the direction of blood flow through your heart. The opening and closing of the heart valves produce the sound of the heartbeat.

Heart valve surgery is open-heart surgery that is done while you are under general anesthesia. A cut is made through the breast bone (sternum). Your blood is routed away from your heart to a heart-lung bypass machine. This machine keeps the blood circulating while your heart is being operated on.

Valves may be repaired or replaced. Replacement heart valves are either natural (biologic) or artificial (mechanical):

- Natural valves are from human donors (cadavers).
- Modified natural valves come from animal donors. (Porcine valves are from pigs, bovine are from cows.) These are placed in synthetic rings.
- Artificial valves are made of metal.

If you receive an artificial valve, you may need to take lifelong medication to prevent blood clots. Natural valves rarely require lifelong medication.

Why the Procedure Is Performed

Heart valve surgery may be recommended for the following conditions:

- Narrowing of the heart valve (stenosis)
- Leaking of the heart valve (regurgitation)

Valve problems may be caused by:

- birth defects;
- calcium deposits (calcification);
- infections such as rheumatic fever;
- medications.

Defective valves may cause congestive heart failure and infections (infective endocarditis).

Risks

The risks for any anesthesia include:

- problems breathing;
- reactions to medications.

The risks for any surgery include:

- bleeding;
- infection.

The risks for cardiac surgery include:

- death;
- heart attack;
- irregular heartbeat (arrhythmia);
- kidney failure;
- stroke;
- temporary confusion after surgery due to the heart-lung machine.

It is very important to take steps to prevent valve infections. You may need to take antibiotics indefinitely, or before dental work and other invasive procedures.

After the Procedure

The success rate of heart valve surgery is high. The operation can relieve your symptoms and prolong your life.

The death rate averages 2% to 5%, depending on the heart valve. About two of every three patients who received an artificial mitral valve are still alive 9 years after the surgery.

The clicking of the mechanical heart valve may be heard in the chest. This is normal.

Outlook (Prognosis)

You will stay in an intensive care unit for the first 2 or 3 days following the operation. Your heart functions will be monitored constantly. The average hospital stay is 1 to 2 weeks. Complete recovery will take a few weeks to several months, depending on your health before surgery.

Chapter 58

Coronary Angioplasty

Coronary angioplasty is a medical procedure in which a balloon is used to open a blockage in a coronary (heart) artery narrowed by atherosclerosis. This procedure improves blood flow to the heart.

Atherosclerosis is a condition in which a material called plaque builds up on the inner walls of the arteries. This can happen in any artery, including the coronary arteries. The coronary arteries carry oxygen-rich blood to your heart. When atherosclerosis affects the coronary arteries, the condition is called coronary artery disease (CAD).

Angioplasty is a common medical procedure. It may be used to do the following:

- Improve symptoms of CAD, such as angina and shortness of breath

- Reduce damage to the heart muscle from a heart attack

- Reduce the risk of death in some patients

A heart attack occurs when blood flow through a coronary artery is completely blocked. Angioplasty is used during a heart attack to open the blockage and restore blood flow through the artery.

Angioplasty is done on more than 1 million people a year in the United States. Serious complications don't occur often, but can happen no matter how careful your doctor is or how well he or she does the procedure.

Excerpted from "Angioplasty," by the National Heart, Lung, and Blood Institute (NHLBI, www.nhlbi.nih.gov), part of the National Institutes of Health, January 2009.

Research on angioplasty is ongoing to make it safer and more effective, to prevent treated arteries from closing again, and to make the procedure an option for more people.

Other Names for Coronary Angioplasty

- Percutaneous coronary intervention (PCI)
- Percutaneous intervention
- Percutaneous transluminal angioplasty
- Percutaneous transluminal coronary angioplasty (PTCA)
- Balloon angioplasty
- Coronary artery angioplasty

Who Needs Coronary Angioplasty?

Coronary angioplasty is used to restore blood flow to the heart when the coronary arteries have become narrowed or blocked due to coronary artery disease (CAD).

When medicines and lifestyle changes, such as following a healthy diet, quitting smoking, and getting more physical activity, don't improve your CAD symptoms, your doctor will talk to you about other treatment options. These options include angioplasty and coronary artery bypass grafting (CABG), a type of open-heart surgery.

Your doctor will take into account a number of factors when recommending the best procedure for you. These factors include how severe your blockages are, where they're located, and other diseases you may have.

Angioplasty is often used when there is less severe narrowing or blockage in your arteries, and when the blockage can be reached during the procedure.

CABG might be chosen if you have severe heart disease, multiple arteries that are blocked, or if you have diabetes or heart failure.

Compared with CABG, some advantages of angioplasty are:

- It has fewer risks than CABG.
- It isn't surgery, so it won't require a large cut.
- It is done with medicines that numb you and help you relax.
- Unlike CABG, you won't be put to sleep for a short time.
- It has a shorter recovery time.

Angioplasty also is used as an emergency procedure during a heart attack. As plaque builds up in the coronary arteries, it can burst, causing a blood clot to form on its surface. If the clot becomes large enough, it can mostly or completely block blood flow to part of the heart muscle.

Quickly opening a blockage lessens the damage to the heart during a heart attack and restores blood flow to the heart muscle. Angioplasty can quickly open the artery and is the best approach during a heart attack.

A disadvantage of angioplasty as compared with CABG is that the artery may narrow again over time. The chance of this happening is lower when stents are used, especially medicine-coated stents. However, these stents aren't without risk. In some cases, blood clots can form in the medicine-coated stents and cause a heart attack.

Your doctor will discuss with you the treatment options and which procedure is best for you.

How Coronary Angioplasty Is Done

Before coronary angioplasty is done, your doctor will need to know whether your coronary arteries are blocked. If one or more of your arteries are blocked, your doctor will need to know where and how severe the blockages are.

To find out, your doctor will do an angiogram and take an x-ray picture of your arteries. During an angiogram, a small tube called a catheter with a balloon at the end is put into a large blood vessel in the groin (upper thigh) or arm. The catheter is then threaded to the coronary arteries. A small amount of dye is injected into the coronary arteries and an x-ray picture is taken.

This picture will show any blockages, how many, and where they're located. Once your doctor has this information, the angioplasty can proceed. Your doctor will blow up (inflate) the balloon in the blockage and push the plaque outward against the artery wall. This opens the artery more and improves blood flow.

A small mesh tube called a stent is usually placed in the newly widened part of the artery. The stent holds up the artery and lowers the risk of the artery renarrowing. Stents are made of metal mesh and look like small springs.

Some stents, called drug-eluting stents, are coated with medicines that are slowly and continuously released into the artery. These medicines help prevent the artery from becoming blocked again from scar tissue that grows around the stent.

In some cases, plaque is removed during angioplasty. In a procedure called atherectomy, a catheter with a rotating shaver on its tip is inserted into the artery to cut away plaque. Lasers also are used to dissolve or break up the plaque. These procedures are now rarely done because angioplasty gives better results for most patients.

What to Expect before Coronary Angioplasty

Meeting with Your Doctor

A cardiologist (a doctor who treats people with heart conditions) performs coronary angioplasty at a hospital. If your angioplasty isn't done as emergency treatment, you'll meet with your cardiologist before the procedure. Your doctor will go over your medical history (including the medicines you take), do a physical exam, and talk about the procedure with you. Your doctor also will order some routine tests, including the following:

- Blood tests
- An EKG (electrocardiogram)
- A chest x-ray

When the procedure is scheduled, you will be advised on the following:

- When to begin fasting (not eating or drinking) before the procedure (often you have to stop eating or drinking by midnight the night before the procedure)
- What medicines you should and shouldn't take on the day of the angioplasty
- When to arrive at the hospital and where to go

Even though angioplasty takes 1 to 2 hours, you will likely need to stay in the hospital overnight. In some cases, you will need to stay in the hospital longer. Your doctor may advise you not to drive for a certain amount of time after the procedure, so you may have to arrange for a ride home.

What to Expect during Coronary Angioplasty

Coronary angioplasty is performed in a special part of the hospital called the cardiac catheterization laboratory. The "cath lab" has special video screens and x-ray machines. Your doctor uses this equipment to see enlarged pictures of the blocked areas in your coronary arteries.

Preparation

In the cath lab, you will lie on a table. An intravenous (IV) line will be placed in your arm to give you fluids and medicines. The medicines will relax you and prevent blood clots from forming. These medicines may make you feel sleepy or as though you're floating or numb.

Here is what usually happens to prepare for the procedure:

- The area where the catheter will be inserted, usually the arm or groin (upper thigh), will be shaved.

- The shaved area will be cleaned to make it germ free and then numbed. The numbing medicine may sting as it's going in.

Steps in Angioplasty

When you're comfortable, the doctor will begin the procedure. You will be awake but sleepy.

A small cut is made in your arm or groin into which a tube called a sheath is put. The doctor then threads a very thin guide wire through the artery in your arm or groin toward the area of the coronary artery that's blocked.

Your doctor puts a long, thin, flexible tube called a catheter through the sheath and slides it over the guide wire and up to the heart. Your doctor moves the catheter into the coronary artery to the blockage. He or she takes out the guide wire once the catheter is in the right spot.

A small amount of dye may be injected through the catheter into the bloodstream to help show the blockage on x-ray. This x-ray picture of the heart is called an angiogram.

Next, your doctor slides a tube with a small deflated balloon inside it through the catheter and into the coronary artery where the blockage is.

When the tube reaches the blockage, the balloon is inflated. The balloon pushes the plaque against the wall of the artery and widens it. This helps to increase the flow of blood to the heart.

The balloon is then deflated. Sometimes the balloon is inflated and deflated more than once to widen the artery. Afterward, the balloon and tube are removed.

In some cases, plaque is removed during angioplasty. A catheter with a rotating shaver on its tip is inserted into the artery to cut away hard plaque. Lasers also may be used to dissolve or break up the plaque.

If your doctor needs to put a stent (small mesh tube) in your artery, another tube with a balloon will be threaded through your artery. A stent is wrapped around the balloon. Your doctor will inflate the balloon, which will cause the stent to expand against the wall of the artery. The balloon is then deflated and pulled out of the artery with the tube. The stent stays in the artery.

After the angioplasty is done, your doctor pulls back the catheter and removes it and the sheath. The hole in the artery is either sealed with a special device, or pressure is put on it until the blood vessel seals.

During angioplasty, strong antiplatelet medicines are given through the IV to prevent blood clots from forming in the artery or on the stent. These medicines help thin your blood. They're usually started just before the angioplasty and may continue for 12–24 hours afterward.

What to Expect after Coronary Angioplasty

After coronary angioplasty, you will be moved to a special care unit, where you will stay for a few hours or overnight.

While you recover in this area, you must lie still for a few hours to allow the blood vessels in your arm or groin (upper thigh) to seal completely. While you recover, nurses will check your heart rate and blood pressure. They also will check your arm or groin for bleeding. After a few hours, you will be able to walk with help.

The place where the tube was inserted may feel sore or tender for about a week.

Chapter 59

Coronary Artery Bypass Grafting

Coronary artery bypass grafting (CABG) is a type of surgery called revascularization, used to improve blood flow to the heart in people with severe coronary artery disease (CAD).

CAD occurs when the arteries that supply blood to the heart muscle (the coronary arteries) become blocked due to the buildup of a material called plaque on the inside of the blood vessels. If the blockage is severe, chest pain (also called angina), shortness of breath, and, in some cases, heart attack can occur.

CABG is one treatment for CAD. During CABG, a healthy artery or vein from another part of the body is connected, or grafted, to the blocked coronary artery. The grafted artery or vein bypasses (that is, it goes around) the blocked portion of the coronary artery. This new passage routes oxygen-rich blood around the blockage to the heart muscle. As many as four major blocked coronary arteries can be bypassed during one surgery.

Overview

CABG is the most common type of open-heart surgery in the United States, with more than 500,000 surgeries performed each year. Doctors called cardiothoracic surgeons perform this surgery.

Excerpted from text by the National Heart, Lung, and Blood Institute (NHLBI, www.nhlbi.nih.gov), part of the National Institutes of Health, March 2007.

CABG isn't used for everyone with CAD. Many people with CAD can be treated by other means, such as lifestyle changes, medicines, and another revascularization procedure called angioplasty.

CABG may be an option if you have severe blockages in the large coronary arteries that supply a major part of the heart muscle with blood—especially if the heart's pumping action has already been weakened.

CABG may also be an option if you have blockages in the heart that can't be treated with angioplasty. In these situations, CABG is considered more effective than other types of treatment.

If you're a candidate for CABG, the goals of having the surgery are the following:

- Improve your quality of life and decrease angina and other symptoms of CAD

- Resume a more active lifestyle

- Improve the pumping action of the heart if it has been damaged by a heart attack

- Lower the chances of a heart attack (in some patients, such as those with diabetes)

- Improve your chance of survival

Repeat surgery may be needed if grafted arteries or veins become blocked, or if new blockages develop in arteries that weren't blocked before. Taking medicines as prescribed and making lifestyle changes that your doctor recommends can lower the chance of a graft becoming blocked.

In people who are candidates for the surgery, the results are usually excellent, with 85 percent of people having significantly reduced symptoms, less risk for future heart attacks, and a decreased chance of dying within 10 years following the surgery.

Types of Coronary Artery Bypass Grafting

Traditional Coronary Artery Bypass Grafting

This is the most common type of coronary artery bypass grafting (CABG). It's used when at least one major artery needs to be bypassed. During the surgery, the chest bone is opened to access the heart. Medicines are given to stop the heart, and a heart-lung machine is used to keep blood and oxygen moving throughout the body during surgery.

This allows the surgeon to operate on a still heart. After surgery, the heart is restarted using mild electric shocks.

Off-Pump Coronary Artery Bypass Grafting

This type of CABG is similar to traditional CABG in that the chest bone is opened to access the heart. However, the heart isn't stopped, and a heart-lung machine isn't used. Off-pump CABG is sometimes called beating heart bypass grafting. This type of surgery may reduce complications that can occur when a heart-lung machine is used, and it may speed up recovery time after surgery.

Minimally Invasive Direct Coronary Artery Bypass Grafting

This surgery is similar to off-pump, but instead of a large incision to open the chest bone, several small incisions are made on the left side of the chest between the ribs. This type of surgery is used mainly for bypassing the vessels in front of the heart. It's a fairly new procedure, which is performed less often than the other types. This type of surgery is not for everybody, especially if more than one or two coronary arteries need to be bypassed.

Other Names for Coronary Artery Bypass Grafting

- Bypass surgery
- Coronary artery bypass surgery
- Heart bypass surgery

When Coronary Artery Bypass Grafting Is Needed

Coronary artery bypass grafting (CABG) is only used to treat people who have severe coronary artery disease (CAD) that could lead to a heart attack.

Your doctor may recommend CABG if other treatments, such as lifestyle changes or medicines, haven't worked. He or she also may recommend CABG if you have severe blockages in the large coronary arteries that supply a major part of the heart muscle with blood—especially if your heart's pumping action has already been weakened.

CABG also may be a treatment option if you have blockages in the heart that can't be treated with angioplasty.

Your doctor will determine if you're a candidate for CABG based on a number of factors. These include the presence and severity of CAD symptoms, the severity and location of blockages in your coronary arteries, your response to other treatments, your quality of life, and any other medical problems you may have.

In some cases, CABG may be performed on an emergency basis, such as pending or during a heart attack.

What to Expect before Coronary Artery Bypass Grafting

Tests may be done to prepare you for coronary artery bypass grafting, including blood tests, EKG, echocardiogram, chest x-ray, cardiac catheterization, and angiography.

Your doctor will give you specific instructions about how to prepare for surgery. There will be instructions about what to eat or drink, what medicines to take, and what activities to stop (such as smoking). You will likely be admitted to the hospital on the same day as the surgery.

What to Expect during Coronary Artery Bypass Grafting

Coronary artery bypass grafting (CABG) requires a team of experts. A cardiothoracic surgeon performs the surgery with support from an anesthesiologist, perfusionist (heart-lung machine specialist), other surgeons, and nurses.

There are several different types of CABG. They range from traditional surgery in which the chest is opened to reach the heart, to a nontraditional surgery in which small incisions are made to bypass the narrowed artery.

Traditional Coronary Artery Bypass Grafting

This type of surgery usually lasts 3 to 5 hours, depending on the number of arteries being bypassed. Numerous steps take place during traditional CABG.

Anesthesia is given to put you to sleep. During the surgery, the anesthesiologist monitors your heartbeat, blood pressure, oxygen levels, and breathing. A breathing tube is placed in your lungs through your throat, and connected to a ventilator (breathing machine).

An incision is made down the center of your chest. The chest bone is then cut and your ribcage is opened so that the surgeon can get to your heart.

Medicines are used to stop your heart, which allows the surgeon to operate on it while it's not beating. A heart-lung machine keeps oxygen-rich blood moving throughout your body. An artery or vein is taken from a different part of your body, such as your chest or leg, and prepared to be used as a graft for the bypass. In surgery with several bypasses, a combination of both artery and vein grafts is commonly used.

- **Artery grafts:** These grafts are much less likely than vein grafts to become blocked over time. The left internal mammary artery is most commonly used for an artery graft. It's located inside the chest close to the heart. Arteries from the arm or other places in the body are sometimes used as well.

- **Vein grafts:** Although veins are commonly used as grafts, they're more likely than artery grafts to develop plaque and become blocked over time. The saphenous vein—a long vein running along the inner side of the leg—is typically used.

After the grafting is complete, your heart is restarted using mild electric shocks. You're disconnected from the heart-lung machine. Tubes are inserted into your chest to drain fluid.

The surgeon uses wires that stay in your body permanently to close your chest bone and stitches or staples to close the skin incision. The breathing tube is removed when you're able to breathe without it.

Nontraditional Coronary Artery Bypass Grafting

Nontraditional CABG includes off-pump CABG and minimally invasive CABG.

Off-pump coronary artery bypass grafting: This type of surgery can be used to bypass any of the coronary arteries. Off-pump CABG also is called beating heart bypass grafting because the heart isn't stopped and a heart-lung machine isn't used. Instead, the part of the heart where grafting is being done is steadied with a mechanical device.

Off-pump CABG may reduce complications that can occur when a heart-lung machine is used, especially in people who have had a stroke or mini-strokes in the past, who are over age 70, and who have diabetes, lung disease, or kidney disease.

Other advantages of this type of bypass surgery include the following:

- Reduced bleeding during surgery and a lower chance of needing a blood transfusion

- A lower chance of infection, stroke, and kidney complications

- A lower chance of complications such as memory loss, difficulty concentrating, or difficulty thinking clearly

- Faster recovery from the surgery

Minimally invasive direct coronary artery bypass grafting: There are several types of minimally invasive direct coronary artery bypass (MIDCAB) grafting. These types of surgery differ from traditional bypass surgery because they only require small incisions rather than opening the chest bone to get to the heart. These procedures sometimes use a heart-lung machine.

- **MIDCAB procedure:** This procedure is used when only one or two coronary arteries need to be bypassed. A series of small incisions is made between your ribs on the left side of your chest, directly over the artery to be bypassed. The incisions are usually about 3 inches long. (The incisions made in traditional CABG are at least 6 to 8 inches long.) The left internal mammary artery is most often used for the graft. A heart-lung machine isn't used during this procedure.

- **Port-access coronary artery bypass procedure:** This procedure is performed through small incisions (ports) made in your chest. Artery or vein grafts are used. The heart-lung machine is used during this procedure.

- **Robot-assisted technique:** This type of procedure allows for even smaller, keyhole-sized incisions. A small video camera is inserted in one incision to show the heart, while the surgeon uses remotely controlled surgical instruments to perform the surgery. The heart-lung machine is sometimes used during this procedure.

Advantages of minimally invasive CABG include smaller incisions, smaller scars, shorter recovery and hospital stay, less bleeding, less chance for infection, and less pain.

What to Expect after Coronary Artery Bypass Grafting

Recovery in the Hospital

After surgery, you will typically spend 1 or 2 days in an intensive care unit. Your heart rate and blood pressure will be continuously monitored during this time. Intravenous medicines (medicines injected through a vein) are often given to regulate blood circulation and blood pressure. You will then be moved to a less intensive care area of the hospital for 3 to 5 days before going home.

Recovery at Home

Your doctor will give you specific instructions for recovering at home, especially concerning the following issues:

- How to care for your healing incisions
- How to recognize signs of infection or other complications
- When to call the doctor immediately
- When to make followup appointments

You may also receive instructions on how to deal with common after-effects from surgery. After-effects often go away within 4 to 6 weeks after surgery, but may include the following:

- Discomfort or itching from healing incisions
- Swelling of the area where an artery or vein was taken for grafting
- Muscle pain or tightness in the shoulders and upper back
- Fatigue (tiredness), mood swings, or depression
- Difficulty sleeping or loss of appetite
- Constipation
- Chest pain around the site of the chest bone incision (more frequent with the traditional surgery)

Full recovery from traditional CABG may take 6 to 12 weeks or more. Less recovery time is needed for nontraditional CABG.

Your doctor will provide instructions on resuming physical activity. This varies from person to person, but there are some typical timeframes. Most people can resume sexual activity within about 4 weeks and driving after 3 to 8 weeks.

Returning to work after 6 weeks is common unless the job involves specific and demanding physical activity. Some people may need to find less physically demanding types of work or work a reduced schedule at first.

Chapter 60

Carotid Endarterectomy

Carotid endarterectomy, or CEA, is surgery to remove plaque from the carotid arteries. These are the two large arteries on each side of your neck. They supply oxygen-rich blood to your brain.

CEA is used to prevent stroke, or "brain attack," in people who have carotid artery disease. Carotid artery disease occurs when plaque builds up in the carotid arteries.

Plaque is made up of fat, cholesterol, calcium, and other substances found in the blood. Over time, plaque hardens and narrows the arteries. This limits or blocks the flow of oxygen-rich blood to your brain, which can lead to a stroke.

A stroke also can occur if the plaque in an artery cracks or ruptures. Blood cells called platelets stick to the site of the injury and may clump together to form blood clots. Blood clots can partly or fully block a carotid artery.

Overview

CEA and carotid angioplasty are the two treatments used to reduce blockages in the carotid arteries. CEA can lower the risk of stroke in people who have narrowed or blocked carotid arteries and symptoms suggesting stroke or transient ischemic attack (TIA). During a TIA, or "mini-stroke," you may have some or all of the symptoms of

Excerpted from text by the National Heart, Lung, and Blood Institute (NHLBI, www.nhlbi.nih.gov), part of the National Institutes of Health, February 2009.

stroke. However, the symptoms usually go away on their own within 24 hours.

CEA also can lower the risk of stroke in people who have severely blocked carotid arteries, even if they don't have stroke symptoms.

Carotid angioplasty is another common treatment for carotid artery disease. For this procedure, a thin tube with a balloon on the end is threaded to the narrowed or blocked artery.

Once in place, the balloon is inflated to push the plaque outward against the wall of the artery. Usually, the doctor then places a small metal stent in the artery to reduce the risk that it will become blocked again.

Antiplatelet medicines also may be used to treat people who have carotid artery disease. These medicines help reduce blood clotting and lower the risk of stroke.

Outlook

CEA can greatly reduce the risk of stroke in people who have carotid artery disease. The surgery is fairly safe when done by a surgeon who has experience with it. However, serious complications, such as stroke and death, can occur. If you have carotid artery disease, talk to your doctor about whether CEA is an option for you.

If you've already had a CEA, you can take steps to lower your risk of future strokes. For example, get ongoing care, treat other conditions (such as high blood pressure and high blood cholesterol), and don't smoke.

Other Names for Carotid Endarterectomy

Carotid endarterectomy also is called carotid artery surgery.

When Carotid Endarterectomy Is Needed

Your doctor may recommend carotid endarterectomy (CEA) if you have carotid artery disease. CEA can help prevent strokes in people who have this condition.

CEA is most helpful for people who have carotid artery disease and one or more of the following:

- A prior stroke

- A prior transient ischemic attack (TIA), or "mini-stroke"

- Severely blocked carotid arteries (even if you don't have stroke symptoms)

What to Expect before Carotid Endarterectomy

Your doctor will talk to you about how to prepare for carotid endarterectomy (CEA). Before CEA, you may have one or more tests to examine your carotid arteries.

These tests can show whether your arteries are narrowed or blocked, and how severe your condition is.

What to Expect during Carotid Endarterectomy

Carotid endarterectomy (CEA) is done in a hospital. The surgery usually takes about 2 hours.

You will have anesthesia during the surgery so you don't feel pain. General anesthesia temporarily puts you to sleep. Local anesthesia numbs only certain areas of your body.

Your surgeon may choose to give you local anesthesia so he or she can talk to you during the surgery. This allows the surgeon to check your brain's reaction to the decrease in blood flow that occurs during the surgery.

During CEA, your surgeon will make an incision (cut) in your neck to expose the blocked section of the carotid artery. He or she will put a clamp on your artery to stop blood flow through it.

During the procedure, your brain gets blood from the carotid artery on the other side of your neck. However, your surgeon also may use a tube called a shunt to move blood around the narrowed or blocked carotid artery.

Next, your surgeon will make a cut in the blocked part of the artery. To remove the plaque, he or she will remove the inner lining of the artery where the blockage is.

Finally, your surgeon will close the artery with stitches and stop any bleeding. He or she will then close the incision in your neck.

What to Expect after Carotid Endarterectomy

After carotid endarterectomy (CEA) surgery, you may stay in the hospital for 1 to 2 days. This allows your doctor to watch for any signs of complications.

If your surgery takes place early in the day and you're doing well, you may be able to go home the same day.

Chapter 61

Total Artificial Heart Surgery

A total artificial heart (TAH) is a device that replaces the two lower chambers of the heart. These chambers are called ventricles. You may benefit from a TAH if both of your ventricles don't work due to end-stage heart failure.

Heart failure is a condition in which the heart is damaged or weakened and can't pump enough blood to meet the body's needs. "End stage" means the condition has become so severe that all treatments, except heart transplant, have failed.

Overview

You may need a TAH for one of two reasons:

- To keep you alive while you wait for a heart transplant
- If you're not eligible for a heart transplant, but you have end-stage heart failure in both ventricles

The TAH is attached to your heart's upper chambers—the atria. Between the TAH and the atria are mechanical valves that work like the heart's own valves. Valves control the flow of blood in the heart.

Currently, there are two types of TAH. They're known by their brand names: the CardioWest and the AbioCor. The main difference

Excerpted from "Total Artificial Heart," by the National Heart, Lung, and Blood Institute (NHLBI, www.nhlbi.nih.gov), part of the National Institutes of Health, September 2008.

between these TAHs is that the CardioWest is connected to an outside power source and the AbioCor isn't.

The CardioWest has tubes that, through holes in the abdomen, connect from inside the chest to an outside power source.

The AbioCor TAH is completely contained inside the chest. A battery powers this TAH. The battery is charged through the skin with a special magnetic charger.

Energy from the external charger reaches the internal battery through an energy transfer device called transcutaneous energy transmission, or TET.

An implanted TET device is connected to the implanted battery. An external TET coil is connected to the external charger. Also, an implanted controller monitors and controls the pumping speed of the heart.

Outlook

A TAH usually extends life for months beyond what is expected with end-stage heart failure. If you're waiting for a heart transplant, a TAH can keep you alive while you wait for a donor heart. It also can improve your quality of life. However, a TAH is a very complex device. It's challenging for surgeons to implant, and it can cause complications.

Currently, TAHs are used only in a small number of people. Researchers are working to make even better TAHs that will allow people to live longer and have fewer complications.

Other Names for a Total Artificial Heart

- Artificial heart
- AbioCor
- CardioWest

When a Total Artificial Heart Is Needed

You may benefit from a total artificial heart (TAH) if both of your ventricles don't work due to end-stage heart failure.

If you're waiting for a heart transplant, a TAH can help you survive longer. It also can improve your quality of life. If your life expectancy is less than 30 days and you're not eligible for a heart transplant, a TAH may extend your life beyond the expected 30 days.

A TAH is a "last resort" device. This means only people who have tried every other type of treatment, except heart transplant, can get it. The TAH isn't used for people who may benefit from medicines or other procedures.

TAHs also have a size limit. These devices are fairly large and can only fit into large chest areas. Currently, no TAHs are available that can fit into children's chests. However, researchers are trying to make smaller models.

The United States Food and Drug Administration (FDA) has approved the TAH for certain types of patients. Your doctor will discuss with you whether you meet the conditions for getting a TAH.

If you and your doctor decide that a TAH is a good option for you, you also will discuss which of the two types of TAH will work best for you.

What to Expect before Total Artificial Heart Surgery

Before you get a total artificial heart (TAH), you will likely spend at least a week in the hospital to prepare for the surgery. You might already be in the hospital getting treatment for heart failure.

During this time, you will learn about the TAH and how to live with it. You and your loved ones will spend time with your surgeons, cardiologist (heart specialist), and nurses to make sure you have all the information you need before surgery. You can ask to see what the device looks like and how it will be attached inside your body.

Your doctors will make sure that your body is strong enough for the surgery. If your doctors think your body is too weak, you may need to get extra nutrition through a feeding tube before surgery.

You also will have tests to make sure you're ready for surgery. These tests include the following:

- **A chest CT scan:** This test is used to make sure the TAH will fit in your chest. Current TAHs are fairly large. Before you have surgery, your doctor will make sure there's enough room in your chest for the device.

- **Blood tests:** These tests are used to check how well your liver and kidneys are working. Blood tests also are used to check the levels of blood cells and important chemicals in your blood.

- **Chest x-ray:** This test is used to create pictures of the inside of your chest to help your doctors prepare for surgery.

- **EKG (electrocardiogram):** This test is used to check how well your heart is working before the ventricles are replaced by the TAH.

What to Expect during Total Artificial Heart Surgery

Total artificial heart (TAH) surgery is complex and can take between 5 and 9 hours. It requires many experts and assistants. As many as 15 people may be in the operating room during surgery.

The team for TAH surgery includes the following:

- Surgeons who do the operation

- Surgical nurses who assist the surgeons

- Anesthesiologists who are in charge of the medicine that makes you sleep during surgery

- Perfusionists who are in charge of the heart-lung machine that keeps blood flowing through your body while the TAH is put in your chest

- Engineers who are trained to assemble the TAH and make sure it's working properly

Before the surgery, you're given anesthesia to make you sleep. During the surgery, the anesthesiologist checks your heartbeat, blood pressure, oxygen levels, and breathing. A breathing tube is placed in your windpipe through your throat. This tube is connected to a ventilator (a machine that helps you breathe).

A cut is made down the center of your chest. The chest bone is then cut and your ribcage is opened so that the surgeon can get to your heart.

Medicines are used to stop your heart. This allows the surgeon to operate on your heart while it's not beating. A heart-lung machine keeps oxygen-rich blood moving through your body.

The surgeons remove your heart's ventricles and attach the TAH to the upper chambers of your heart. When everything is attached properly, the heart-lung machine is switched off and the TAH starts pumping.

What to Expect after Total Artificial Heart Surgery

Recovery in the Hospital

Recovery time after total artificial heart (TAH) surgery depends a lot on your condition before the surgery.

If you had severe heart failure for a while before getting the TAH, your body may be weak and your lungs may not work very well. Thus, you may still need a ventilator (a machine that helps you breathe) after surgery. You also may need to continue getting nutrition through a feeding tube.

Your hospital stay could last a month or longer after TAH surgery.

Right after surgery, you'll be in the hospital's intensive care unit. An intravenous (IV) line will be inserted into a vein in your arm to give you fluids and nutrition. You'll also have a tube in your bladder to drain urine.

After a few days or more, depending on how quickly your body recovers, you'll move to a regular hospital room. Nurses who have experience with TAHs and similar devices will take care of you.

The nurses will help you get out of bed, sit, and walk around. As you get stronger, you'll be able to go to the bathroom and have a regular diet. The feeding and urine tubes will be removed. You'll also be able to take a shower. You'll learn how to do this while taking care of your TAH device.

Nurses and physical therapists will help you gain your strength through a slow increase in activity. You'll also learn how to care for your TAH device at home.

Having family or friends visit you at the hospital can be very helpful. They can help you with various activities. They also can learn about caring for the TAH device so they can help when you go home.

Going Home

Activity level: When you go home after TAH surgery, you'll likely be able to do more activities than you could before. You'll probably be able to get out of bed, get dressed, and move around the house. You may even be able to drive. Your health care team will advise you on the level of activity that's right for you.

Bathing: If you have an AbioCor TAH, you can shower or swim, as long as the device is charged.

If you have a CardioWest TAH, you will have tubes connected to a power source outside of your body. The tubes go through an opening in your skin. This opening can let in bacteria and increase your risk for infections.

You will need to take special steps before you bathe to make sure the tubes going through your abdomen don't get wet. Your health care team will explain how to do this.

Chapter 62

Heart Transplants

A heart transplant is surgery to remove a person's diseased heart and replace it with a healthy heart from a deceased donor. Ninety percent of heart transplants are done on patients who have end-stage heart failure.

Heart failure is a condition in which the heart is damaged or weakened and can't pump enough blood to meet the body's needs. End-stage means the condition has become so severe that all treatments, other than heart transplant, have failed.

Overview

Heart transplants are done as a life-saving measure for end-stage heart failure when medical treatment and less drastic surgery have failed.

Because donor hearts are in short supply, patients who need a heart transplant go through a careful selection process. They need to be sick enough to need a new heart, yet healthy enough to receive it.

Survival rates for people receiving heart transplants have improved over the past 5 to 10 years, especially in the first year after the transplant.

About 88 percent of patients survive the first year after transplant surgery, and 72 percent survive for 5 years. The 10-year survival rate

Excerpted from "Heart Transplant," by the National Heart, Lung, and Blood Institute (NHLBI, www.nhlbi.nih.gov), part of the National Institutes of Health, October 2009.

is close to 50 percent, and 16 percent of heart transplant patients survive 20 years.

After the surgery, most heart transplant recipients (about 90 percent) can come close to resuming their normal lifestyles. However, fewer than 40 percent return to work for many different reasons.

The Heart Transplant Process

The heart transplant process starts when doctors refer patients who have end-stage heart failure to a heart transplant center for evaluation. Patients found to be eligible for a heart transplant are placed on a waiting list for a donor heart.

Heart transplant surgery is done in a hospital when a suitable donor heart is found. After the transplant, patients are started on a lifelong health care plan. The plan involves multiple medicines and frequent medical checkups.

When a Heart Transplant Is Needed

Referral to a Heart Transplant Center

Most patients referred to a heart transplant center have end-stage heart failure. Of these patients, close to half have heart failure as a result of coronary heart disease (also called coronary artery disease).

Others have heart failure caused by hereditary conditions, viral infections of the heart, or damaged heart valves and muscles. (Some medicines, alcohol, and pregnancy can damage the heart valves and muscles.)

Most patients considered for a heart transplant have tried other, less drastic treatments and have been hospitalized a number of times for heart failure.

Eligibility for a Heart Transplant

The heart transplant specialists at the heart transplant center will determine whether a patient is eligible for a transplant. Specialists often include the following:

- Cardiologist (a doctor who specializes in diagnosing and treating heart problems)

- Cardiovascular surgeon (a doctor who does the transplant surgery)

- Transplant coordinator (a person who makes arrangements for the surgery, such as transportation of the donor heart)
- Social worker
- Dietitian
- Psychiatrist

In general, patients selected for heart transplants have severe end-stage heart failure, but are healthy enough to have the transplant. Heart failure is considered end stage when all possible treatments—such as medicine, implanted devices, and surgery—have failed.

Patients who have the following conditions might not be candidates for heart transplant surgery because the procedure is less likely to be successful.

- Advanced age
- Poor blood circulation throughout the body, including the brain
- Kidney, lung, or liver diseases that can't be reversed
- History of cancer or malignant tumors
- Inability or unwillingness to follow lifelong medical instructions after a transplant
- Pulmonary hypertension (high blood pressure in the lungs) that can't be reversed
- Active infection throughout the body

Although there's no widely accepted upper age limit for a heart transplant, most transplant surgery is done on patients younger than 70 years old.

What to Expect before a Heart Transplant

The Heart Transplant Waiting List

Patients who are eligible for a heart transplant are placed on a waiting list for a donor heart. This waiting list is part of a national allocation system for donor organs run by the Organ Procurement and Transplantation Network (OPTN).

OPTN has policies in place to make sure donor hearts are given out fairly. These policies are based on urgency of need, the organs that are available for transplant, and the location of the patient who is receiving the heart (the recipient).

Organs are matched for blood type and size of donor and recipient.

The Donor Heart

Guidelines on how a donor heart is selected require that the donor meet the legal requirement for brain death and that the appropriate consent forms are signed.

Guidelines suggest that the donor be younger than 65 years old, have little or no history of heart disease or trauma to the chest, and not be exposed to hepatitis or HIV. The guidelines also recommend that the donor heart not be without blood circulation for more than 4 hours.

Waiting Times

Approximately 3,000 people in the United States are on the waiting list for a heart transplant on any given day. About 2,000 donor hearts are available each year. Wait times vary from days to several months and will depend on a recipient's blood type and condition.

A person may be taken off the list for some time if he or she has a serious medical event such as a stroke, infection, or kidney failure.

Time spent on the waiting list plays a part in who receives a donor heart. For example, if a donor heart becomes available and two recipients have equal need, the recipient who has been waiting longer usually will get the heart.

Ongoing Medical Treatment

Patients on the waiting list for a donor heart receive ongoing treatment for heart failure and other medical conditions.

Treating arrhythmias (irregular heartbeats), for example, is very important because they can cause sudden cardiac arrest in people who have heart failure.

As a result, many transplant centers will place implantable cardioverter defibrillators (ICDs) in patients before surgery. An ICD is a small device that's placed in the chest or abdomen to help control life-threatening arrhythmias.

Another treatment that may be recommended to waiting list patients is an implanted mechanical pump called a ventricular assist device (VAD). This device helps the heart pump blood.

Regular outpatient care for waiting list patients may include frequent exercise testing, assessing the strength of the heartbeat, and right cardiac catheterization (a test to measure blood pressure in the right side of the heart).

Contact with the Transplant Center during the Wait

People on the waiting list often are in close contact with their transplant centers. Most donor hearts must be transplanted within 4 hours after removal from the donor.

At some heart transplant centers, recipients get a pager so the center can contact them at any time. They're asked to tell the transplant center staff if they're going out of town. Recipients often need to be prepared to arrive at the hospital within 2 hours of being notified about a donor heart.

Not all patients who are called to the hospital will get a heart transplant. Sometimes, at the last minute, doctors find that a donor heart isn't suitable for a patient. Other times, patients from the waiting list are called to come in as possible substitutes, in case something happens with the selected recipient.

What to Expect during a Heart Transplant

Just before the heart transplant surgery, patients will get general anesthesia. The term "anesthesia" refers to a loss of feeling and awareness. General anesthesia temporarily puts you to sleep.

A bypass machine is hooked up to the arteries and veins of the heart. The machine pumps blood through the patient's lungs and body while the diseased heart is removed and the donor heart is sewn into place.

What to Expect after a Heart Transplant

In the Hospital

The amount of time a heart transplant recipient spends in the hospital will vary with each person. It often involves 1 to 2 weeks in the hospital and 3 months of monitoring by the transplant team at the heart transplant center.

Monitoring may include frequent blood tests, lung function tests, EKGs (electrocardiograms), echocardiograms, and biopsies of the heart tissue.

A heart biopsy is a standard test used to see whether your body is rejecting the new heart. It might be done often in the weeks after a transplant.

During a heart biopsy, a tiny grabbing device is inserted into a vein in the neck or groin (upper thigh). The device is threaded through the vein to the right atrium of the new heart to take a small tissue sample. The tissue sample is checked for signs of rejection.

While in the hospital, your health care team may recommend that you start a cardiac rehabilitation (rehab) program. Cardiac rehab is a medically supervised program that helps improve the health and well-being of people who have heart problems.

Cardiac rehab includes counseling, education, and exercise training to help you recover. Rehab may start with a member of the rehab team helping you sit up in a chair or take a few steps. Over time, you'll increase your activity level.

Watching for Signs of Rejection

The new heart is a foreign body that your immune system may attack if you're not getting enough medicine to suppress your immune system after the surgery.

You and the transplant team will work together to protect the new heart by watching for signs of rejection. These signs include the following:

- Shortness of breath
- Fever
- Fatigue (tiredness)
- Weight gain (retaining fluid in the body)
- Reduced amounts of urine (problems in the kidneys can cause this)

You and the team also will work together to manage the transplant medicines and their side effects, prevent infections, and continue treatment of ongoing medical conditions.

You may be asked to check your temperature, blood pressure, and pulse when you go home.

Preventing Rejection

You'll need to take medicine to suppress your immune system so that it doesn't reject the new heart.

These transplant medicines are called immunosuppressants. They're a combination of medicines that are tailored to your situation. Often, they include cyclosporine, tacrolimus, MMF (mycophenolate mofetil), and steroids such as prednisone.

Your doctors may need to change or adjust your transplant medicines if they aren't working well or if you have too many side effects.

Managing Transplant Medicines and Their Side Effects

You'll have to manage multiple medicines. It's helpful to set up a routine for taking medicines at the same time each day and for refilling prescriptions. It's crucial to never run out of medicine. Always using the same pharmacy may help.

Keep a list of all your medicines with you at all times in case of an accident. When traveling, keep extra doses of medicine with you, not packed in your luggage. Bring your medicines with you to all doctor visits.

Side effects from medicines can be serious. Side effects include risk of infection, diabetes, osteoporosis (thinning of the bones), high blood pressure, kidney disease, and cancer—especially lymphoma and skin cancer.

Discuss any side effects of the medicines with your transplant team. Your doctors may change or adjust your medicines if you're having problems. Make sure your doctors know all of the medicines you're taking.

Preventing Infection

Some transplant medicines can increase your risk of infection. You may be asked to watch for signs of infection, including fever, sore throat, cold sores, and flu-like symptoms.

Signs of possible chest or lung infections could include shortness of breath, cough, and a change in the color of sputum (spit).

The incision (cut) from your surgery must be checked for redness, swelling, or drainage. It's especially important to look for signs of infection because transplant medicines often can mask these signs.

Talk to your doctor about what steps you should take to reduce your risk of infection. For example, your doctor may recommend that you avoid contact with animals or crowds of people in the first few months after your transplant.

Regular dental care also is important. Your doctor may prescribe antibiotics before any dental work to prevent infections.

Pregnancy

Many successful pregnancies have occurred after heart transplant surgeries; however, special care is important. If you've had a heart transplant, talk with your doctor before planning a pregnancy.

Emotional Issues and Support

Having a heart transplant may cause fear, anxiety, and stress. While you're waiting for a heart transplant, you may worry that you won't live long enough to get a new heart. After surgery, you may feel overwhelmed, depressed, or worried about complications.

All of these feelings are normal for someone going through major heart surgery. It's important to talk about how you feel with your health care team. Talking to a professional counselor also can help. If you're feeling very depressed, your health care team or counselor may prescribe medicines to make you feel better.

Support from family and friends also can help relieve stress and anxiety. Let your loved ones know how you feel and what they can do to help you.

Risks of a Heart Transplant

Although heart transplant surgery is a life-saving measure, it has many risks. Careful monitoring, treatment, and regular medical care can prevent or help manage some of these risks.

Risks of heart transplant include the following:

- Failure of the donor heart
- Complications from medicines
- Infection
- Cancer
- Problems that arise from not following a lifelong health care plan

Failure of the Donor Heart

Over time, the new heart may fail due to the same reasons that caused the original heart to fail. Failure of the donor heart also can occur if your body rejects the donor heart or if cardiac allograft vasculopathy (CAV) develops. CAV is a blood vessel disease.

Patients who have a heart transplant that fails can be considered for another transplant (called a retransplant).

Primary Graft Dysfunction

The most frequent cause of death in the first 30 days after transplant is primary graft dysfunction. This occurs if the new donor heart fails and isn't able to function.

Factors such as shock or trauma to the donor heart or narrowed blood vessels in the recipient's lungs can cause primary graft dysfunction. Medicines (for example, inhaled nitric oxide and intravenous nitrates) may be used to treat this condition.

Rejection of the Donor Heart

Rejection is one of the leading causes of death in the first year after transplant. The recipient's immune system sees the new heart as a foreign body and attacks it.

During the first year, 25 percent of heart transplant patients have signs of a possible rejection at least once. Half of all possible rejections happen in the first 6 weeks after surgery, and most happen within 6 months of surgery.

Cardiac Allograft Vasculopathy

CAV is a chronic (ongoing) disease in which the walls of the coronary arteries in the new heart become thick, hard, and lose their elasticity. CAV can destroy blood circulation in the new heart and cause serious damage.

CAV is a leading cause of donor heart failure and death in the years following transplant surgery. CAV can cause heart attack, heart failure, dangerous arrhythmias, and sudden cardiac arrest.

To detect CAV, your doctor may recommend coronary angiography yearly and other tests, such as stress echocardiography or intravascular ultrasound.

Complications from Medicines

Taking daily medicines that stop the immune system from attacking the new heart is absolutely critical, even though the medicine combinations have serious side effects.

Cyclosporine and other medicines can cause kidney damage. Kidney damage affects more than 25 percent of patients in the first year after transplant. Five percent of transplant patients will develop end-stage kidney disease within 7 years.

Infection

When the immune system—the body's defense system—is suppressed, the risk of infection increases. Infection is a major cause of hospital admission for heart transplant patients and a leading cause of death in the first year after transplant.

Cancer

Suppressing the immune system leaves patients at risk of cancers and malignancies. Malignancies are a major cause of late death in heart transplant patients, accounting for nearly 25 percent of heart transplant deaths 3 years after transplant.

The most common malignancies are tumors of the skin and lips (patients at highest risk are older, male, and fair-skinned) and malignancies in the lymph system, such as non-Hodgkin lymphoma.

Other Complications

High blood pressure develops in more than 70 percent of heart transplant patients in the first year after transplant and in nearly 95 percent of patients within 5 years.

High levels of cholesterol and triglycerides in the blood develop in more than 50 percent of heart transplant patients in the first year after transplant and in 84 percent of patients within 5 years.

Osteoporosis can develop or worsen in heart transplant patients. This condition thins and weakens the bones.

Complications from Not Following a Lifelong Health Care Plan

Not following a lifelong health care plan increases the risk of all heart transplant complications. Heart transplant patients are asked to closely follow their doctors' instructions and check their own health status throughout their lives.

Lifelong health care includes taking multiple medicines on a strict schedule, watching for signs and symptoms of complications, keeping all medical appointments, and stopping unhealthy behaviors (such as smoking).

Chapter 63

Cardiac Rehabilitation

Cardiac rehabilitation (rehab) is a medically supervised program that helps improve the health and well-being of people who have heart problems.

Rehab programs include exercise training, education on heart-healthy living, and counseling to reduce stress and help you return to an active life.

Cardiac rehab helps people who have heart problems do the following:

- Recover after a heart attack or heart surgery

- Prevent future hospital stays, heart problems, and death related to heart problems

- Address risk factors that lead to coronary heart disease (also called coronary artery disease) and other heart problems

- Adopt healthy lifestyle changes

- Improve their health and quality of life

Each patient will have a program that's designed to meet his or her needs.

Excerpted from "Cardiac Rehabilitation," by the National Heart, Lung, and Blood Institute (NHLBI, www.nhlbi.nih.gov), part of the National Institutes of Health, August 2009.

The Cardiac Rehabilitation Team

Cardiac rehab involves a long-term commitment from the patient and a team of health care providers.

The cardiac rehab team may include doctors (such as a family doctor, a heart specialist, and a surgeon), nurses, exercise specialists, physical and occupational therapists, dietitians or nutritionists, and psychologists or other mental health specialists. In some cases, a case manager will help track the patient's care.

Working with the team is an important part of cardiac rehab. The patient should share questions and concerns with the team. This will help the patient reach his or her goals.

Outlook

People of all ages can benefit from cardiac rehab. The lifestyle changes made during rehab have few risks. These changes can improve your overall health and prevent future heart problems and even death.

Exercise training as part of cardiac rehab may not be safe for all patients. For example, people who have very high blood pressure or severe heart disease may not be ready to exercise. These patients can still benefit from other parts of the cardiac rehab program.

Ask your doctor whether cardiac rehab can help you prevent a future heart problem and improve your health.

When Cardiac Rehabilitation Is Needed

People of all ages and ethnic backgrounds can benefit from cardiac rehabilitation (rehab). Rehab may help people who have had the following:

- A heart attack
- Angioplasty or coronary artery bypass grafting for coronary heart disease
- Heart valve repair or replacement
- A heart transplant or a lung transplant
- Stable angina
- Heart failure

Cardiac rehab is equally helpful to both men and women. It can improve your overall health and prevent future heart problems and even death.

What to Expect When Starting Cardiac Rehabilitation

Your doctor may refer you to cardiac rehabilitation (rehab) during an office visit or while you're in the hospital recovering from a heart attack or heart surgery. If your doctor doesn't mention it, ask him or her whether cardiac rehab might benefit you.

Rehab activities vary depending on your condition. If you're recovering from major heart surgery, rehab will start with a member of the rehab team helping you sit up in a chair or take a few steps. You'll work on range-of-motion exercises. These include moving your fingers, hands, arms, legs, and feet. Over time, you'll increase your activity level.

Once you leave the hospital, rehab will continue in a rehab center. The rehab center may be part of the hospital or in another place.

Try to find a center close to home that offers services at a convenient time. If no centers are near your home, or if it's too hard to get to them, ask your doctor about home-based rehab.

For the first 2 to 3 months, you'll need to go to rehab regularly to learn how to reduce risk factors and to begin an exercise program. After that, your rehab team may recommend less frequent visits.

Overall, you may work with the rehab team for 12 months or more. The length of time you continue cardiac rehab depends on your situation.

Health Assessment

Before you start your cardiac rehab program, your rehab team will assess your health. This includes taking your medical history and doing a physical exam and tests.

Medical history: A doctor or nurse will ask you about previous heart problems, heart surgery, and any heart-related symptoms you have. He or she also will ask whether you've had medical procedures or other health problems (such as diabetes or kidney disease).

The doctor or nurse may ask questions about the following:

- Whether your family has a history of heart disease
- What medicines you're taking, including over-the-counter medicines and dietary supplements (such as vitamins and herbal remedies)
- Whether you smoke and how much
- How you check your blood sugar level, and how often you do it (if you have diabetes)

- Whether you've ever had hypoglycemia, a condition can occur in people who take medicines to control their blood sugar levels

Your rehab team will ask questions to help them assess your quality of life and well-being.

Physical exam: A doctor or nurse will do a physical exam to check your overall health, including your heart rate, blood pressure, reflexes, and breathing.

Tests: Your doctor may recommend tests to check your heart.

A resting EKG (electrocardiogram) is a simple test that detects and records your heart's electrical activity. The test shows how fast your heart is beating and your heart's rhythm (steady or irregular). An EKG also shows the strength and timing of electrical signals as they pass through each part of your heart.

You also may need tests to measure your cholesterol and blood sugar levels. If you have diabetes, staff also will do an HbA1C test to check your blood sugar control. This test shows how well your diabetes has been managed over time.

What to Expect during Cardiac Rehabilitation

During cardiac rehabilitation (rehab), you'll learn how to do the following:

- Increase your physical activity and exercise safely
- Follow a heart-healthy diet
- Reduce risk factors for future heart problems
- Improve your emotional health

The rehab team will work with you to create a plan that meets your needs. Each part of cardiac rehab will help lower your risk for future heart problems.

Over time, the lifestyle changes you make during rehab will become more routine. They will help you maintain a reduced risk for heart disease.

Support from your family can help make cardiac rehab easier. For example, family members can help you plan healthy meals and do physical activities. The healthy lifestyle changes you learn during cardiac rehab can benefit your entire family.

Increase Physical Activity and Exercise Safely

Physical activity is an important part of a healthy lifestyle. It can strengthen your heart muscle, reduce your risk for heart disease, and improve your muscle strength, flexibility, and endurance.

Your rehab team will assess your physical activity level to learn how active you are at home, at work, and during recreation. If your job includes heavy labor, the team may recreate your workplace conditions to help you practice in a safe setting.

You'll work with the team to find ways to safely add physical activity to your daily routine. For example, you may decide to park farther from building entrances, walk up two or more flights of stairs, or walk for 15 minutes during your lunch break.

Your rehab team also will work with you to create an easy-to-follow exercise plan. It will include time for a warmup, flexibility exercises, and cooling down. It also may include aerobic exercise and muscle-strengthening activities. You'll get a written plan that lists each exercise and explains how often and for how long you should do it.

You're more likely to make exercise a habit if you enjoy the activity. Work with the rehab team to find the types of activity that you enjoy and that are safe for you. If you prefer to exercise with other people, join a group or ask a friend to join you.

Exercise training as part of cardiac rehab may not be safe for all patients. For example, if you have very high blood pressure or severe heart disease, you may not be ready for exercise training. Or, you may only be able to tolerate very light conditioning exercises. The rehab team will help decide what level of exercise is safe for you.

Aerobic exercise: Typically, your rehab team will ask you to do aerobic exercise 3 to 5 days per week for 30 to 60 minutes. The exercise specialist on your team will make sure that your exercise plan is safe and right for you. Examples of aerobic exercise are walking (outside or on a treadmill), cycling, rowing, or climbing stairs.

Muscle-strengthening activities: Typically, your rehab team will ask you to do muscle-strengthening activities 2 or 3 days per week. Your exercise plan will show how many times to repeat each exercise. Muscle-strengthening activities may include lifting weights (hand weights, free weights, or weight machines), using a wall pulley, or using elastic bands to stretch and condition your muscles.

Exercise at the rehab center and at home: When you start cardiac rehab, you'll exercise at the rehab center. Members of your

545

rehab team will carefully watch you to make sure you're exercising safely.

A team member will check your blood pressure several times during exercise training. You also may need an EKG (electrocardiogram) to check your heart's electrical activity during exercise. This test shows how fast your heart is beating and whether its rhythm is steady or irregular.

Your exercise program will change as your health improves. After awhile, you'll add at-home exercises to your plan.

Follow a Heart-Healthy Diet

Your rehab team will help you create and follow a heart-healthy diet. The diet will help you reach your rehab goals, which may include managing your weight, cholesterol levels, blood pressure, diabetes, kidney disease, heart failure, and/or other health problems that your diet can affect.

You'll learn how to plan meals that meet your calorie needs and are low in saturated and trans fats, cholesterol, and sodium (salt).

Your rehab team also may advise you to limit alcohol and other substances. Alcohol can raise your blood pressure and harm your liver, brain, and heart.

Reduce Risk Factors for Future Heart Problems

Your cardiac rehab team will work with you to control your risk factors for heart problems. Risk factors include high blood pressure, high blood cholesterol, overweight or obesity, diabetes, and smoking.

High blood pressure: High blood pressure raises your risk for future heart problems. The rehab team will work with you to reach the blood pressure goal your doctor sets. This goal will depend on factors such as your age and whether you have heart failure, diabetes, or kidney disease.

Exercising, losing weight, limiting how much salt and alcohol you consume, and quitting smoking can help you lower your blood pressure. You may need medicine to lower your blood pressure if lifestyle changes aren't enough.

High blood cholesterol: Too much cholesterol in the blood can cause heart disease. Your rehab team will work with you to lower high blood cholesterol. You can do this by following a heart-healthy diet, losing weight, exercising, quitting smoking, and limiting how much alcohol you drink.

Physical activity also can increase HDL [high-density lipoprotein] cholesterol, which is sometimes called good cholesterol. This is because it helps remove cholesterol from your arteries.

You may need medicine to lower your cholesterol if lifestyle changes aren't enough.

Overweight and obesity: If you're overweight or obese, your rehab team will help you set short- and long-term weight-loss goals. You can reach these goals by following the diet and exercise plans that the team creates for you.

Diabetes: If you have diabetes, your rehab team will work with you to control your blood sugar level. Following a heart-healthy diet, losing weight, and exercising can lower your blood sugar level.

Your doctor may suggest that you test your blood sugar before and after exercising to watch for numbers that are too high or too low. Your doctors will tell you what numbers to look for.

You may need medicine to lower your blood sugar level if lifestyle changes aren't enough.

Smoking: Smoking is a risk factor for heart disease. If you smoke, quitting can help you avoid future heart problems. Quitting can help lower your blood pressure and keep your cholesterol levels healthy.

Talk to your rehab team about programs and products that can help you quit smoking. Also, try to avoid secondhand smoke.

It may help to set a quit date. Some people find it helpful to enroll in smoking cessation programs or to seek counseling. Other people find acupuncture or hypnosis helpful.

Improve Emotional Health

Psychological factors increase the risk of getting heart disease or making it worse. Depression, anxiety, and anger are common among people who have heart disease or have had a heart attack or heart surgery.

Get treatment if you feel sad, anxious, angry, or isolated. These feelings can affect your physical recovery. Depression is linked to complications such as irregular heartbeats, chest pain, a longer recovery time, the need to return to the hospital, and even an increased risk of death.

Seeking help is important. Group or individual counseling helps lower your risk for future heart attacks and death. It also may motivate you to exercise and help you relax and learn how to reduce stress.

People with heart disease who get mental health treatment often show improvements in blood pressure, cholesterol, and other measures of physical health.

The rehab team may include a mental health specialist, or someone from the team may be able to refer you to one. Without help from a professional, these problems may not go away.

Some communities have support groups for people who have had heart attacks or heart surgery. They also may have walking groups or exercise classes. Help with basic needs and transportation also may be available.

Counseling for Sexual Dysfunction

People who have heart problems sometimes have sexual problems. The most common problem is less interest or no interest in sex. Impotence or premature or delayed ejaculation may occur in men.

Depression, medicines, fear of causing a heart attack, or diabetes can contribute to sexual problems.

Sexual activity often is safe for low-risk patients. The maximum heart rate during usual sexual activity is similar to other daily activities, such as walking up one or two flights of stairs.

Talk to your doctor if you're having sexual problems or to find out whether sexual activity is safe for you.

Chapter 64

Getting Back into Your Life after a Heart Attack

How soon can I return to my regular activities?

The amount of activity you can do after a heart attack will be based on the condition of your heart. Your doctor will work with you to develop a recovery plan. Most people can return to work and the activities they enjoy within a few months of having a heart attack. Others may have to limit their activity if the heart muscle is very weak.

You will need to start slowly. For the first few days after your heart attack, you may need to rest and let your heart heal. As your heart heals, you'll be ready to start moving around again. A few days after your heart attack, your doctor may want you to move around more. You may do stretching exercises and get up and walk. You'll then slowly become more active based on advice from your doctor.

Once you've gotten through the early period after a heart attack, your doctor may talk to you about how to be active within your limits. Your doctor will probably want you to do an exercise test, also called a stress test. During this test, your doctor will ask you to exercise (usually walking on a treadmill) while he or she monitors your heart. Based on the results, your doctor will develop an exercise plan for you.

How can I improve my recovery plan?

Your doctor may recommend that you get involved in a cardiac rehabilitation program. Cardiac rehabilitation programs are supervised by exercise specialists. Many hospitals sponsor these programs to get people started with a safe level of exercise after a heart attack. After a while, you'll probably be able to exercise on your own. But if you have any of the symptoms listed below, call your doctor. You may be working too hard.

Exercise alert! Call your doctor right away if you have any of the following symptoms during exercise:

- Shortness of breath for more than about 10 minutes
- Chest pain or pain in your arms, neck, jaw, or stomach
- Dizzy spells
- Pale or splotchy skin
- Very fast heartbeat or an irregular heartbeat
- Cold sweats
- Nausea and vomiting
- Weakness or fainting
- Swelling or pain in your legs

Why is exercise so important?

Exercise strengthens your heart muscle. It can also boost your energy, help you feel more in control of your health, and help you lose weight and keep it off. Exercise may also lower your blood pressure and reduce your cholesterol level.

What kind of exercise is good?

The best types of exercise are those that involve your whole body, such as walking, cycling, jogging, cross-country skiing, or swimming. Your doctor or rehabilitation therapists may also prescribe activities to increase your strength and flexibility.

Risk factors for another heart attack: Taking charge of the things that put you at risk for another heart attack can help you feel better and reduce your risk of future problems. The following factors can put you at risk for another heart attack:

- Not exercising
- Alcohol in excessive amounts
- Being overweight or obese
- High cholesterol level
- High blood sugar level if you have diabetes
- High blood pressure
- Smoking
- Too much stress in your life

How often should I exercise?

This depends on your exercise plan. You'll probably start slowly and gradually add to your routine. Your doctor may want you to exercise three or four times a week for about 10 to 30 minutes at a time. Be sure to warm up before exercising by stretching for 5 minutes or more.

What is a MET?

You may hear your doctor talk about METs when he or she discusses your activity level. METs stands for metabolic equivalents. Different activities are given different MET levels depending on how much energy they take to do (see Table 64.1).

The higher the MET level, the more energy the activity takes. Your doctor may ask you not to do things that take more than 3 or 3.5 METs right after your heart attack.

What can I do to speed my recovery and stay healthy?

Your doctor will probably recommend that you make some changes in your diet, such as cutting back on fat and cholesterol and watching how much salt you eat.

If you smoke, you will have to quit. Your doctor may also suggest that you learn better ways to deal with stress, such as time management, relaxation training, and deep breathing.

When can I go back to work?

Most people go back to work within 1 to 3 months after having a heart attack. The amount of time you are off from work depends on the condition of your heart and how strenuous or stressful your work is. You may have to make some changes in how you do your job or you may have to change jobs, at least for a short time, if your job is too hard on your heart.

What about sex?

You can probably start having sex again in 3 to 4 weeks after your heart attack. As with other types of activity, you may need to start out slowly and work your way back into your normal patterns.

Don't be afraid of sex because of your heart attack. Try different positions if one position seems to make you uncomfortable. Let your partner be on top to reduce the amount of energy you use during sex. Talk with your doctor if you or your partner has any concerns.

Table 64.1. MET Activities

Sitting in a chair	1.0
Sweeping the floor	1.5
Driving a car	2.0
Ironing	3.5
Showering	3.5
Bowling	3.5
Sex	3.7–5.0
Golfing	4.0
Gardening	4.5
Playing tennis	6.0
Lawn mowing	6.5
Shoveling	7.0
Skiing	8.0

Chapter 65

Poststroke Rehabilitation

In the United States more than 700,000 people suffer a stroke each year, and approximately two thirds of these individuals survive and require rehabilitation. The goals of rehabilitation are to help survivors become as independent as possible and to attain the best possible quality of life. Even though rehabilitation does not "cure" stroke in that it does not reverse brain damage, rehabilitation can substantially help people achieve the best possible long-term outcome.

What is poststroke rehabilitation?

Rehabilitation helps stroke survivors relearn skills that are lost when part of the brain is damaged. For example, these skills can include coordinating leg movements in order to walk or carrying out the steps involved in any complex activity. Rehabilitation also teaches survivors new ways of performing tasks to circumvent or compensate for any residual disabilities. Patients may need to learn how to bathe and dress using only one hand, or how to communicate effectively when their ability to use language has been compromised. There is a strong consensus among rehabilitation experts that the most important element in any rehabilitation program is carefully directed, well-focused, repetitive practice—the same kind of practice used by all people when

Excerpted from "Post-Stroke Rehabilitation Fact Sheet," by the National Institute of Neurological Disorders and Stroke (NINDS, www.ninds.nih.gov), part of the National Institutes of Health, October 30, 2009.

they learn a new skill, such as playing the piano or pitching a baseball.

Rehabilitative therapy begins in the acute-care hospital after the patient's medical condition has been stabilized, often within 24 to 48 hours after the stroke. The first steps involve promoting independent movement because many patients are paralyzed or seriously weakened. Patients are prompted to change positions frequently while lying in bed and to engage in passive or active range-of-motion exercises to strengthen their stroke-impaired limbs. (Passive range-of-motion exercises are those in which the therapist actively helps the patient move a limb repeatedly, whereas "active" exercises are performed by the patient with no physical assistance from the therapist.) Patients progress from sitting up and transferring between the bed and a chair to standing, bearing their own weight, and walking, with or without assistance. Rehabilitation nurses and therapists help patients perform progressively more complex and demanding tasks, such as bathing, dressing, and using a toilet, and they encourage patients to begin using their stroke-impaired limbs while engaging in those tasks. Beginning to reacquire the ability to carry out these basic activities of daily living represents the first stage in a stroke survivor's return to functional independence.

For some stroke survivors, rehabilitation will be an ongoing process to maintain and refine skills and could involve working with specialists for months or years after the stroke.

What disabilities can result from a stroke?

The types and degrees of disability that follow a stroke depend upon which area of the brain is damaged. Generally, stroke can cause five types of disabilities: paralysis or problems controlling movement; sensory disturbances including pain; problems using or understanding language; problems with thinking and memory; and emotional disturbances.

Paralysis or problems controlling movement (motor control): Paralysis is one of the most common disabilities resulting from stroke. The paralysis is usually on the side of the body opposite the side of the brain damaged by stroke, and may affect the face, an arm, a leg, or the entire side of the body. This one-sided paralysis is called hemiplegia (one-sided weakness is called hemiparesis). Stroke patients with hemiparesis or hemiplegia may have difficulty with everyday activities such as walking or grasping objects. Some stroke patients have problems with swallowing, called dysphagia, due to damage to the part of the brain that controls the muscles for swallowing. Damage to a lower part of the brain, the cerebellum, can affect the body's ability to coordinate movement, a disability called ataxia, leading to problems with body posture, walking, and balance.

Sensory disturbances including pain: Stroke patients may lose the ability to feel touch, pain, temperature, or position. Sensory deficits may also hinder the ability to recognize objects that patients are holding and can even be severe enough to cause loss of recognition of one's own limb. Some stroke patients experience pain, numbness, or odd sensations of tingling or prickling in paralyzed or weakened limbs, a condition known as paresthesia.

Stroke survivors frequently have a variety of chronic pain syndromes resulting from stroke-induced damage to the nervous system (neuropathic pain). Patients who have a seriously weakened or paralyzed arm commonly experience moderate to severe pain that radiates outward from the shoulder. Most often, the pain results from a joint becoming immobilized due to lack of movement and the tendons and ligaments around the joint become fixed in one position. This is commonly called a frozen joint; passive movement at the joint in a paralyzed limb is essential to prevent painful freezing and to allow easy movement if and when voluntary motor strength returns. In some stroke patients, pathways for sensation in the brain are damaged, causing the transmission of false signals that result in the sensation of pain in a limb or side of the body that has the sensory deficit. The most common of these pain syndromes is called thalamic pain syndrome, which can be difficult to treat even with medications.

The loss of urinary continence is fairly common immediately after a stroke and often results from a combination of sensory and motor deficits. Stroke survivors may lose the ability to sense the need to urinate or the ability to control muscles of the bladder. Some may lack enough mobility to reach a toilet in time. Loss of bowel control or constipation may also occur. Permanent incontinence after a stroke is uncommon. But even a temporary loss of bowel or bladder control can be emotionally difficult for stroke survivors.

Problems using or understanding language (aphasia): At least one-fourth of all stroke survivors experience language impairments, involving the ability to speak, write, and understand spoken and written language. A stroke-induced injury to any of the brain's language-control centers can severely impair verbal communication.

Damage to a language center located on the dominant side of the brain, known as the Broca area, causes expressive aphasia. People with this type of aphasia have difficulty conveying their thoughts through words or writing. They lose the ability to speak the words they are thinking and to put words together in coherent, grammatically correct sentences. In contrast, damage to a language center located in a rear portion of the brain, called the Wernicke area, results in receptive aphasia. People with this condition have difficulty understanding spoken or written language and often have incoherent speech. Although they can form grammatically correct sentences, their utterances are often devoid of meaning. The most severe form of aphasia, global aphasia, is caused by extensive damage to several areas involved in language function. People with global aphasia lose nearly all their linguistic abilities; they can neither understand language nor use it to convey thought. A less severe form of aphasia, called anomic or amnesic aphasia, occurs when there is only a minimal amount of brain damage; its effects are often quite subtle. People with anomic aphasia may simply selectively forget interrelated groups of words, such as the names of people or particular kinds of objects.

Problems with thinking and memory: Stroke can cause damage to parts of the brain responsible for memory, learning, and awareness. Stroke survivors may have dramatically shortened attention spans or may experience deficits in short-term memory. Individuals also may lose their ability to make plans, comprehend meaning, learn new tasks, or engage in other complex mental activities. Two fairly common deficits resulting from stroke are anosognosia, an inability to acknowledge the reality of the physical impairments resulting from stroke, and neglect, the loss of the ability to respond to objects or sensory stimuli located on one side of the body, usually the stroke-impaired side. Stroke survivors who develop apraxia lose their ability to plan the steps involved in a complex task and to carry the steps out in the proper sequence. Stroke survivors with apraxia may also have problems following a set of instructions. Apraxia appears to be caused by a disruption of the subtle connections that exist between thought and action.

Emotional disturbances: Many people who survive a stroke feel fear, anxiety, frustration, anger, sadness, and a sense of grief for their physical and mental losses. These feelings are a natural response to the psychological trauma of stroke. Some emotional disturbances and personality changes are caused by the physical effects of brain damage.

Clinical depression, which is a sense of hopelessness that disrupts an individual's ability to function, appears to be the emotional disorder most commonly experienced by stroke survivors. Signs of clinical depression include sleep disturbances, a radical change in eating patterns that may lead to sudden weight loss or gain, lethargy, social withdrawal, irritability, fatigue, self-loathing, and suicidal thoughts. Poststroke depression can be treated with antidepressant medications and psychological counseling.

Chapter 66

The Future of Cardiovascular Disorder Treatment: Stem Cell Research

American Heart Association (AHA) Policy

The American Heart Association funds meritorious research involving human adult stem cells as part of our scientific research grant program. We do not fund any research involving stem cells derived from human embryos or fetal tissue.

The American Heart Association recognizes the value of all types of stem cell research and supports federal funding of this research. We are committed to supporting medical and scientific research to help us pursue our mission of reducing death and disability from cardiovascular diseases and stroke.

To stay abreast of the benefits and challenges in the area of human stem cell research the American Heart Association Research Committee annually monitors scientific activity in the area and periodically assesses current scientific opinion on the potential impact of embryonic and adult stem cell research on CVD [cardiovascular disease] and stroke.

What are stem cells, and how can they be used?

Stem cells are unspecialized cells within the body that have the potential to develop into one or many kinds of cells. Stem cells potentially

"Stem Cell Research," reprinted with permission. © 2009 American Heart Association, Inc. (www.americanheart.org).

could treat or cure many diseases and conditions, including Parkinson's disease, Alzheimer's disease, diabetes, certain heart diseases, stroke, arthritis, certain birth defects, osteoporosis, spinal cord injury, and burns.

There are essentially two types of human stem cells—embryonic and adult. In order for a stem cell to differentiate into a specialized cell type, such as a cardiac or brain cell, the stem cell must achieve a "pluripotent" state. Pluripotent stem cells can potentially develop into any kind of cell in the body and come from three sources:

- fetal tissue from miscarriages and abortions;

- embryos created for in vitro fertility treatments but not selected for implantation;

- adult cells that have been reprogrammed to embryonic stem cell-like state.

The American Heart Association funds meritorious research involving human adult stem cells.

Adult stem cells are found in a many organs and tissues. An adult stem cell is an undifferentiated cell found among differentiated cells in a tissue or organ, can renew itself, and can differentiate to yield the major specialized cell types of the tissue or organ. The primary roles of adult stem cells in a living organism are to maintain and repair the tissue in which they are found. In their original state they have less ability than embryonic stem cells to differentiate into other types of cells.

Until recently, it was thought that only embryonic stem cells were pluripotent. However, recent research has developed a way to successfully induce adult stem cells into a pluripotent state, which has the potential to create patient-specific cell therapies that could reduce many of the underlying complications seen in therapies with embryonic stem cells.

Even though this new method of inducing adult stem cells could provide an alternative to use of embryonic stem cells, it is still important for research to continue in both cell types. In order to know how induced adult stem cells need to perform, we must know more about the innate function of embryonic stem cells. Therefore, to bring effective and safe stem cell based therapies into reality, research on both cell types continues to be important.

What is the importance of stem cell research to cardiovascular disease and stroke?

Stem cell research offers great promise to treat or cure many diseases and conditions. It could be used to develop dramatic new procedures and techniques to reverse degenerative heart disease. For example, it may help generate new, healthy heart tissue, valves and other vital tissues and structures. About 128 million people suffer from diseases that might be cured or treated through stem cell research. About 58 million of these people suffer from cardiovascular disease.

New discoveries in the field also show potential for being able to study the origins of disease, which could lead to new knowledge related to CVD and stroke prevention. Also, the development of cardiac cells from stem cells provides the unique opportunity for researchers to test new drugs on actual human tissue rather than in animals.

Part Seven

Preventing Disease and Regaining Cardiovascular Health

Chapter 67

Weight Management

The Importance of a Healthy Weight

Being overweight or obese increases your risk for many diseases and conditions. The more you weigh, the more likely you are to suffer from heart disease, high blood pressure, diabetes, gallbladder disease, sleep apnea, and certain cancers. On the other hand, a healthy weight has many benefits: It helps you to lower your risk for developing these problems, helps you to feel good about yourself, and gives you more energy to enjoy life.

Risk for Weight-Related Diseases

Body Mass Index (BMI)

Your BMI accurately estimates your total body fat. And, the amount of fat that you carry is a good indicator of your risk for a variety of diseases.

There are two ways to check your BMI:

- Use a BMI chart. First, find your height in the left-hand column. Then, follow it over until you find your weight. The number on the top of that column is your BMI.

Excerpted from "Facts About Healthy Weight," from the Aim for a Healthy Weight Provider Kit, by the National Heart, Lung, and Blood Institute (NHLBI, www.nhlbi.nih.gov), part of the National Institutes of Health, 2006.

- Use the BMI calculator on the National Heart, Lung, and Blood Institute's (NHLBI's) Web site: http://www.nhlbisupport.com/bmi.

Although BMI can be used for most men and women, it does have some limitations:

- It may overestimate body fat in athletes and others who have a muscular build.

- It may underestimate body fat in older persons and others who have lost muscle.

Waist Circumference Measurement

Your waist circumference is also an important measurement to help you figure out your overall health risks. If most of your fat is around your waist, then you are more at risk for heart disease and diabetes. This risk increases with a waist measurement that is greater than 35 inches for women and greater than 40 inches for men.

Other Risk Factors for Heart Disease

If you have other risk factors for heart disease and are overweight or obese, then you will be at greater risk for health problems. Your doctor will check your BMI, waist circumference, and other risk factors for heart disease:

- If you are overweight (BMI 25–29.9), do not have a high waist circumference, and have less than two risk factors, then it's important that you not gain any more weight.

- If you are overweight (BMI 25–29.9) or have a high waist circumference and have two or more risk factors, then it is important for you to lose weight.

- If you are obese (BMI 30), then it is important for you to lose weight.

Even a small weight loss (just 5–10 percent of your current weight) will help to lower your risk of developing weight-related diseases.

How to Lose Weight and Maintain It

Changing the way you approach weight loss can help you be more successful at losing it. Most people who try to lose weight focus on one thing: weight loss. However, if you set goals, begin to eat healthy foods, become more physically active, and learn how to change behaviors, then you may be more successful at losing weight. Over time, these changes will become routine and part of your everyday life.

Weight Loss Goals

Setting the right goals is an important first step to losing and maintaining weight.

- Losing just 5–10 percent of your current weight over 6 months will lower your risk for heart disease and other conditions.

- Losing 1–2 pounds per week is a reasonable and safe weight loss. Losing weight at this rate will help you to keep off the weight. And it will give you the time to make new healthy lifestyle changes.

- Maintaining a modest weight loss over a longer period of time is better than losing a lot of weight and regaining it. You can think about additional weight loss after you've lost 10 percent of your current body weight and have kept it off for 6 months.

Keeping a Balance

Maintaining a healthy weight calls for keeping a balance . . . a balance of energy. You must balance the calories or energy that you get from food and beverages with the calories that you use to keep your body going and to be physically active.

- The same amount of energy IN and OUT over time = weight stays the same

- More energy IN than OUT over time = weight gain

- More energy OUT than IN over time = weight loss

Your energy IN and OUT doesn't have to balance exactly every day: Balancing energy over time will help you to maintain a healthy weight in the long run.

Calories

Cutting back on calories is part of a healthy eating plan to lose weight. Choose foods that are lower in fats, especially saturated and trans fats, cholesterol, and added sugars. Also, pay attention to portion sizes.

To lose 1–2 pounds a week, daily intake should be reduced by 500 to 1,000 calories. In general:

- Eating plans that contain 1,000–1,200 calories each day will help most women to lose weight safely.

- Eating plans that contain 1,200–1,600 calories each day are suitable for men and may also be appropriate for women who weigh 165 pounds or more or who exercise regularly.

If you eat 1,600 calories a day but do not lose weight, then you may want to cut back to 1,200 calories. If you are hungry on either diet, then you may want to boost your calories by 100 to 200 per day. Very low calorie diets of less than 800 calories per day should not be used unless you are being monitored by your doctor.

Physical Activity

Staying physically active and eating fewer calories will help you lose weight and keep the weight off over time.

How much physical activity should you aim for?

- For overall health and to reduce the risk of disease, aim for at least 30 minutes of moderate physical activity most days of the week.

- To help manage body weight and prevent gradual weight gain, aim for 60 minutes of moderate-to-vigorous physical activity most days of the week.

- To maintain weight loss, aim for at least 60–90 minutes of daily moderate physical activity.

You can break up the amount of time that you do physical activity, such as 15 minutes at a time. If you haven't been physically active for some time, then don't let that stop you. Start slowly and gradually increase your activity. For example, start walking for 10–15 minutes three times a week, then gradually build up to the recommended amount with brisk walking.

Other Weight Loss Options

Weight loss drugs and weight loss surgery may be options for some people who are at high risk from overweight or obesity or who have been unsuccessful at making lifestyle changes. If you think that you may benefit from weight loss drugs or surgery, then talk to your doctor.

Tips to Weight Loss Success

Maintaining long-term weight loss can be difficult. Three keys to success are setting realistic goals, following a healthy diet, and aiming for 60–90 minutes of physical activity most days of the week.

Other tips for weight loss success include the following:

- Set specific, realistic goals that are forgiving (less than perfect). To start, try walking 30 minutes, 3 days a week.

- Ask for encouragement from your health care provider(s) via telephone or e-mail; friends and family can help. You can also join a support group.

- Keep a record of your food intake and the amount of physical activity that you do. This is an easy way to track how you are doing. A record can also inspire you. For example, when it shows that you've been more active, you'll be encouraged to keep it up.

- Change your surroundings to avoid overeating. For example, don't eat while watching television. Plan to meet a friend in a nonfood setting.

- Reward your success but not with food. Instead, choose rewards that you'll enjoy, such as a movie, music CD, an afternoon off from work, a massage, or personal time.

Chapter 68

Physical Activity and Heart Health

Physical Activity

Physical activity is any body movement that works your muscles and uses more energy than you use when you're resting. Walking, running, dancing, swimming, yoga, and gardening are examples of physical activity.

According to the Department of Health and Human Services' "2008 Physical Activity Guidelines for Americans," physical activity generally refers to bodily movement that enhances health.

Exercise is a type of physical activity that's planned and structured. Lifting weights, taking an aerobics class, and playing on a sports team are examples of exercise.

Physical activity is good for many parts of your body. This text focuses on the benefits of physical activity for your heart and lungs.

Types of Physical Activity

The four main types of physical activity are aerobic, muscle-strengthening, bone-strengthening, and stretching. Aerobic activity is the type that benefits your heart and lungs the most.

This chapter contains text excerpted from "Physical Activity," by the National Heart, Lung, and Blood Institute (NHLBI, www.nhlbi.nih.gov), part of the National Institutes of Health, May 2009, and from "Physical Activity and Weight Affect Coronary Heart Disease Risk," by the National Institutes of Health (NIH, www.nih.gov), May 12, 2008.

Aerobic Activity

Aerobic activity moves your large muscles, such as those in your arms and legs. Running, swimming, walking, bicycling, dancing, and doing jumping jacks are examples of aerobic activity. Aerobic activity also is called endurance activity.

Aerobic activity makes your heart beat faster than usual. You also breathe harder during this type of activity. Over time, regular aerobic activity makes your heart and lungs stronger and able to work better.

Other Types of Physical Activity

The other types of physical activity—muscle-strengthening, bone-strengthening, and stretching—benefit your body in other ways.

Muscle-strengthening activities improve the strength, power, and endurance of your muscles. Doing pushups and sit-ups, lifting weights, climbing stairs, and digging in the garden are examples of muscle-strengthening activities.

With bone-strengthening activities, your feet, legs, or arms support your body's weight, and your muscles push against your bones. This helps make your bones strong. Running, walking, jumping rope, and lifting weights are examples of bone-strengthening activities.

Muscle-strengthening and bone-strengthening activities also can be aerobic, depending on whether they make your heart and lungs work harder than usual. For example, running is both an aerobic activity and a bone-strengthening activity.

Stretching helps improve your flexibility and your ability to fully move your joints. Touching your toes, doing side stretches, and doing yoga exercises are examples of stretching.

Levels of Intensity in Aerobic Activity

You can do aerobic activity with light, moderate, or vigorous intensity. Moderate- and vigorous-intensity aerobic activities are better for your heart than light-intensity activities. However, even light-intensity activities are better than no activity at all.

The level of intensity depends on how hard you have to work to do the activity. To do the same activity, people who are less fit usually have to work harder than people who are more fit. So, for example, what is light-intensity activity for one person may be moderate-intensity for another.

Light- and moderate-intensity activities: Light-intensity activities are common daily activities that don't require much effort.

Moderate-intensity activities make your heart, lungs, and muscles work harder than light-intensity activities do.

On a scale of 0 to 10, moderate-intensity activity is a 5 or 6 and produces noticeable increases in breathing and heart rate. A person doing moderate-intensity activity can talk but not sing.

Vigorous-intensity activities: Vigorous-intensity activities make your heart, lungs, and muscles work hard. On a scale of 0 to 10, vigorous-intensity activity is a 7 or 8. A person doing vigorous-intensity activity can't say more than a few words without stopping for a breath.

Examples of Aerobic Activities

Below are examples of aerobic activities. Depending on your level of fitness, they can be light, moderate, or vigorous in intensity:

- Pushing a grocery cart around a store
- Gardening, such as digging or hoeing that causes your heart rate to go up
- Walking, hiking, jogging, running
- Water aerobics or swimming laps
- Bicycling, skateboarding, inline skating, and jumping rope
- Ballroom dancing and aerobic dancing
- Tennis, soccer, hockey, and basketball

Benefits of Physical Activity

Physical activity, especially aerobic activity, is good for your heart and lungs in many ways. The benefits of physical activity apply to people of all ages and races and both sexes.

Physical Activity Strengthens Your Heart and Improves Lung Function

Moderate- and vigorous-intensity physical activity done regularly strengthens your heart muscle. This improves your heart muscle's ability to pump blood to your lungs and throughout your body. As a result, more blood flows to your muscles, and oxygen levels in your blood rise.

Capillaries, your body's tiny blood vessels, also widen. This allows them to deliver more oxygen to your body and carry away waste products, such as carbon dioxide and lactic acid.

Physical Activity Reduces Coronary Heart Disease Risk Factors

Moderate- and vigorous-intensity aerobic activity done regularly can lower your risk for coronary heart disease (CHD), also called coronary artery disease. CHD is a condition in which a fatty material called plaque builds up inside your coronary arteries. These arteries supply oxygen-rich blood to your heart.

Plaque narrows the coronary arteries and reduces blood flow to the heart. It also makes it more likely that blood clots will form in your arteries. Blood clots can partly or completely block blood flow. This can lead to a heart attack.

Certain traits, conditions, or habits may raise your risk for CHD. Physical activity can help control some of these risk factors:

- Physical activity can lower blood pressure.

- Physical activity helps improve and manage levels of cholesterol and other fats in the blood. Physical activity can lower triglyceride levels. Triglycerides are a type of fat. Physical activity also can raise high-density lipoprotein (HDL), or "good," cholesterol levels.

- Physical activity improves your body's ability to manage blood sugar and insulin levels. This lowers your risk for type 2 diabetes.

- Physical activity reduces levels of C-reactive protein (CRP) in your body. This protein is a sign of inflammation. High levels of CRP may raise your risk for CHD.

- Physical activity helps reduce overweight and obesity when combined with reduced calorie intake. Physical activity also helps you maintain a healthy weight over time.

- Physical activity may help people quit smoking. Smoking is a major risk factor for CHD.

Inactive people are nearly twice as likely to develop CHD as people who are physically active. Studies suggest that like high blood cholesterol, high blood pressure, and smoking, inactivity is a major risk factor for CHD.

Physical Activity Reduces the Risk of Heart Attack

In people who have CHD, aerobic activity done regularly helps the heart work better. It also may reduce the risk of a second heart attack in people who already have had a heart attack.

Vigorous aerobic activity may not be safe for people who have CHD. Talk to your doctor about what type of activity is safe for you.

Risks of Physical Activity

In general, the benefits of regular physical activity far outweigh risks to the heart and lungs.

Rarely, heart problems, such as arrhythmia, sudden cardiac arrest, or heart attack, occur during physical activity. These events generally happen to people who already have heart conditions.

In youth and young adults, the risk for heart problems due to physical activity is higher in people who have underlying congenital heart problems. These are heart problems that have been present since birth.

Congenital heart problems include hypertrophic cardiomyopathy, congenital heart defects, and myocarditis (inflammation of the heart muscle). People who have these conditions should talk to their doctors about which physical activities are safe for them.

In middle-aged and older adults, the risk for heart problems due to physical activity is related to coronary heart disease (CHD). People who already have CHD are more likely to have a heart attack when they're exercising vigorously than when they're not.

The risk for heart problems due to physical activity is related to your fitness level and the intensity of the activity you're doing. For example, someone who doesn't do physical activity regularly is at higher risk for heart attack during vigorous activity than a person who is physically fit and regularly active.

If you have a heart problem or chronic (ongoing) disease, such as heart disease, diabetes, or high blood pressure, talk to your doctor about what types of physical activity are safe for you. You also should talk to your doctor about safe physical activities if you have symptoms such as chest pain or dizziness. Discuss ways that you can slowly and safely build physical activity into your daily routine.

Recommendations for Physical Activity

The U.S. Department of Health and Human Services (DHHS) has released new physical activity guidelines for all Americans aged 6 and older.

The "2008 Physical Activity Guidelines for Americans" explains that regular physical activity improves health. They encourage people to be as active as possible.

The guidelines provide specific recommendations about the types and amounts of physical activity that children, adults, older adults, and other groups should do. The guidelines also provide suggestions for how to fit physical activity into your daily life.

The information in this portion of text is based on the new guidelines from DHHS.

Guidelines for Children and Youth

For children and youth, the guidelines advise the following:

- They do 60 minutes or more of physical activity every day. These activities should vary and be a good fit for their age and physical development. Children are naturally active, especially when they're involved in unstructured play (like recess). Any type of activity counts toward the advised 60 minutes or more.

- Most physical activity should be moderate-intensity aerobic activity. Examples include walking, running, skipping, playing on the playground, playing basketball, and biking.

- Vigorous-intensity aerobic activity should be included at least 3 days a week. Examples include running, doing jumping jacks, and fast swimming.

- Muscle-strengthening activities should be included at least 3 days a week. Examples include climbing trees, playing tug-of-war, and doing pushups and pull-ups.

- Bone-strengthening activities should be included at least 3 days a week. Examples include hopping, skipping, doing jumping jacks, playing volleyball, and working with resistance bands.

Children and youth who have disabilities should work with their doctors to find out what types and amounts of physical activity are safe for them. When possible, these children should meet the recommendations in the guidelines.

Some experts also advise that children and youth reduce screen time because it limits time for physical activity. They recommend that children aged 2 and older should spend no more than 2 hours a day watching television or using a computer (except for school work).

Guidelines for Adults

For adults, the guidelines advise:

- Some physical activity is better than none. Inactive adults should gradually increase their level of activity. People gain some health benefits from as little as 60 minutes of moderate-intensity aerobic activity per week.

- For major health benefits, do at least 150 minutes (2 hours and 30 minutes) of moderate-intensity aerobic activity or 75 minutes (1 hour and 15 minutes) of vigorous-intensity aerobic activity each week. Another option is to do a combination of both. A general rule is that 2 minutes of moderate-intensity activity counts the same as 1 minute of vigorous-intensity activity.

- When doing aerobic activity, do it for at least 10 minutes at a time. Spread the activity throughout the week.

- For more health benefits, do 300 minutes (5 hours) of moderate-intensity aerobic activity or 150 minutes (2 hours and 30 minutes) of vigorous-intensity activity each week (or a combination of both). More physical activity will increase your health benefits.

- Muscle-strengthening activities that are moderate or high intensity should be included 2 or more days a week. These activities should work all of the major muscle groups (legs, hips, back, chest, abdomen, shoulders, and arms). Examples include lifting weights, working with resistance bands, doing sit-ups and push-ups, doing yoga, and doing heavy gardening.

Guidelines for Older Adults

For older adults, the guidelines advise:

- All older adults should avoid inactivity. Older adults who do any amount of physical activity gain some health benefits. If inactive, older adults should gradually increase their activity levels and avoid vigorous activity at first. You should follow the guidelines for adults, if possible.

- Older adults should do a variety of activities, including walking. Walking has been shown to provide health benefits and a low risk of injury.

- If you can't do 150 minutes (2 hours and 30 minutes) of activity each week, be as physically active as your abilities and condition allow.

- You should do balance exercises if you're at risk for falls. Examples include walking backward or sideways, standing on one leg, and standing from a sitting position several times in a row.

- If you have a chronic (ongoing) condition, such as heart disease, lung disease, or diabetes, talk to your doctor about whether you can do physical activity. Ask your doctor which activities are safe for you.

Guidelines for Women during Pregnancy and Soon after Delivery

For pregnant women and women who have recently given birth, the guidelines advise:

- You should talk to your doctor about safe physical activities to do during pregnancy and after delivery.

- If you're healthy but not already very active, do at least 150 minutes (2 hours and 30 minutes) of moderate-intensity aerobic activity each week. If possible, spread this activity across the week.

- If you're already very active, you can continue being active as long as you stay healthy and talk to your doctor about your activity level throughout your pregnancy.

- After the first 3 months of pregnancy, you shouldn't do exercises that involve lying on your back.

- You shouldn't do activities in which you might fall or hurt yourself, such as horseback riding, downhill skiing, soccer, and basketball.

Guidelines for Other Groups

The guidelines also have recommendations for other groups, including people who have disabilities and people who have certain chronic conditions, such as osteoarthritis, diabetes, and cancer.

Physical Activity and Weight Affect Coronary Heart Disease Risk

Researchers have long known that both physical activity and excess weight affect the risk of coronary heart disease. However, it's been hard to tease apart how much each contributes. A study found that being physically active can considerably, but not completely, lower the risk of cardiovascular disease associated with being overweight or obese.

The research stems from the Women's Health Study, begun in 1992 by NIH's National Cancer Institute (NCI) and National Heart, Lung, and Blood Institute (NHLBI). Its original goals were to evaluate the effects of vitamin E and low-dose aspirin on cardiovascular disease and cancer in healthy women. Recognizing the value of the data they were collecting, the researchers extended the study to do more follow-up and evaluate other cardiovascular risk factors.

Dr. Amy Weinstein at the Beth Israel Deaconess Medical Center in Boston and colleagues at Brigham and Women's Hospital analyzed data collected in the Women's Health Study on almost 39,000 women who were 45 and older. They compared the participants' body mass index (BMI—a ratio of weight to height) and physical activity levels at the start of the study with cardiovascular outcomes (such as heart attacks) over an average of 11 years of follow-up.

In the April 28, 2008, issue of *Archives of Internal Medicine*, the researchers reported that the group had 948 cases of coronary heart disease during the follow-up period. The risk of coronary heart disease, they found, increased as BMI increased. Obese women were over twice as likely to have a coronary event as women in the normal weight category.

Overall, the women who were physically active were 31% less likely to have coronary heart disease than those who weren't active. After the researchers adjusted the data to account for other known influences—such as alcohol use, smoking, and diet—the physically active women still had an 18% lower risk of coronary heart disease. In particular, the researchers found that physical activity significantly reduced the risk of coronary heart disease in the overweight and obese women.

The researchers also looked at the time the women spent walking and found that the more the women walked, the lower their risk for coronary heart disease. The greatest drop, for each weight category, was between those who didn't walk for exercise or recreation and those who walked 1–1.5 hours per week.

This study adds to a growing body of evidence showing that physical activity can help you live longer, regardless of whether you have excess weight. A half hour of moderate physical activity every day significantly reduces your risk of chronic disease, and more than 30 minutes further reduces the risk.

Although walking and physical activity significantly reduced the risk of coronary heart disease among the overweight and obese women in this study, their risk didn't drop as low as normal-weight women. Both weight control and physical activity are important for preventing coronary heart disease.

Chapter 69

Nutrition and Cardiovascular Health

Chapter Contents

Section 69.1

What Is Heart-Healthy Eating?

Excerpted from "Heart Healthy Eating," by the Office of
Women's Health (www.womenshealth.gov), January 1, 2008.

Why do I need to be concerned about heart healthy eating?

What you eat affects your risk for having heart disease and poor
blood circulation, which can lead to a heart attack or stroke. Heart
disease is the number one killer and stroke is the number three killer
of American women and men.

In the main type of heart disease, a fatty substance called plaque
builds up in the arteries that bring oxygen-rich blood to the heart.
Over time, this buildup causes the arteries to narrow and harden.
When this happens, the heart does not get all the blood it needs to
work properly. The result can be chest pain or a heart attack.

Most cases of stroke occur when a blood vessel bringing blood to
the brain becomes blocked. The underlying condition for this type of
blockage is having fatty deposits lining the vessel walls.

What foods should I eat to help prevent heart disease and stroke?

You should eat mainly the following:

- Fruits and vegetables

- Grains (at least half of your grains should be whole grains,
  such as whole wheat, whole oats, oatmeal, whole-grain corn,
  brown rice, wild rice, whole rye, whole-grain barley, buckwheat,
  bulgur, millet, quinoa, and sorghum)

- Fat-free or low-fat versions of milk, cheese, yogurt, and other
  milk products

- Fish, skinless poultry, lean meats, dry beans, eggs, and nuts

- Polyunsaturated and monounsaturated fats (found in fish, nuts,
  and vegetable oils)

Also, you should limit the amount of foods you eat that contain the following:

- Saturated fat (found in foods such as fatty cuts of meat, whole milk, cheese made from whole milk, ice cream, sherbet, frozen yogurt, butter, lard, cakes, cookies, doughnuts, sausage, regular mayonnaise, coconut, palm oil)

- Trans fat (found mainly in processed foods such as cakes, cookies, crackers, pies, stick or hard margarine, potato chips, corn chips)

- Cholesterol (found in foods such as liver, chicken and turkey giblets, pork, sausage, whole milk, cheese made from whole milk, ice cream, sherbet, frozen yogurt)

- Sodium (found in salt and baking soda)

- Added sugars (such as corn syrup, corn sweetener, fructose, glucose, sucrose, dextrose, lactose, maltose, honey, molasses, raw sugar, invert sugar, malt syrup, syrup, caramel, and fruit juice concentrates)

Eating lots of saturated fat, trans fat, and cholesterol may cause plaque buildup in your arteries. Eating lots of sodium may cause you to develop high blood pressure, also called hypertension. Eating lots of added sugars may cause you to develop type 2 diabetes. Both hypertension and diabetes increase your risk of heart disease and stroke.

How can I tell how much saturated fat, trans fat, and other substances are in the foods I eat?

Prepared foods that come in packages—such as breads, cereals, canned and frozen foods, snacks, desserts, and drinks—have a Nutrition Facts label on the package. The label states how many calories and how much saturated fat, trans fat, and other substances are in each serving. For information on how to read a Nutrition Facts label, see the Fitness and Nutrition section of womenshealth.gov.

For food that does not have a Nutrition Facts label, such as fresh salmon or a raw apple, you can use the U.S. Department of Agriculture (USDA) National Nutrient Database. This is a bit harder than using the Nutrition Facts label. But by comparing different foods you can get an idea if a food is high or low in saturated fat, sodium, and other substances. To compare lots of different foods at one time, check out the Nutrient Lists.

What is a calorie?

When talking about a calorie in food, it is a measure of the energy that the food supplies to your body. When talking about burning calories during physical activity, a calorie is a measure of the energy used by your body. To maintain the same body weight, the number of food calories you eat during the day should be about the same as the number of calories your body uses.

The number of calories you should eat each day depends on your age, sex, body size, how physically active you are, and other conditions. For instance, a woman between the ages of 31 and 50 who is of normal weight and moderately active should eat about 2,000 calories each day.

I've heard that eating fish is good for my heart. Why is that?

Fish and shellfish contain a type of fat called omega-3 fatty acids. Research suggests that eating omega-3 fatty acids lowers your chances of dying from heart disease. Fish that naturally contain more oil (such as salmon, trout, herring, mackerel, anchovies, and sardines) have more omega-3 fatty acids than lean fish (such as cod, haddock, and catfish). Be careful, though, about eating too much shellfish. Shrimp is a type of shellfish that has a lot of cholesterol.

You can also get omega-3 fatty acids from plant sources, such as the following:

- Canola oil
- Soybean oil
- Walnuts
- Ground flaxseed (linseed) and flaxseed oil

Is drinking alcohol bad for my heart?

Drinking too much alcohol can, over time, damage your heart and raise your blood pressure. If you drink alcohol, you should do so moderately. For women, moderate drinking means one drink per day. For men, it means two drinks per day. One drink counts as:

- 5 ounces of wine;
- 12 ounces of beer; or
- 1.5 ounces of 80-proof hard liquor.

Research suggests that moderate drinkers are less likely to develop heart disease than people who don't drink any alcohol or who drink too much. Red wine drinkers in particular seem to be protected to some degree against heart disease. Red wine contains flavonoids, which are thought to prevent plaque buildup.

Flavonoids also are found in the following:

- Red grapes
- Berries
- Apples
- Broccoli

On the other hand, drinking more than one drink per day increases the risks of certain cancers, including breast cancer. And if you are pregnant, could become pregnant, or have another health condition that could make alcohol use harmful, you should not drink.

With the help of your doctor, decide whether moderate drinking to lower heart attack risk outweighs the possible increased risk of breast cancer or other medical problems.

I need help working out an eating plan that's right for me. Who can I ask for help?

You may want to talk with a registered dietitian. A dietitian is a nutrition expert who can give you advice about what foods to eat and how much of each type. Ask your doctor to recommend a dietitian. You also can contact the American Dietetic Association.

Besides eating healthy foods, what else can I do to keep my heart healthy?

To reduce your risk of heart disease, try the following:

- Quit smoking—talk with your doctor or nurse if you need help quitting.
- Get at least 2 hours and 30 minutes of moderate aerobic physical activity each week. For more information on physical activity, see the Fitness and Nutrition section of womenshealth.gov.
- Lose weight if you are overweight, and keep a healthy weight.
- Get your blood pressure, cholesterol, and blood sugar levels checked regularly.

Section 69.2

Lower Blood Pressure with the DASH Eating Plan

Excerpted from "In Brief: Your Guide to Lowering Your Blood Pressure With DASH," from the National Heart, Lung, and Blood Institute (NHLBI, www.nhlbi.nih.gov), U.S. Department of Health and Human Services, and the National Institutes of Health, June 2007.

What you eat affects your chances of developing high blood pressure (hypertension). Research shows that high blood pressure can be prevented—and lowered—by following the Dietary Approaches to Stop Hypertension (DASH) eating plan, which includes eating less salt and sodium.

High blood pressure, which is blood pressure higher than 140/90 mmHg [millimeters of mercury], affects more than 65 million—or one out of every three—American adults. Another 59 million Americans have prehypertension, which is blood pressure between 120/80 and 140/89 mmHg. This increases their chances of developing high blood pressure and its complications.

High blood pressure is dangerous because it makes your heart work too hard, hardens the walls of your arteries, and can cause the brain to hemorrhage or the kidneys to function poorly or not at all. If not controlled, high blood pressure can lead to heart and kidney disease, stroke, and blindness.

But high blood pressure can be prevented—and lowered—if you take these steps:

- Follow a healthy eating plan, such as DASH, that includes foods lower in salt and sodium.

- Maintain a healthy weight.

- Be moderately physically active for at least 30 minutes on most days of the week.

- If you drink alcoholic beverages, do so in moderation.

If you already have high blood pressure and your doctor has prescribed medicine, take your medicine, as directed, and also follow these steps.

The DASH Eating Plan

The DASH eating plan is rich in fruits, vegetables, fat-free or low-fat milk and milk products, whole grains, fish, poultry, beans, seeds, and nuts. It also contains less salt and sodium; sweets, added sugars, and sugar-containing beverages; fats; and red meats than the typical American diet. This heart healthy way of eating is also lower in saturated fat, trans fat, and cholesterol and rich in nutrients that are associated with lowering blood pressure—mainly potassium, magnesium, and calcium, protein, and fiber.

How Do I Make the DASH?

The DASH eating plan requires no special foods and has no hard-to-follow recipes. It simply calls for a certain number of daily servings from various food groups.

The number of servings depends on the number of calories you're allowed each day. Your calorie level depends on your age and, especially, how active you are. Think of this as an energy balance system—if you want to maintain your current weight, you should take in only as many calories as you burn by being physically active. If you need to lose weight, eat fewer calories than you burn or increase your activity level to burn more calories than you eat.

Choose and prepare foods with less salt, and don't bring the salt shaker to the table. Be creative—try herbs, spices, lemon, lime, vinegar, wine, and salt-free seasoning blends in cooking and at the table. And, because most of the salt, or sodium, that we eat comes from processed foods, be sure to read food labels to check the amount of sodium in different food products. Aim for foods that contain 5 percent or less of the Daily Value of sodium. Foods with 20 percent or more Daily Value of sodium are considered high. These include baked goods, certain cereals, soy sauce, some antacids—the range is wide.

DASH Tips for Gradual Change

Make these changes over a couple of days or weeks to give yourself a chance to adjust and make them part of your daily routine:

- Add a serving of vegetables at lunch one day and dinner the next, and add fruit at one meal or as a snack.

- Increase your use of fat-free and low-fat milk products to three servings a day.

- Limit lean meats to 6 ounces a day—3 ounces a meal, which is about the size of a deck of cards. If you usually eat large portions of meats, cut them back over a couple of days—by half or a third at each meal.

- Include two or more vegetarian-style, or meatless, meals each week.

- Increase servings of vegetables, brown rice, whole wheat pasta, and cooked dry beans. Try casseroles and stir-fry dishes, which have less meat and more vegetables, grains, and dry beans.

- For snacks and desserts, use fruits or other foods low in saturated fat, trans fat, cholesterol, sodium, sugar, and calories—for example, unsalted rice cakes; unsalted nuts or seeds, raisins; graham crackers; fat-free, low-fat, or frozen yogurt; popcorn with no salt or butter added; or raw vegetables.

- Use fresh, frozen, or low-sodium canned vegetables and fruits.

DASH Hints

- Be aware that DASH has more servings of fruits, vegetables, and whole-grain foods than you may be used to eating. These foods are high in fiber and may cause some bloating and diarrhea. To avoid these problems, gradually increase the amount of fruit, vegetables, and whole-grain foods that you eat over several weeks.

- If you have trouble digesting milk products, try taking lactase-enzyme pills (available at drug stores and groceries) with milk products. Or buy lactose-free milk, which includes the lactase enzyme.

- If you don't like or are allergic to nuts, use seeds or legumes (cooked dried beans or peas).

- If you take medicines to control your high blood pressure, keep taking them. But tell your doctor that you are now eating the DASH way.

Other Lifestyle Changes

Making other lifestyle changes while following the DASH eating plan is the best way to prevent and control high blood pressure.

Lose Weight, If Necessary, while Following DASH

DASH is rich in lower calorie foods, such as fruits and vegetables, so it can easily be changed to support weight loss. You can reduce calories even more by replacing higher calorie foods, such as sweets, with more fruits and vegetables.

The best way to take off pounds is to do it slowly, over time, by getting more physical activity and eating fewer calories. To develop a weight-loss or weight-maintenance program that's tailored for you, talk to your doctor or registered dietitian.

Be Physically Active while Following the DASH Eating Plan

Combining DASH with a regular physical activity program, such as walking or swimming, will help you shed pounds and stay trim for the long term. Start with a simple 15-minute walk during your favorite time of day and gradually increase the amount of time you are active. You can do an activity for 30 minutes at one time, or choose shorter periods of at least 10 minutes each. The important thing is to total about 30 minutes of moderate activity on most days. To avoid weight gain or sustain weight loss, try for 60 minutes of moderate-to-vigorous activity each day.

Make the DASH for Life

DASH can help you prevent and control high blood pressure. It can also help you lose weight, if you need to. It meets your nutritional needs and has other health benefits for your heart. So get started today and make the DASH for a healthy life.

Chapter 70

Dietary Supplements and Cardiovascular Health

Chapter Contents

Section 70.1

Omega-3 Fatty Acids

American Heart Association (AHA) Recommendation

Omega-3 fatty acids benefit the heart of healthy people, and those at high risk of—or who have—cardiovascular disease.

We recommend eating fish (particularly fatty fish) at least two times a week. Fish is a good source of protein and doesn't have the high saturated fat that fatty meat products do. Fatty fish like mackerel, lake trout, herring, sardines, albacore tuna, and salmon are high in two kinds of omega-3 fatty acids, eicosapentaenoic acid (EPA) and docosahexaenoic acid (DHA).

To learn about omega-3 levels for different types of fish—as well as mercury levels, which can be a concern—see our Encyclopedia entry on Fish, Levels of Mercury and Omega-3 Fatty Acids [http://www.americanheart.org/presenter.jhtml?identifier=3013797].

We also recommend eating tofu and other forms of soybeans, canola, walnut and flaxseed, and their oils. These contain alpha-linolenic acid (LNA), which can become omega-3 fatty acid in the body. The extent of this modification is modest and controversial, however. More studies are needed to show a cause-and-effect relationship between alpha-linolenic acid and heart disease.

Table 70.1 is a good guide to use for consuming omega-3 fatty acids.

Patients taking more than 3 g of omega-3 fatty acids from capsules should do so only under a physician's care. High intakes could cause excessive bleeding in some people.

Background

In 2002, the American Heart Association released a scientific statement, "Fish Consumption, Fish Oil, Omega-3 Fatty Acids and Cardiovascular Disease," on the effects of omega-3 fatty acids on heart function (including antiarrhythmic effects), hemodynamics (cardiac mechanics), and arterial endothelial function. The link between omega-3 fatty acids and CVD risk reduction are still being studied, but research has shown that omega-3 fatty acids:

- decrease risk of arrhythmias, which can lead to sudden cardiac death;
- decrease triglyceride levels;
- decrease growth rate of atherosclerotic plaque;
- lower blood pressure (slightly).

What do epidemiological and observational studies show? Epidemiologic and clinical trials have shown that omega-3 fatty acids reduce CVD incidence. Large-scale epidemiologic studies suggest that people at risk for coronary heart disease benefit from consuming omega-3 fatty acids from plants and marine sources.

The ideal amount to take isn't clear. Evidence from prospective secondary prevention studies suggests that taking EPA+DHA ranging from 0.5 to 1.8 g per day (either as fatty fish or supplements) significantly reduces deaths from heart disease and all causes. For alpha-linolenic acid, a total intake of 1.5–3 g per day seems beneficial.

Randomized clinical trials have shown that omega-3 fatty acid supplements can reduce cardiovascular events (death, nonfatal heart attacks, nonfatal strokes). They can also slow the progression of atherosclerosis in coronary patients. However, more studies are needed to confirm and further define the health benefits of omega-3 fatty acid supplements for preventing a first or subsequent cardiovascular event.

Table 70.1. Summary of Recommendations for Omega-3 Fatty Acid Intake

Population	Recommendation
Patients without documented coronary heart disease (CHD)	Eat a variety of (preferably fatty) fish at least twice a week. Include oils and foods rich in alpha-linolenic acid (flaxseed, canola and soybean oils, flaxseed, and walnuts).
Patients with documented CHD	Consume about 1 g of EPA+DHA per day, preferably from fatty fish. EPA+DHA in capsule form could be considered in consultation with the physician.
Patients who need to lower triglycerides	2 to 4 g of EPA+DHA per day provided as capsules under a physician's care.

For example, placebo-controlled, double-blind, randomized clinical trials are needed to document the safety and efficacy of omega-3 fatty acid supplements in high-risk patients (those with type 2 diabetes, dyslipidemia, hypertension, and smokers) and coronary patients on drug therapy. Mechanistic studies on their apparent effects on sudden death also are needed.

Increasing omega-3 fatty acid intake through foods is preferable. However, coronary artery disease patients may not be able to get enough omega-3 by diet alone. These people may want to talk to their doctor about taking a supplement. Supplements also could help people with high triglycerides, who need even larger doses. The availability of high-quality omega-3 fatty acid supplements, free of contaminants, is an important prerequisite to their use.

Section 70.2

Cardiovascular Benefits of Fish Oil Canceled by High-Fat Diet

"Benefits of fish oil cancelled by high-fat diet in lab study of heart failure," reprinted with permission. © 2009 American Heart Association, Inc. (www.americanheart.org).

Study highlights:

- In an animal study of heart failure, fish oil supplementation was helpful to animals on a low-fat diet, but not to those on a high-fat diet.

- Researchers think that a high-fat diet may block the heart cells' ability to absorb the omega-3 fatty acids in fish oil.

Fish oil (EPA & DHA [eicosapentaenoic acid and docosahexaenoic acid]) supplementation helped the heart when paired with a low-fat diet, but not when added to a high saturated-fat diet fed to rats with heart failure, according to a [July 2009] study in *Hypertension: Journal of the American Heart Association*.

A group of six researchers from different institutions, led by William C. Stanley, PhD, from the University of Maryland-Baltimore, hypothesized that when the heart is stressed, such as in heart failure, a high-fat diet may block the heart cells' ability to absorb the heart-healthy omega-3 polyunsaturated fatty acids (PUFAs) found in fish oil.

The investigators found that heart size—measured by left ventricular mass (LV mass)—increased in rats fed low- and high saturated-fat diets without fish oil by 40 percent and 42 percent respectively. On a low-fat plus fish oil diet, LV mass increased just 4 percent, while the group fed high saturated-fat diet with fish oil saw a 36 percent LV mass increase.

The scientists also found that certain genes associated with heart failure did not get "switched on" in the group fed a low-fat diet supplemented with fish oil.

The researchers conclude, "This suggests that in order to maximize the benefit from fish oil supplementation, patients at risk for heart failure should not consume a high saturated fat diet."

As part of an overall healthy diet, the American Heart Association recommends limiting saturated fat in the diet to 7 percent or less of calories and consuming fish, especially oily fish, two times per week. Author disclosures are on the manuscript. The National Institutes of Health funded the study.

Section 70.3

Garlic and Cholesterol

From "Garlic for LDL Cholesterol," National Center for
Complementary and Alternative Medicine (NCCAM, www
.nccam.nih.gov), part of the National Institutes of Health, 2007.

LDL (low-density lipoprotein) cholesterol is widely known as "bad cholesterol" and is believed to be a leading contributor to heart disease. This 2007 study's results cast doubt on garlic's effectiveness in lowering LDL cholesterol levels in adults with moderately high cholesterol.

Dr. Gardner and his team conducted a randomized, placebo-controlled trial studying whether three different formulations of garlic could lower LDL cholesterol. The study participants were randomly divided into four groups to receive either raw garlic, a powdered garlic supplement, an aged extract supplement, or a placebo.

The 169 participants who completed the study had their cholesterol levels checked monthly during the 6-month trial. None of the formulations of garlic had a statistically significant effect on the LDL cholesterol levels. The authors caution that their results should not be generalized for all populations or all health effects. An accompanying editorial in the *Archives of Internal Medicine* points out that LDL cholesterol levels are only one factor contributing to heart disease and that this trial did not investigate garlic's effects on other risk factors, such as high blood pressure.

Gardner CD, Lawson LD, Block E, et al. Effect of raw garlic vs. commercial garlic supplements on plasma lipid concentrations in adults with moderate hypercholesterolemia: a randomized clinical trial. *Archives of Internal Medicine.* 2007;167(4):346–353.

Section 70.4

Vitamin D and Heart Disease

"Lack of vitamin D may increase heart disease risk,"
reprinted with permission. © 2009 American Heart Association, Inc.
(www.americanheart.org).

The same vitamin D deficiency that can result in weak bones now has been associated with an increased risk of cardiovascular disease, Framingham Heart Study researchers report in *Circulation: Journal of the American Heart Association* [2008].

"Vitamin D deficiency is associated with increased cardiovascular risk, above and beyond established cardiovascular risk factors," said Thomas J. Wang, MD, assistant professor of medicine at Harvard Medical School in Boston, Massachusetts. "The higher risk associated with vitamin D deficiency was particularly evident among individuals with high blood pressure."

In a study of 1,739 offspring from Framingham Heart Study participants (average age 59, all Caucasian), researchers found that those with blood levels of vitamin D below 15 nanograms per milliliter (ng/mL) had twice the risk of a cardiovascular event such as a heart attack, heart failure, or stroke in the next 5 years compared to those with higher levels of vitamin D.

When researchers adjusted for traditional cardiovascular risk factors such as high cholesterol, diabetes, and high blood pressure, the risk remained significant with a 62 percent higher risk of a cardiovascular event in participants with low levels of vitamin D compared to those with higher levels.

Researchers observed the highest rate of cardiovascular disease events in subset analyses dividing 688 participants according to high blood pressure status. After researchers adjusted for conventional cardiovascular risk factors, participants with hypertension and a vitamin D deficiency had about two times the risk of having a cardiovascular disease event in 5 years.

Researchers also found an increase in cardiovascular risk with each level of vitamin D deficiency.

"We found that people with low vitamin D levels had a higher rate of cardiovascular events over the 5-year follow-up period," Wang said.

597

"These results are intriguing and suggestive but need to be followed up with further study."

Study participants had no prior cardiovascular disease and were tested for vitamin D status and then followed for an average of 5.4 years.

The participants attended the offspring examinations between 1996 and 2001. Researchers obtained medical history, physical examinations and laboratory assessments of vascular risk factors. They also obtained medical records related to cardiovascular disease.

Overall, 28 percent of individuals had levels of vitamin D below 15 ng/mL and 9 percent had levels below 10 ng/mL. Although levels above 30 ng/mL are considered optimal for bone metabolism, only 10 percent of the study sample had levels in this range, researchers said.

During follow-up:

- 120 participants developed a first cardiovascular event including fatal and nonfatal coronary heart disease;

- 28 participants had fatal or nonfatal cerebrovascular events such as nonhemorrhagic stroke;

- 19 participants were diagnosed with heart failure; and

- 8 had occurrences of claudication, fatigue in the legs during activity.

"Low levels of vitamin D are highly prevalent in the United States, especially in areas without much sunshine," Wang said. "Twenty to 30 percent of the population in many areas has moderate to severe vitamin D deficiency."

Most of this is attributed to lack of sun exposure, pigmented skin that prevents penetration of the sun's rays, and inadequate dietary intake of vitamin D enriched foods, researchers said.

"A growing body of evidence suggests that low levels of vitamin D may adversely affect the cardiovascular system," Wang said. "Vitamin D receptors have a broad tissue distribution that includes vascular smooth muscle and endothelium, the inner lining of the body's vessels. Our data raise the possibility that treating vitamin D deficiency via supplementation or lifestyle measures could reduce cardiovascular risk.

"What hasn't been proven yet is that vitamin D deficiency actually causes increased risk of cardiovascular disease. This would require a large randomized trial to show whether correcting the vitamin D deficiency would result in a reduction in cardiovascular risk."

Therefore, Wang doesn't recommend physicians check for vitamin D deficiency or that those with a known vitamin D deficiency be treated to prevent heart disease at this time.

During the past decade, researchers have studied several other vitamins that initially showed promise in reducing heart disease. But the vitamins didn't reduce heart disease in subsequent large randomized trials.

"On the flip side, just because other vitamins haven't succeeded doesn't preclude the possibility of finding vitamins that might prevent cardiovascular disease," Wang said. "This is always an area of great interest. Vitamins are easy to administer and in general have few toxic effects."

The American Heart Association recommends that healthy people get adequate nutrients by eating a variety of foods in moderation, rather than by taking supplements. Food sources of vitamin D include milk, salmon, mackerel, sardines, cod liver oil, and some fortified cereals. Vitamin or mineral supplements aren't a substitute for a balanced, nutritious diet that limits excess calories, saturated fat, trans fat, sodium, and dietary cholesterol. This dietary approach has been shown to reduce coronary heart disease risk in healthy people and those with coronary disease.

Co-authors are: Michael J. Pencina, PhD; Sarah L. Booth, PhD; Paul F. Jacques, DSc; Erik Ingelsson, MD, PhD; Katherine Lanier, BS; Emelia J. Benjamin, MD; Ralph B. D'Agostino, PhD; Myles Wolf, MD; and Ramachandran S. Vasan, MD.

The National Institute of Health, U.S. Department of Agriculture, and American Heart Association funded the study.

Statements and conclusions of study authors that are published in the American Heart Association scientific journals are solely those of the study authors and do not necessarily reflect association policy or position. The American Heart Association makes no representation or warranty as to their accuracy or reliability.

Section 70.5

Vitamin E

Excerpted from "Vitamin E Fact Sheet," by the Office of
Dietary Supplements (ODS, ods.od.nih.gov), part of the National
Institutes of Health, May 4, 2009.

Vitamin E is found naturally in some foods, added to others, and available as a dietary supplement. Vitamin E is the collective name for a group of fat-soluble compounds with distinctive antioxidant activities.

Antioxidants protect cells from the damaging effects of free radicals, which are molecules that contain an unshared electron. Free radicals damage cells and might contribute to the development of cardiovascular disease and cancer. Unshared electrons are highly energetic and react rapidly with oxygen to form reactive oxygen species (ROS). The body forms ROS endogenously when it converts food to energy, and antioxidants might protect cells from the damaging effects of ROS. The body is also exposed to free radicals from environmental exposures, such as cigarette smoke, air pollution, and ultraviolet radiation from the sun. ROS are part of signaling mechanisms among cells.

Vitamin E is a fat-soluble antioxidant that stops the production of ROS formed when fat undergoes oxidation. Scientists are investigating whether, by limiting free-radical production and possibly through other mechanisms, vitamin E might help prevent or delay the chronic diseases associated with free radicals.

In addition to its activities as an antioxidant, vitamin E is involved in immune function and, as shown primarily by in vitro studies of cells, cell signaling, regulation of gene expression, and other metabolic processes. Vitamin E inhibits the activity of protein kinase C, an enzyme involved in cell proliferation and differentiation in smooth muscle cells, platelets, and monocytes. Vitamin-E–replete endothelial cells lining the interior surface of blood vessels are better able to resist blood-cell components adhering to this surface. Vitamin E also increases the expression of two enzymes that suppress arachidonic acid metabolism, thereby increasing the release of prostacyclin from the endothelium, which, in turn, dilates blood vessels and inhibits platelet aggregation.

Vitamin E and Coronary Heart Disease

Evidence that vitamin E could help prevent or delay coronary heart disease (CHD) comes from several sources. In vitro studies have found that the nutrient inhibits oxidation of low-density lipoprotein (LDL) cholesterol, thought to be a crucial initiating step for atherosclerosis. Vitamin E might also help prevent the formation of blood clots that could lead to a heart attack or venous thromboembolism.

Several observational studies have associated lower rates of heart disease with higher vitamin E intakes. One study of approximately 90,000 nurses found that the incidence of heart disease was 30% to 40% lower in those with the highest intakes of vitamin E, primarily from supplements. Among a group of 5,133 Finnish men and women followed for a mean of 14 years, higher vitamin E intakes from food were associated with decreased mortality from CHD.

However, randomized clinical trials cast doubt on the efficacy of vitamin E supplements to prevent CHD. For example, the Heart Outcomes Prevention Evaluation (HOPE) study, which followed almost 10,000 patients at high risk of heart attack or stroke for 4.5 years, found that participants taking 400 IU [international units]/day of natural vitamin E experienced no fewer cardiovascular events or hospitalizations for heart failure or chest pain than participants taking a placebo. In the HOPE-TOO followup study, almost 4,000 of the original participants continued to take vitamin E or placebo for an additional 2.5 years. HOPE-TOO found that vitamin E provided no significant protection against heart attacks, strokes, unstable angina, or deaths from cardiovascular disease or other causes after 7 years of treatment. Participants taking vitamin E, however, were 13% more likely to experience, and 21% more likely to be hospitalized for, heart failure, a statistically significant but unexpected finding not reported in other large studies.

The HOPE and HOPE-TOO trials provide compelling evidence that moderately high doses of vitamin E supplements do not reduce the risk of serious cardiovascular events among men and women over 50 years of age with established heart disease or diabetes. These findings are supported by evidence from the Women's Angiographic Vitamin and Estrogen study, in which 423 postmenopausal women with some degree of coronary stenosis took supplements with 400 IU vitamin E (type not specified) and 500 mg vitamin C twice a day or placebo for more than 4 years. Not only did the supplements provide no cardiovascular benefits, but all-cause mortality was significantly higher in the women taking the supplements.

The latest published clinical trial of vitamin E's effects on the heart and blood vessels of women included almost 40,000 healthy women 45 years of age and older who were randomly assigned to receive either 600 IU of natural vitamin E on alternate days or placebo and who were followed for an average of 10 years. The investigators found no significant differences in rates of overall cardiovascular events (combined nonfatal heart attacks, strokes, and cardiovascular deaths) or all-cause mortality between the groups. However, the study did find two positive and significant results for women taking vitamin E: They had a 24% reduction in cardiovascular death rates, and those 65 years of age or older had a 26% decrease in nonfatal heart attack and a 49% decrease in cardiovascular death rates.

The most recent published clinical trial of vitamin E and men's cardiovascular health included almost 15,000 healthy physicians 50 years of age or older who were randomly assigned to receive 400 IU synthetic alpha-tocopherol [vitamin E] every other day, 500 mg vitamin C daily, both vitamins, or placebo. During a mean followup period of 8 years, intake of vitamin E (and/or vitamin C) had no effect on the incidence of major cardiovascular events, myocardial infarction, stroke, or cardiovascular morality. Furthermore, use of vitamin E was associated with a significantly increased risk of hemorrhagic stroke.

In general, clinical trials have not provided evidence that routine use of vitamin E supplements prevents cardiovascular disease or reduces its morbidity and mortality. However, participants in these studies have been largely middle-aged or elderly individuals with demonstrated heart disease or risk factors for heart disease. Some researchers have suggested that understanding the potential utility of vitamin E in preventing CHD might require longer studies in younger participants taking higher doses of the supplement.

Further research is needed to determine whether supplemental vitamin E has any protective value for younger, healthier people at no obvious risk of CHD.

Chapter 71

Quitting Smoking: Why to Quit and How to Get Help

What health problems are caused by smoking?

Smoking harms nearly every organ of the body and diminishes a person's overall health. Smoking is a leading cause of cancer and of death from cancer. It causes cancers of the lung, esophagus, larynx (voice box), mouth, throat, kidney, bladder, pancreas, stomach, and cervix, as well as acute myeloid leukemia.

Smoking also causes heart disease, stroke, lung disease (chronic bronchitis and emphysema), hip fractures, and cataracts. Smokers are at higher risk of developing pneumonia and other airway infections.

A pregnant smoker is at higher risk of having her baby born too early and with an abnormally low weight. A woman who smokes during or after pregnancy increases her infant's risk of death from sudden infant death syndrome (SIDS).

Millions of Americans have health problems caused by smoking. Cigarette smoking and exposure to tobacco smoke cause an estimated average of 438,000 premature deaths each year in the United States. Of these premature deaths, about 40 percent are from cancer, 35 percent are from heart disease and stroke, and 25 percent are from lung disease. Smoking is the leading cause of premature, preventable death in this country.

Regardless of their age, smokers can substantially reduce their risk of disease, including cancer, by quitting.

Excerpted from text by the National Cancer Institute (NCI, www.cancer.gov), part of the National Institutes of Health, August 17, 2007.

603

Does tobacco smoke contain harmful chemicals?

Yes. Tobacco smoke contains chemicals that are harmful to both smokers and nonsmokers. Breathing even a little tobacco smoke can be harmful. Of the 4,000 chemicals in tobacco smoke, at least 250 are known to be harmful. The toxic chemicals found in smoke include hydrogen cyanide (used in chemical weapons), carbon monoxide (found in car exhaust), formaldehyde (used as an embalming fluid), ammonia (used in household cleaners), and toluene (found in paint thinners).

Of the 250 known harmful chemicals in tobacco smoke, more than 50 have been found to cause cancer. These chemicals include the following:

- Arsenic (a heavy metal toxin)
- Benzene (a chemical found in gasoline)
- Beryllium (a toxic metal)
- Cadmium (a metal used in batteries)
- Chromium (a metallic element)
- Ethylene oxide (a chemical used to sterilize medical devices)
- Nickel (a metallic element)
- Polonium-210 (a chemical element that gives off radiation)
- Vinyl chloride (a toxic substance used in plastics manufacture)

What are the immediate benefits of quitting smoking?

The immediate health benefits of quitting smoking are substantial. Heart rate and blood pressure, which were abnormally high while smoking, begin to return to normal. Within a few hours, the level of carbon monoxide in the blood begins to decline. (Carbon monoxide, a colorless, odorless gas found in cigarette smoke, reduces the blood's ability to carry oxygen.) Within a few weeks, people who quit smoking have improved circulation, don't produce as much phlegm, and don't cough or wheeze as often. Within several months of quitting, people can expect significant improvements in lung function.

What are the long-term benefits of quitting smoking?

Quitting smoking reduces the risk of cancer and other diseases, such as heart disease and lung disease, caused by smoking. People who quit smoking, regardless of their age, are less likely than those who continue to smoke to die from smoking-related illness.

Studies have shown that quitting at about age 30 reduces the chance of dying from smoking-related diseases by more than 90 percent. People who quit at about age 50 reduce their risk of dying prematurely by 50 percent compared with those who continue to smoke. Even people who quit at about age 60 or older live longer than those who continue to smoke.

How can I help someone I know quit smoking?

It's understandable to be concerned about someone you know who currently smokes. It's important to find out if this person wants to quit smoking. Most smokers say they want to quit. If they don't want to quit, try to find out why.

Here are some things you can do to help:

- Express things in terms of your own concern about the smoker's health ("I'm worried about . . .").

- Acknowledge that the smoker may get something out of smoking and may find it difficult to quit.

- Be encouraging and express your faith that the smoker can quit for good.

- Suggest a specific action, such as calling a smoking quitline, for help in quitting smoking.

- Ask the smoker for ways you can provide support.

Here are two things you should not do:

- Don't send quit smoking materials to smokers unless they ask for them.

- Don't criticize, nag, or remind the smoker about past failures.

Chapter 72

Alcohol and Heart Disease: Learning Healthier Behaviors

Most people don't think of alcohol as a drug but it is. Alcohol abuse has destroyed more lives, broken apart more families, caused more diseases, and contributed to more auto fatalities than any other drug. It is the major contributing factor in the growing epidemic of domestic violence.

More than half of all adults drink, but, not everyone who drinks is an alcoholic. Alcoholism is a complex psychosocial disease. Those who drink risk becoming an alcoholic. It impairs your judgment and affects the way you think, feel, and communicate.

The cause of alcoholism is unknown, but, like heart disease, there are both controllable and uncontrollable risk factors. Having an alcoholic parent is an uncontrollable risk. You are at risk if you are angry, lonely, or sad or have few or no friends. Those who are poor or under great stress are also at risk for alcoholism.

Alcohol addiction has four characteristics:

1. Alcoholism carries an overwhelming urge to repeat the experience of getting high on alcohol. At times, this urge

"Alcohol and Heart Disease," http://www.womensheart.org/content/Heart Disease/alcohol_and_heart_disease.asp. © 2007 Women's Heart Foundation (www.womensheart.org). Reprinted with permission. Women's Heart Foundation is the only non-governmental nonprofit organization implementing heart disease prevention and wellness programs in schools and is dedicated to improving survival and quality of life. Founded June 11, 1992.

will go beyond the strength of a person's will to resist, no matter how much risk or harm may be involved.

2. Satisfying the urge to drink becomes the top priority in the alcoholic's life. This urge can become stronger than sexual needs, stronger than the need to satisfy hunger, stronger even than the need for survival.

3. The urge to get high with alcohol becomes linked to all other aspects of life. Tension, depression, anger, and excitement can all trigger the desire to take a drink.

4. No matter how long an alcoholic has been sober, he or she will always be at risk for alcohol abuse. As time passes with sobriety, the urge to drink weakens and occurs less often, but it can return with ferocious and overpowering strength at any time.

Do you wonder if drinking may be a problem for you? Take this quiz to find out.

- Do you calm yourself down with a drink when under pressure at work?
- Do you ever have hangovers?
- Do family quarrels usually occur after you have had a drink or two?
- Does your family think you drink too much?
- Have you ever injured yourself or other persons after drinking?
- Are you often on, and off, the wagon?
- Have you ever driven while intoxicated?
- Do you avoid situations where it would be difficult for you to get a drink if you wanted one?
- When giving yourself a second or third drink, do you reassure yourself that you deserve it?
- If you know that you have to drive home in an hour, do you ever have a second drink anyway?

If you answered **yes** to any of these questions, you need to look carefully at how alcohol is affecting your life and your relationships with others. Discuss your concerns with your primary care doctor.

How much alcohol is "safe" to drink on a daily basis? For some, no amount of alcohol is safe to take in. It is highly addictive and, as tolerance level increases, control decreases.

Alcohol's Effect on the Heart

Numerous studies suggest that moderate alcohol consumption helps protect against heart disease by raising HDL ([high-density lipoprotein] good) cholesterol and reducing plaque accumulations in your arteries. Alcohol also has a mild anti-coagulating effect, keeping platelets from clumping together to form clots. Both actions can reduce risk of heart attack but exactly how alcohol influences either one still remains unclear.

On the other hand, drinking more than three drinks a day has a direct toxic effect on the heart. Heavy drinking, particularly over time, can damage the heart and lead to high blood pressure, alcoholic cardiomyopathy, (enlarged and weakened heart), congestive heart failure, and stroke. Heavy drinking puts more fat into the circulation in your body, raising your triglyceride level. That's why doctors will tell you "If you don't drink, don't start." There are other, healthier ways to reduce your risk of heart disease like eating right, getting regular exercise, and maintaining a healthy weight.

What's "Moderate Drinking" for one may be legally drunk for another. By nature's design, a woman's body metabolizes alcohol differently so that one alcoholic beverage in a woman is equal to two in a man. Alcohol remains in a woman's body longer than in a man's. Also, the older you are, the less efficient the body can metabolize alcohol. Many states have revised their drunk-driving laws and 0.08 percent is considered to be intoxicated. Women, especially women of small stature, must be alert to these laws and metabolic differences when drinking, and limit their alcohol intake accordingly.

Other Medical Consequences of Alcoholism

Studies show that alcoholics have a worse outcome after undergoing surgical procedures. The reasons for this are not entirely clear. Poorer outcomes may be attributed to a poorer general state of health with malnutrition and the depressant effects of alcohol. Binge drinking (consuming large amounts of alcohol infrequently, such as on weekends) places one at risk for atrial fibrillation which may also be a factor in surviving surgery. Still another factor is that heavy drinking affects the body's ability to stop bleeding. A liver damaged by alcohol has trouble making clotting proteins.

Alcohol interacts with many drugs—both prescription and non-prescription. Mixing alcohol with your medicine can lead to serious untoward effects.

Alcoholism increases risk of cancers, including breast cancer, lung cancer, and cancer of the liver.

Long-term heavy use of alcohol destroys the cerebellum of the brain, causing irreversible brain damage and resulting in slowed thinking, an unsteady walk, and slurred speech.

Alcoholism contributes to many diseases, including hepatitis, cirrhosis, malnutrition, pancreatitis, stomach ulcer, fetal alcohol syndrome, and heart disease, just to name a few.

The Twelve Steps

1. We admitted that we were powerless over alcohol—that our lives had become unmanageable.

2. Came to believe that a power greater than ourselves could restore us to sanity.

3. Made a decision to turn our will and our lives over to the care of God as we understood Him.

4. Made a searching and fearless moral inventory of ourselves.

5. Admitted to God, to ourselves, and to another human being the exact nature of our wrongs.

6. Were entirely ready to have God remove all these defects of character.

7. Humbly asked Him to remove our shortcomings.

8. Made a list of all persons we had harmed, and became willing to make amends to them all.

9. Made direct amends to such people wherever possible, except when to do so would injure them or others.

10. Continued to take personal inventory and when we were wrong promptly admitted it.

11. Sought through prayer and meditation to improve our conscious contact with God as we understood Him, praying only for knowledge of His will for us and the power to carry that out.

12.   Having had a spiritual awakening as the result of these steps, we tried to carry this message to alcoholics, and to practice these principles in all our affairs.

Learning Healthier Behaviors

Cutting back on drinking or abstaining altogether isn't easy. If you have a physical dependence on alcohol, you most likely need medical assistance to help you to break the habit. If you feel you just drink too much as a pattern of behavior you've slipped into, then, here are some tips to replace drinking behaviors with more healthful ones:

- **When you eat out, order up a glass of water and some food.** Drink the water right away so that you are not drinking alcohol just to quench a thirst. Having food to eat will slow the absorption rate of the alcohol and keep your hands busy.

- **Discover new places.** Sports bars usually have other activities you can busy yourself with while socializing. You can throw darts, play a game of pool, or challenge a friend to an air hockey match. There's lots you can do besides just sitting at a bar and drinking.

- **Order up a non-alcoholic drink.** If you just ask for a glass of white grape juice in a wine glass, or you get a non-alcoholic beer in a beer mug, no one is the wiser but you.

- **Find supportive friends.** What do you have in common with your current friends besides drinking? What would you do or talk about if you weren't drinking? If you don't know, then it's time to move on.

- **Get involved.** Women must give up their caregiving role as their children mature and leave home. This time period is often referred to as the empty nest. Rather than allowing an empty feeling to creep in, why not give of your time and energy to a worthy cause?

- **Relax at home with a sparkling ginger ale or tonic water with cranberry juice.** It's festive, fun, and refreshing.

If you or someone you care about has a drinking problem, you can obtain information from the Yellow Pages by looking under Social Service Organizations for Alcoholic Anonymous. Al-Anon and Alateen are support groups for those living with an alcoholic. Read books and talk to your family physician or minister. Alcoholism is treatable but only if the person who is drinking is willing to admit she has a problem and is willing to accept help. Alcoholism is a disease that is characterized by denial, so, while you may not be able to change the behavior of someone you love, you still need to get help for yourself because alcoholism becomes a family illness.

Note: Moderate drinking is defined as no more than one drink a day for women and two drinks a day for men. A drink, according to guidelines from the U.S. Department of Health and Human Services, is roughly 1/2 ounce of absolute alcohol, a 5-ounce glass of wine, a 12-ounce bottle of beer, or 1/2 ounce distilled spirits (80 proof). Each contains about the same amount of alcohol.

Sources

1. Spence, W.R., *The Medical Consequences of Alcoholism*, Health Edco®, '96.

2. DeWitt, D.E., Romaine, D.S., *Guide to a Happy, Healthy Heart*, Alpha Books, '98.

Chapter 73

Stress Management

What are some of the most common causes of stress?

Stress can arise for a variety of reasons. Stress can be brought about by a traumatic accident, death, or emergency situation. Stress can also be a side effect of a serious illness or disease.

There is also stress associated with daily life, the workplace, and family responsibilities. It's hard to stay calm and relaxed in our hectic lives. With all we have going on in our lives, it seems almost impossible to find ways to de-stress. But it's important to find those ways. Your health depends on it.

What are some early signs of stress?

Stress can take on many different forms and can contribute to symptoms of illness. Common symptoms include headache, sleep disorders, difficulty concentrating, short temper, upset stomach, job dissatisfaction, low morale, depression, and anxiety.

How does stress affect my body and my health?

Everyone has stress. We have short-term stress, like getting lost while driving or missing the bus. Even everyday events, such as planning a

Excerpted from "Stress and Your Health," by the Office on Women's Health (www.womenshealth.gov), part of the U.S. Department of Health and Human Services, August 1, 2005.

meal or making time for errands, can be stressful. This kind of stress can make us feel worried or anxious.

Other times, we face long-term stress, such as racial discrimination, a life-threatening illness, or divorce. These stressful events also affect your health on many levels. Long-term stress is real and can increase your risk for some health problems, like depression.

Both short- and long-term stress can have effects on your body. Research is starting to show the serious effects of stress on our bodies. Stress triggers changes in our bodies and makes us more likely to get sick. It can also make problems we already have worse. It can play a part in these problems:

- Trouble sleeping
- Headaches
- Constipation
- Diarrhea
- Irritability
- Lack of energy
- Lack of concentration
- Eating too much or not at all
- Anger
- Sadness
- Higher risk of asthma and arthritis flare-ups
- Tension
- Stomach cramping
- Stomach bloating
- Skin problems, like hives
- Depression
- Anxiety
- Weight gain or loss
- Heart problems
- High blood pressure
- Irritable bowel syndrome
- Diabetes
- Neck and/or back pain

- Less sexual desire
- Harder to get pregnant

What are some of the most stressful life events?

Any change in our lives can be stressful—even some of the happiest ones like having a baby or taking a new job. Here are some of life's most stressful events (from the Holmes and Rahe Scale of Life Events, 1967):

- Death of a spouse
- Divorce
- Marital separation
- Spending time in jail
- Death of a close family member
- Personal illness or injury
- Marriage
- Pregnancy
- Retirement

How can I help handle my stress?

Don't let stress make you sick. Often we aren't even aware of our stress levels. Listen to your body, so that you know when stress is affecting your health. Here are ways to help you handle your stress.

- **Relax.** It's important to unwind. Each person has her own way to relax. Some ways include deep breathing, yoga, meditation, and massage therapy. If you can't do these things, take a few minutes to sit, listen to soothing music, or read a book.

- **Make time for yourself.** It's important to care for yourself. Think of this as an order from your doctor, so you don't feel guilty. No matter how busy you are, you can try to set aside at least 15 minutes each day in your schedule to do something for yourself, like taking a bubble bath, going for a walk, or calling a friend.

- **Sleep.** Sleeping is a great way to help both your body and mind. Your stress could get worse if you don't get enough sleep. You also can't fight off sickness as well when you sleep poorly.

With enough sleep, you can tackle your problems better and lower your risk for illness. Try to get 7 to 9 hours of sleep every night.

- **Eat right.** Try to fuel up with fruits, vegetables, and proteins. Good sources of protein can be peanut butter, chicken, or tuna salad. Eat whole-grains, such as wheat breads and wheat crackers. Don't be fooled by the jolt you get from caffeine or sugar. Your energy will wear off.

- **Get moving.** Believe it or not, getting physical activity not only helps relieve your tense muscles, but helps your mood too! Your body makes certain chemicals, called endorphins, before and after you work out. They relieve stress and improve your mood.

- **Talk to friends.** Talk to your friends to help you work through your stress. Friends are good listeners. Finding someone who will let you talk freely about your problems and feelings without judging you does a world of good. It also helps to hear a different point of view. Friends will remind you that you're not alone.

- **Get help from a professional if you need it.** Talk to a therapist. A therapist can help you work through stress and find better ways to deal with problems. For more serious stress-related disorders, therapy can be helpful. There also are medications that can help ease symptoms of depression and anxiety and help promote sleep.

- **Compromise.** Sometimes, it's not always worth the stress to argue. Give in once in awhile.

- **Write down your thoughts.** Have you ever typed an e-mail to a friend about your lousy day and felt better afterward? Why not grab a pen and paper and write down what's going on in your life. Keeping a journal can be a great way to get things off your chest and work through issues. Later, you can go back and read through your journal and see how you've made progress.

- **Help others.** Helping someone else can help you. Help your neighbor or volunteer in your community.

- **Get a hobby.** Find something you enjoy. Make sure to give yourself time to explore your interests.

- **Set limits.** When it comes to things like work and family, figure out what you can really do. There are only so many hours in the day. Set limits with yourself and others. Don't be afraid to say **no** to requests for your time and energy.

- **Plan your time.** Think ahead about how you're going to spend your time. Write a to-do list. Figure out what's most important to do.

- **Don't deal with stress in unhealthy ways.** This includes drinking too much alcohol, using drugs, smoking, or overeating.

I heard deep breathing could help my stress. How do I do it?

Deep breathing is a good way to relax. Try it a couple of times every day. Here's how to do it.

- Lie down or sit in a chair.
- Rest your hands on your stomach.
- Slowly count to four and inhale through your nose. Feel your stomach rise. Hold it for a second.
- Slowly count to four while you exhale through your mouth. To control how fast you exhale, purse your lips like you're going to whistle. Your stomach will slowly fall.
- Repeat five to 10 times.

Part Eight

Additional Help
and Information

Chapter 74

Glossary of Terms Related to Cardiovascular Disease

aneurysm: A thin or weak spot in an artery that balloons out and can burst.[1]

angina: A recurring pain or discomfort in the chest that happens when some part of the heart does not receive enough blood. It is a common symptom of coronary heart disease, which occurs when vessels that carry blood to the heart become narrowed and blocked due to atherosclerosis.[1]

angioplasty: A medical procedure in which a balloon is used to open a blockage in a coronary artery narrowed by atherosclerosis. This procedure improves blood flow to the heart.[2]

aorta: The major artery coming out of the heart that supplies blood to the body.[2]

arrhythmia: A problem with the rate or rhythm of the heartbeat. During an arrhythmia, the heart can beat too fast, too slow, or with an irregular rhythm.[2]

Definitions in this chapter were compiled from documents published by several public domain sources. Terms marked 1 are from publications by the Office on Women's Health (www.womenshealth.gov); terms marked 2 are from publications by the National Heart, Lung, and Blood Institute (NHLBI, www.nhlbi.nih.gov); and terms marked 3 are from publications by the National Institute of Neurological Disorders and Stroke (NINDS, www.ninds.nih.gov).

arteries: Blood vessels that carry oxygen and blood to the heart, brain, and other parts of the body.[1]

atherosclerosis: A disease in which fatty material is deposited on the wall of the arteries. This fatty material causes the arteries to become narrow and eventually restricts blood flow.[1]

atria: The two upper chambers of the heart. The atria receive and collect blood.[2]

atrial fibrillation: When rapid, disorganized electrical signals cause the atria to fibrillate, or contract very fast and irregularly.[2]

automated external defibrillators (AEDs): Special defibrillators that untrained bystanders can use to restore a person's heart rhythm in an emergency. AEDs are programmed to give an electric shock if they detect a dangerous arrhythmia.[2]

blood pressure: The force of blood pushing against the walls of the arteries as the heart pumps out blood.[2]

body mass index: A measure of body fat based on a person's height and weight.[1]

bradycardia: A heartbeat that is too slow.[2]

cardiac rehabilitation: A medically supervised program that helps improve the health and well-being of people who have heart problems. Rehab programs include exercise training, education on heart-healthy living, and counseling to reduce stress and help a person return to an active life.[2]

cardiogenic shock: A state in which a weakened heart isn't able to pump enough blood to meet the body's needs. It is a medical emergency and is fatal if not treated right away. The most common cause of cardiogenic shock is damage to the heart muscle from a severe heart attack.[2]

cardiomyopathy: Diseases of the heart muscle that cause it to become enlarged, thick, or rigid. In rare cases, the muscle tissue in the heart is replaced with scar tissue. As cardiomyopathy worsens, the heart becomes weaker.[2]

cardiopulmonary resuscitation (CPR): Emergency procedure performed when a person's breathing or heartbeat has stopped.[2]

cardiovascular diseases: Disease of the heart and blood vessels.[1]

carotid artery disease: A condition in which a fatty material called plaque builds up inside the carotid arteries.[2]

carotid endarterectomy: Surgery to remove plaque from the carotid arteries.[2]

cerebrovascular disease: Disease of the blood vessels in the brain.[1]

cholesterol: A fatty substance present in all parts of the body. It is a component of cell membranes and is used to make vitamin D and some hormones. Some cholesterol in the body is produced by the liver and some is derived from food, particularly animal products. A high level of cholesterol in the blood can help cause atherosclerosis and coronary artery disease. In the blood, cholesterol is bound to chemicals called lipoproteins. Cholesterol attached to low-density lipoprotein (LDL) harms health and is often called bad cholesterol. Cholesterol attached to high-density lipoprotein (HDL) is good for health and is often called good cholesterol.[1]

congenital heart disease: Abnormalities of the heart's structure and function caused by abnormal or disordered heart development before birth.[1]

coronary angiography: A test that uses dye and special x-rays to show the inside of the coronary arteries.[2]

coronary artery bypass grafting: A type of surgery used to improve blood flow to the heart in people with severe coronary artery disease (CAD). During this surgery, a healthy artery or vein from another part of the body is connected, or grafted, to the blocked coronary artery. The grafted artery or vein bypasses the blocked portion of the coronary artery. This new passage routes oxygen-rich blood around the blockage to the heart muscle.[2]

coronary artery disease: Also called coronary heart disease. It is the most common type of heart disease that results from atherosclerosis, the gradual buildup of plaques in the coronary arteries, the blood vessels that bring blood to the heart.[1]

coronary microvascular disease: A condition in which a fatty material called plaque builds up in the heart's smallest arteries.[2]

deep vein thrombosis: A blood clot that forms in a vein deep in the body.[2]

echocardiography (echo): A painless test that uses sound waves to create pictures of the heart.[2]

electrocardiogram (ECG or EKG): An external, noninvasive test that records the electrical activity of the heart.[1]

endocarditis: An infection of the inner lining of the heart chambers and valves called the endocardium.[2]

event monitors: Devices that record problems with the heart's rhythm when symptoms occur.[2]

heart block: An arrhythmia that occurs when the electrical signal is slowed or disrupted as it moves through the heart.[2]

heart disease: A number of abnormal conditions affecting the heart and the blood vessels in the heart. The most common type of heart disease is coronary artery disease, which is the gradual buildup of plaques in the coronary arteries.[1]

heart failure: A condition in which the heart can't pump blood the way it should. In some cases, the heart can't fill with enough blood. In other cases, the heart can't send blood to the rest of the body with enough force.[2]

heart murmur: An extra or unusual sound heard during a heartbeat. Murmurs range from very faint to very loud. They sometimes sound like a whooshing or swishing noise.[2]

heart transplant: Surgery to remove a person's diseased heart and replace it with a healthy heart from a deceased donor.[2]

heart valve disease: A condition in which one or more of the heart's four valves don't work properly.[2]

Holter monitors: Devices that record heart rhythm continuously for 24 to 48 hours.[2]

hypertension: Also called high blood pressure, it is having blood pressure greater than 140 over 90 mmHg (millimeters of mercury). Long-term high blood pressure can damage blood vessels and organs, including the heart, kidneys, eyes, and brain.[1]

hypotension: Low blood pressure.[1]

ischemia: Decrease in the blood supply to a an organ, tissue, or other part caused by the narrowing or blockage of the blood vessels.[1]

ischemic stroke: A blockage of blood vessels supplying blood to the brain, causing a decrease in blood supply.[1]

long QT syndrome: A disorder of the heart's electrical activity that causes a person to develop a sudden, uncontrollable, and dangerous arrhythmia in response to exercise or stress.[2]

metabolic syndrome: A group of risk factors—including large waistline, abnormal blood fat levels, higher than normal blood pressure, and higher than normal blood sugar levels—linked to overweight and obesity that raise the chance for heart disease and other health problems such as diabetes and stroke.[2]

mitral valve prolapse: A condition in which one of the heart's valves don't close tightly.[2]

obesity: Having too much body fat. People with a body mass index of 30 or higher are obese.[1]

pacemaker: A small device that's placed under the skin of the chest or abdomen to help control abnormal heart rhythms. This device uses electrical pulses to prompt the heart to beat at a normal rate.[2]

palpitations: Feelings that the heart is skipping a beat, fluttering, or beating too hard or fast. They can occur during activity or even when sitting still or lying down.[2]

pericarditis: A condition in which the membrane, or sac, around the heart, called the pericardium, is inflamed.[2]

peripheral arterial disease: A condition in which plaque builds up in the arteries that carry blood to the head, organs, and limbs, often causing pain and numbness in the lower body.[2]

plaque: A buildup of fat, cholesterol, and other substances that accumulate in the walls of the arteries.[1]

poststroke rehabilitation: Therapy to help stroke survivors relearn skills that are lost when part of the brain is damaged.[3]

Raynaud syndrome: A rare disorder that affects the arteries, causing reduced blood flow to the fingers and toes.[2]

septum: A wall of tissue that divides the right and left sides of the heart.[2]

sleep apnea: A condition that causes a person to stop breathing for short periods during sleep.[2]

stent: A small mesh tube that's used to treat narrowed or weakened arteries in the body. A stent is placed in a weakened artery to improve blood flow and to help prevent the artery from bursting. Stents usually are made of metal mesh, but sometimes they're made of fabric. Fabric stents, also called stent grafts, are used in larger arteries.[2]

stress test (treadmill test): A test that gives doctors information about how the heart works during physical stress. During a stress test, a person exercises (walks or runs on a treadmill or pedals a bicycle) to make the heart work hard and beat fast. Tests are done on the heart during exercise.[2]

stroke: Stoppage of blood flow to an area of the brain, causing permanent damage to nerve cells in that region. A stroke can occur either because an artery is clogged by a blood clot (called ischemic stroke) or an artery tears and bleeds into the brain. A stroke can cause symptoms such as loss of consciousness, problems with movement, and loss of speech.[1]

sudden cardiac arrest (SCA): A condition in which the heart suddenly and unexpectedly stops beating. When this happens, blood stops flowing to the brain and other vital organs.[2]

tachycardia: A heartbeat that is too fast.[2]

total artificial heart: A device that replaces the two lower chambers of the heart. These chambers are called ventricles.[2]

transient ischemic attack (TIA): A "mini-stroke" where there is a short-term reduction in blood flow to the brain usually resulting in temporary stoke symptoms. Does not cause damage to the brain, but puts a person at higher risk of having a full stroke.[1]

triglyceride: A type of fat in the blood stream and fat tissue. High triglyceride levels (above 200) can contribute to the hardening and narrowing of arteries.[1]

ultrasound: A painless, harmless test that uses sound waves to produce images of the organs and structures of the body on a screen. Also called sonography.[1]

varicose veins: Swollen, twisted veins that be seen just under the surface of the skin. These veins usually occur in the legs.[2]

vasculitis: A condition that involves inflammation in the blood vessels.[2]

ventricles: The two lower chambers of the heart. The ventricles pump blood out of the heart into the circulatory system to other parts of the body.[2]

Chapter 75

Directory of Organizations That Provide Information about Cardiovascular Disease

Government Agencies That Provide Information about Cardiovascular Disease

Agency for Healthcare Research and Quality
Office of Communications and Knowledge Transfer
540 Gaither Road, Second Floor
Rockville, MD 20850
Phone: 301-427-1364
Fax: 301-427-1873
Website: www.ahrq.gov

Centers for Disease Control and Prevention
1600 Clifton Road
Atlanta, GA 30333
Toll-Free: 800-CDC-INFO (232-4636)
Phone: 404-639-3311
Website: www.cdc.gov
E-mail: cdcinfo@cdc.gov

Centers for Medicare and Medicaid Services
7500 Security Boulevard
Baltimore, MD 21244-1850
Toll-Free: 800-633-4227
Website: www.medicare.gov

Healthfinder®
National Health Information Center
P.O. Box 1133
Washington, DC 20013-1133
Toll-Free: 800-336-4797
Phone: 301-565-4167
Fax: 301-984-4256
Website: www.healthfinder.gov
E-mail: healthfinder@nhic.org

Resources in this chapter were compiled from several sources deemed reliable; all contact information was verified and updated in October 2009.

627

National Cancer Institute
Cancer Information Service
6116 Executive Boulevard
Room 3036A
Bethesda, MD 20892-8322
Toll-Free: 800-4-CANCER
(422-6237)
TTY Toll-Free: 800-332-8615
Website: www.cancer.gov
E-mail:
cancergovstaff@mail.nih.gov

*National Center for
Complementary and
Alternative Medicine*
National Institutes of Health
NCCAM Clearinghouse
P.O. 7923
Gaithersburg, MD 20898-7923
Toll-Free: 888-644-6226
TTY: 866-464-3615
Fax: 866-464-3616
Website: nccam.nih.gov
E-mail: info@nccam.nih.gov

*National Heart, Lung, and
Blood Institute*
P.O. Box 30105
Bethesda, MD 20824-0105
Phone: 301-592-8573
Fax: 301-592-8563
Website: www.nhlbi.nih.gov
E-mail: nhlbiinfo@nhlbi.nih.gov

*National Human Genome
Research Institute*
Building 31, Room 4B09
31 Center Drive, MSC 2152
9000 Rockville Pike
Bethesda, MD 20892-2152
Phone: 301-402-0911
Fax: 301-402-4831
Website: www.genome.gov

*National Institute of
Arthritis and Musculoskel-
etal and Skin Diseases*
National Institutes of Health
1 AMS Circle
Bethesda, MD 20892-3675
Toll Free: 877-22-NIAMS
(226-4267)
TTY: 301–565–2966
Phone: 301-495-4484
Fax: 301-718-6366
Website: www.niams.nih.gov
E-mail:
NIAMSinfo@mail.nih.gov

*National Institute of
Diabetes, Digestive and
Kidney Diseases*
Building 31, Rm. 9A06
31 Center Drive, MSC 2560
Bethesda, MD 20892-2560
Phone: 301-496-3583
Website: www.niddk.nih.gov

National Institute of Neurological Disorders and Stroke
NIH Neurological Institute
P.O. Box 5801
Bethesda, MD 20824
Toll-Free: 800-352-9424
Phone: 301-496-5751
TTY: 301-468-5981
Website: www.ninds.nih.gov
E-mail: braininfo@ninds.nih.gov

National Institutes of Health
9000 Rockville Pike
Bethesda, MD 20892
Phone: 301-496-4000
TTY: 301-402-9612
Website: www.nih.gov
E-mail: NIHinfo@od.nih.gov

National Institute on Aging
Building 31, Room 5C27
31 Center Drive, MSC 2292
Bethesda, MD 20892
Phone: 301-496-1752
Fax: 301-496-1072
Website: www.nia.nih.gov

National Women's Health Information Center
8270 Willow Oaks Corporate Drive
Fairfax, VA 22031
Toll-Free: 800-994-9662
TDD: 888-220-5446
Website:
www.womenshealth.gov

Office of Minority Health
Resource Center
P.O. Box 37337
Washington, DC 20013-7337
Toll-Free: 800-444-6472
Fax: 301-251-2160
Website: www.omhrc.gov
E-mail: info@omhrc.gov

U.S. Department of Health and Human Services
200 Independent Avenue, SW
Washington, DC 20201
Toll-Free: 877-696-6775
Website: www.hhs.gov

U.S. Food and Drug Administration
10903 New Hampshire Avenue
Silver Spring, MD 20903
Toll-Free: 888-463-6332
Website: www.fda.gov

U.S. National Library of Medicine
8600 Rockville Pike
Bethesda, MD 20894
Toll-Free: 888-346-3656
Phone: 301-594-5983
TDD: 800-735-2258
Fax: 301-402-1384
Website: www.nlm.nih.gov
E-mail: custserv@nlm.nih.gov

Private Agencies That Provide Information about Cardiovascular Disease

American Academy of Family Physicians
11400 Tomahawk Creek Parkway
Leawood, KS 66211-2680
Toll-Free: 800-274-2237
Fax: 913-906-6075
Website: www.aafp.org

American Academy of Pediatrics
141 Northwest Point Boulevard
Elk Grove Village, IL 60007-1098
Phone: 847-434-4000
Fax: 847-434-8000
Website: www.aap.org
E-mail: kidsdocs@aap.org

American Academy of Physical Medicine and Rehabilitation
330 North Wabash Avenue
Suite 2500
Chicago, IL 60611-7617
Phone: 312-464-9700
Fax: 312-464-0227
Website: www.aapmr.org
E-mail: info@aapmr.org

American Association for Clinical Chemistry
1850 K Street NW, Suite 625
Washington, DC 20006
Toll-Free: 800-892-1400
Fax: 202-887-5093
Website: www.aacc.org

American Association of Cardiovascular and Pulmonary Rehabilitation
401 North Michigan Avenue
Suite 2200
Chicago, IL 60611
Phone: 312-321-5146
Fax: 312-673-6924
Website: www.aacvpr.org
E-mail: aacvpr@aacvpr.org

American Behçet's Disease Foundation
Office Correspondence
P.O. Box 869
Smithtown, NY 11787-0869
Donations and Memberships
P.O. Box 80576
Rochester, MI 48308
Toll-Free: 800-723-4287
Phone: 631-656-0537
Fax: 480-247-5377
Website: www.behcets.com
E-mail: smcelgunn@behcets.com
or mburke@behcets.com

American College of Cardiology
Heart House
2400 N Street NW
Washington, DC 20037
Toll-Free: 800-253-4636
Phone: 202-375-6000
Fax: 202-375-7000
Website: www.acc.org

American College of Chest Physicians
3300 Dundee Road
Northbrook, IL 60062-2348
Toll-Free: 800-343-2227
Phone: 847-498-1400
Website: www.chestnet.org

American College of Emergency Physicians
1125 Executive Circle
Irving, TX 75038-2522
Toll-Free: 800-798-1822
Phone: 972-550-0911
Fax: 972-580-2816
Website: www.acep.org
E-mail: membership@acep.org

American College of Physicians
190 North Independence Mall West
Philadelphia, PA 19106-1572
Toll-Free: 800-523-1546
Phone: 215-351-2400
Website: www.acponline.org

American College of Sports Medicine
401 West Michigan Street
Indianapolis, IN 46202-3233
Phone: 317-637-9200
Fax: 317-634-7817
Website: www.acsm.org

American Council on Exercise
4851 Paramount Drive
San Diego, CA 92123
Phone: 858-279-8227
Fax: 858-279-8064
Website: www.acefitness.org
E-mail: support@acefitness.org

American Diabetes Association
1701 North Beauregard Street
Alexandria, VA 22311
Toll-Free: 800-342-2383
Website: www.diabetes.org
E-mail: AskADA@diabetes.org

American Dietetic Association
120 South Riverside Plaza
Suite 2000
Chicago, IL 60606-6995
Toll-Free: 800-877-1600
Website: www.eatright.org

American Lung Association
1301 Pennsylvania Avenue NW
Suite 800
Washington, DC 20004
Toll-Free: 800-LUNGUSA
(586-4872)
Website: www.lungusa.org

American Heart Association
National Center
7272 Greenville Avenue
Dallas, TX 75231
Toll-Free: 800-AHA-USA-1
(242-8721)
Website: www.americanheart.org

**American Medical
Association**
515 N. State Street
Chicago, IL 60654
Toll-Free: 800-621-8335
Website: www.ama-assn.org

**American Medical Women's
Association**
100 North 20th Street, 4th Floor
Philadelphia, PA 19103
Phone: 215-320-3716
Fax: 215-564-2175
Website: www.amwa-doc.org

**American Psychological
Association**
750 First Street NE
Washington, DC 20002-4242
Toll-Free: 800-374-2721
Phone: 202-336-5500
Website: www.apa.org

**American Society of
Echocardiography**
2100 Gateway Centre Boulevard
Suite 310
Morrisville, NC 27560
Phone: 919-861-5574
Fax: 919-882-9900
Website: www.asecho.org

**American Society of
Hypertension, Inc.**
148 Madison Avenue
Fifth Floor
New York, NY 10016
Phone: 212-696-9099
Fax: 212-696-0711
Website: www.ash-us.org
E-mail: ash@ash-us.org

**American Society of
Nuclear Cardiology**
4550 Montgomery Avenue
Suite 780 North
Bethesda, MD 20814-3304
Phone: 301-215-7575
Fax: 301-215-7113
Website: www.asnc.org
E-mail: info@asnc.org

**American Stroke
Association**
7272 Greenville Avenue
Dallas, TX 75231
Toll-Free: 888-478-7653
Website:
www.strokeassociation.org

**Brain Aneurysm
Foundation, Inc.**
269 Hanover Street, Building 3
Hanover, MA 02339
Toll-Free 888-272-4602
Phone: 781-826-5556
Website: www.bafound.org
E-mail: office@bafound.org

**Children's Cardiomyopathy
Foundation**
P.O. Box 547
Tenafly, NJ 07670
Phone: 866-808-2873
Fax: 201-227-7016
Website: www
.childrenscardiomyopathy.org
E-mail: info
@childrenscardiomyopathy.org

Children's Hemiplegia and Stroke Association (CHASA)
4101 W. Green Oaks
Suite 305 #149
Arlington, TX 76016
Phone: 817-492-4325
Website: www.chasa.org

Cleveland Clinic
9500 Euclid Avenue
Cleveland, OH 44195
Toll-Free: 866-594-2091
Phone: 216-444-2200
TTY: 216-444-0261
Website: www.clevelandclinic.org

Congenital Heart Information Network
101 N Washington Avenue
Suite 1A
Margate City, NJ 08402-1195
Phone: 609-822-1572
Fax: 609-822-1574
Website: www.tchin.org

Endocrine Society
8401 Connecticut Avenue
Suite 900
Chevy Chase, MD 20815
Toll-Free: 888-363-6274
Phone: 301-941-0200
Website: www.endo-society.org

Howard Gilman Institute for Valvular Heart Disease
635 Madison Avenue, Third Floor
New York, NY 10022
Phone: 212-289-7777
Website: www.gilmanheartvalve.us
E-mail: info@gilmanheartvalve.us

Heart Failure Society of America
Court International—Suite 240 S
2550 University Avenue West
Saint Paul, MN 55114
Phone: 651-642-1633
Fax: 651-642-1502
Website: www.hfsa.org
E-mail: info@hfsa.org

Heart Rhythm Society
1400 K Street, NW, Suite 500
Washington, DC 20005
Phone: 202-464-3400
Fax: 202-464-3401
Website: www.hrsonline.org
E-mail: info@hrsonline.org

Hypertrophic Cardiomyopathy Association
328 Green Pond Road
P.O. Box 306
Hibernia, NJ 07842
Phone: 973-983-7429
Fax: 973-983-7870
Website: www.4hcm.org
E-mail: support@4hcm.org

March of Dimes
1275 Mamaroneck Avenue
White Plains, NY 10605
Phone: 914-997-4488
Website:
www.marchofdimes.com

Mayo Clinic
Website: www.mayoclinic.org

Mended Hearts, Inc.
7272 Greenville Avenue
Dallas, TX 75231-4596
Toll-Free: 888-432-7899
Phone: 214-360-6149
Fax: 214-360-6145
Website: www.mendedhearts.org
E-mail: info@mendedhearts.org

Minneapolis Heart Institute Foundation
920 East 28th Street, Suite 100
Minneapolis, MN 55407
Phone: 612-863-3833
Fax: 612-863-3801
Toll-Free: 877-800-2729
Website: www.mplsheart.org
E-mail: info@mhif.org

National Hypertension Association
324 East 30th Street
New York, NY 10016
Phone: 212-889-3557
Fax: 212-447-7032
Website:
www.nathypertension.org
E-mail:
nathypertension@aol.com

National Stroke Association
9707 E Easter Lane Building B
Centennial, CO 80112
Toll-Free: 800-STROKES
(787-6537)
Fax: 303-649-1328
Website: www.stroke.org
E-mail: info@stroke.org

Nemours Foundation Center for Children's Health Media
1600 Rockland Road
Wilmington, DE 19803
Phone: 302-651-4000
Website: www.kidshealth.org
E-mail: info@kidshealth.org

Society for Vascular Surgery
633 N. St. Clair, 24th Floor
Chicago, IL 60611
Toll-Free: 800-258-7188
Phone: 312-334-2300
Fax: 312-334-2320
Website:
www.vascularsociety.org
E-mail:
vascular@vascularsociety.org

Society of Interventional Radiology
3975 Fair Ridge Drive
Suite 400 North
Fairfax, VA 22033
Toll-Free: 800-488-7284
Phone: 703-691-1805
Fax: 703-691-1855
Website: www.scvir.org

Society of Thoracic Surgeons
633 N. Saint Clair Street
Suite 2320
Chicago, IL 60611
Phone: 312-202-5800
Fax: 312-202-5801
Website: www.sts.org
E-mail: sts@sts.org

Sudden Arrhythmia Death Syndromes Foundation
508 E. South Temple, Suite 202
Salt Lake City, UT 84102
Toll-Free: 800-STOP-SAD
(786-7723)
Website: www.sads.org

Sudden Cardiac Arrest Association
1133 Connecticut Ave NW
11th Floor
Washington, DC 20036
Toll-Free: 866-972-7222
Fax: 202-719-8983
Website:
www.suddencardiacarrest.org
E-mail:
info@suddencardiacarrest.org

Texas Heart Institute
6770 Bertner Avenue
Houston, TX 77030
Phone: 832-355-4011
Website: www.texasheart.org

Vascular Disease Foundation
1075 South Yukon, Suite 320
Lakewood, CO 80226
Toll-Free: 888-833-4463
Phone: 303-989-0500
Fax: 303-989-0200
Website: www.vdf.org

WomenHeart: The National Coalition for Women with Heart Disease
818 18th Street NW, Suite 1000
Washington, DC 20006
Toll-Free: 877-771-0030
Phone: 202-728-7199
Fax: 888-343-0764
Website: www.womenheart.org
E-mail: mail@womenheart.org

Women's Heart Foundation
1901 North Olden Avenue
Suite 6A
Trenton, NJ 08618
Phone: 609-771-9600
Fax: 609-771-3778
Website: www.womensheart.org

Index

Index

Page numbers followed by 'n' indicate a footnote. Page numbers in *italics* indicate a table or illustration.

"Heart Failure Before Age 50
Substantially More Common in
Blacks" (NIH) 322n
Heart Failure Society of America,
contact information 633
heart-healthy diet
cardiac rehabilitation 546
overview 582–85
see also diet and nutrition
"Heart Healthy Eating" (Office
of Women's Health) 582n
heart MRI *see* magnetic resonance
imaging
"Heart Murmur" (NHLBI) 327n
heart murmurs
defined 624
heart valve disease 191
overview 327–30
heart palpitations
defined 625
overview 86–89
heart rate, age factor 79–81
Heart Rhythm Society, contact
information 633
"Heart Surgery" (NHLBI) 496n
heart surgery, overview 496–504
see also surgical procedures
"Heart Transplant" (NHLBI) 531n
heart transplantation
cardiogenic shock 147
defined 624
described 499–500
overview 531–40
heart valve disease
defined 624
overview 186–92
see also mitral valve prolapse;
rheumatic heart disease
"Heart Valve Disease" (NHLBI) 186n
heart valves
depicted 5
described 3, 6
see also aortic valve; mitral valve;
pulmonary valve; tricuspid valve
"Heart Valve Surgery" (A.D.A.M.,
Inc.) 504n
heart valve surgery, overview 504–6
hematocrit, blood tests 342
hemiparesis, described 554

hemiplegia, described 554
hemoglobin, blood tests 342
hemorrhagic stroke, described 90,
247–48
Henoch-Schönlein purpura,
described 277
heparin
arrhythmias 172
deep vein thrombosis 287
described 451
heredity
cardiomyopathy 156, 159
cholesterol levels 39
congenital heart defects 335
coronary artery disease 106
hypertension 31
long QT syndrome 183
myxomas 215
sudden cardiac arrest 138
see also family history
HHS *see* US Department of
Health and Human Services
hibernation, stroke research 250
"High Blood Cholesterol" (NHLBI) 37n
high blood pressure *see* hypertension
"High Blood Pressure" (NHLBI) 27n
"High Blood Pressure - Medicines to
Help You" (FDA) 429n
high-density lipoprotein (HDL)
cholesterol
blood tests 344
categories *41*
coronary artery disease 70–71
described 21, 37–38, 449
diabetes mellitus 55
metabolic syndrome 56
high sensitivity C-reactive protein
blood tests 344
research 349–50
His-Purkinje system, described 10–11
HMG-CoA reductase inhibitors
see statin medications
Hodes, Richard J. 70
"Holter and Event Monitors"
(NHLBI) 373n
Holter monitors
defined 624
electrocardiograms 363
overview 373–81

indapamide *439*
Inderal (propranolol) *432*
infarction, ischemic stroke 246
infections
  arrhythmias 171
  endocarditis 203–4
  heart transplantation 537, 539
  heart valve disease 189
  mitral valve prolapse 196
  pericarditis 209
  peripheral artery disease 261
infective endocarditis, described 196,
  203
inferior vena cava, described 4
inflammation
  coronary artery disease 106
  rheumatic heart disease 199
innocent heart murmurs,
  described 328
INR *see* international
  normalized ratio
insulin, described 23, 51–52
insulin resistance
  atherosclerosis 224, 241
  carotid artery disease 232, 233
  coronary artery disease 105
  metabolic syndrome 56–57
interarterial septum, described 6
intermittent claudication,
  described 264
"International Effort Finds New
  Genetic Variants Associated with
  Lipid Levels, Risk for Coronary
  Artery Disease" (NIA) 69n
international normalized ratio (INR),
  described 425
interstitial keratitis, described 274
interventricular septum, described 6
intra-aortic balloon pump,
  cardiogenic shock 146–47
intravenous drug users,
  endocarditis 205
INVEST study 59–60
ion channels,
  long QT syndrome 183
irbesartan *436*
ischemia
  defined 624
  described 245

ischemic heart disease
  described 104
  thyroid disease 63–64
ischemic stroke
  defined 624
  described 90, 246–47
  tissue plasminogen activator 91
ISH *see* isolated systolic hypertension
isolated systolic hypertension (ISH)
  age factor 30
  described 29
Isoptin (verapamil) *432*
isosorbide dinitrate 197
isradipine *432*

J

Jacobs, David 60
joints, vasculitis 281
journals (diaries)
  event monitors 379
  stress management 616

K

Kawasaki disease, described 276
Kerlone (betaxolol) *432*
kidney disorders
  blood tests 343
  endocarditis 206
  heart transplantation 539
  hypertension 28, 29, 32
"Know Stroke. Know the Signs.
  Act in Time." (NINDS) 90n

L

labetalol *432*
"Lack of vitamin D may increase
  heart disease risk" (American
  Heart Association) 597n
Lakatta, Edward 77
laser therapy, varicose veins 298–99
Lasix (furosemide; indapamide) *439*
LDL cholesterol *see* low-density
  lipoprotein (LDL) cholesterol
leaflets, described 6, 7

rheumatic fever
  heart murmurs 329
  heart valve disease 189
rheumatic heart disease
  atrial fibrillation 176
  overview 199–201
"Rheumatic Heart Disease/
  Rheumatic Fever" (American
  Heart Association) 199n
right-side heart failure,
  described 149–50
risk factors
  aneurysms 256–57
  angina 118–19
  arrhythmias 170–71
  atherosclerosis 223–25, 241–42
  atrial fibrillation 175–76
  cardiogenic shock 144–45
  cardiomyopathy 159–60
  carotid artery disease 233–34
  coronary artery disease 105–6,
    133–34
  coronary microvascular
    disease 242
  deep vein thrombosis 284
  endocarditis 203–4, 206–7
  heart attack 128
  heart disease 15, 19–26, 54
  heart failure 152–53
  heart valve disease 191
  high blood cholesterol 41–42
  hypertension 30–31
  metabolic syndrome 56
  mitral valve prolapse 195
  pericarditis 210–11
  peripheral artery
    disease 263–64
  sudden cardiac arrest 138
  vasculitis 280–81
rosuvastatin 450
Rubenfire, Melvyn 316–17

S

Sacco, Ralph 59
Saluron (hydroflumethiazide) *439*
SA node *see* sinoatrial node
sarcoidosis, heart block 180

SCA *see* sudden cardiac arrest
Schelssinger, David 72
sclerotherapy, varicose veins 297–99
secondary Raynaud,
  described 268–69
Sectral (acebutolol) *432*
Sedrakyan, Art 493
septal defects, described 329
septal rupture, described 147
septum
  defined 625
  described 6, 329
serum myoglobin tests,
  heart attack 131
sestamibi stress test 367, 371
sexual activity
  cardiac rehabilitation 548
  heart attack 552
shock, described 141–42
sick sinus syndrome, atrial
  fibrillation 176
side effects
  angiotensin converting
    enzyme inhibitors 430
  angiotensin II antagonists 435–36
  anticoagulant medications 422
  beta-blockers 431
  calcium channel blockers 433
  centrally-acting alpha
    adrenergics 437
  digoxin 441–42
  diuretics 439
  implantable cardioverter
    defibrillator 472–73
  overview 435
  peripherally acting alpha-
    adrenergic blockers 434
  rejection medications 537
  renin inhibitors 440
silent heart attack, described 128
simvastatin 450
single-photon emission computed
  tomography (SPECT), nuclear
  heart scan 408–9
sinoatrial node (SA node)
  described 10, 164
  heart block 179
  pacemaker 79
skin, vasculitis 281

Health Reference Series

Complete Catalog

List price $93 per volume. School and library price $84 per volume.

Adolescent Health Sourcebook, 3rd Edition

Basic Consumer Health Information about Adolescent Growth and Development, Puberty, Sexuality, Reproductive Health, and Physical, Emotional, Social, and Mental Health Concerns of Teens and Their Parents, Including Facts about Nutrition, Physical Activity, Weight Management, Acne, Allergies, Cancer, Diabetes, Growth Disorders, Juvenile Arthritis, Infections, Substance Abuse, and More

Along with Information about Adolescent Safety Concerns, Youth Violence, a Glossary of Related Terms, and a Directory of Resources

Edited by Amy L. Sutton. 600 pages. 2010. 978-0-7808-1140-9.

Adult Health Concerns Sourcebook

Basic Consumer Health Information about Medical and Mental Concerns of Adults, Including Facts about Choosing Healthcare Providers, Navigating Insurance Options, Maintaining Wellness, Preventing Cancer, Heart Disease, Stroke, Diabetes, and Osteoporosis, and Understanding Aging-Related Health Concerns, Including Menopause, Cognitive Changes, and Changes in the Coronary and Vascular Systems

Along with Tips on Caring for Aging Parents and Dealing with Health-Related Work and Travel Issues, a Glossary, and a Directory of Resources for Additional Help and Information

Edited by Sandra J. Judd. 648 pages. 2008. 978-0-7808-0999-4.

"Provides a thorough list of topics that are important to adult health and for caregivers."
—*CHOICE, Nov '08*

"Written in easy-to-understand language... the content is well-organized and is intended to aid adults in making health care-related decisions."
—*AORN Journal, Dec '08*

AIDS Sourcebook, 4th Edition

Basic Consumer Health Information about Human Immunodeficiency Virus (HIV) and Acquired Immunodeficiency Syndrome (AIDS), Featuring Updated Statistics and Facts about Risks, Prevention, Screening, Diagnosis, Treatments, Side Effects, and Complications, and Including a Section about the Impact of HIV/AIDS on the Health of Women, Children, and Adolescents

Along with Tips on Managing Life with AIDS, Reports on Current Research Initiatives and Clinical Trials, a Glossary of Related Terms, and Resource Directories for Further Help and Information

Edited by Ivy L. Alexander. 680 pages. 2008. 978-0-7808-0997-0.

SEE ALSO *Contagious Diseases Sourcebook, 2nd Edition*

Alcoholism Sourcebook, 3rd Edition

Basic Consumer Health Information about Alcohol Use, Abuse, and Dependence, Featuring Facts about the Physical, Mental, and Social Health Effects of Alcohol Addiction, Including Alcoholic Liver Disease, Pancreatic Disease, Cardiovascular Disease, Neurological Disorders, and the Effects of Drinking during Pregnancy

Along with Information about Alcohol Treatment, Medications, and Recovery Programs, in Addition to Tips for Reducing the Prevalence of Underage Drinking, Statistics about Alcohol Use, a Glossary of Related Terms, and Directories of Resources for More Help and Information

Edited by Joyce Brennfleck Shannon. 600 pages. 2010. 978-0-7808-1141-6.

SEE ALSO *Drug Abuse Sourcebook, 3rd Edition*

Allergies Sourcebook, 3rd Edition

Basic Consumer Health Information about Allergic Disorders, Such as Anaphylaxis,

Hives, Eczema, Rhinitis, Sinusitis, and Conjunctivitis, and Their Triggers, Including Pollen, Mold, Dust Mites, Animal Dander, Insects, Chemicals, Food, Food Additives, and Medications

Along with Advice about the Diagnosis and Treatment of Allergy Symptoms, a Glossary of Related Terms, a Directory of Resources for Help and Information, and Suggestions for Additional Reading

Edited by Amy L. Sutton. 588 pages. 2007. 978-0-7808-0950-5.

SEE ALSO Asthma Sourcebook, 2nd Edition

Alzheimer Disease Sourcebook, 4th Edition

Basic Consumer Health Information about Alzheimer Disease, Other Dementias, and Related Disorders, Including Multi-Infarct Dementia, Dementia with Lewy Bodies, Frontotemporal Dementia (Pick Disease), Wernicke-Korsakoff Syndrome (Alcohol-Related Dementia), AIDS Dementia Complex, Huntington Disease, Creutzfeldt-Jacob Disease, and Delirium

Along with Information about Coping with Memory Loss and Forgetfulness, Maintaining Skills, and Long-Term Planning for People with Dementia, and Suggestions Addressing Common Caregiver Concerns, Updated Information about Current Research Efforts, a Glossary of Related Terms, and Directories of Sources for Additional Help and Information

Edited by Karen Bellenir. 603 pages. 2008. 978-0-7808-1001-3.

"An invaluable resource for persons who have received a diagnosis, for caregivers, and for family members dealing with this insidious disease. It is recommended for public, community college, and ready-reference sections in academic libraries."
—American Reference Books Annual, 2009

SEE ALSO Brain Disorders Sourcebook, 3rd Edition

Arthritis Sourcebook, 3rd Edition

Basic Consumer Health Information about the Risk Factors, Symptoms, Diagnosis, and Treatment of Osteoarthritis, Rheumatoid Arthritis, Juvenile Arthritis, Gout, Infectious Arthritis, and Autoimmune Disorders Associated with Arthritis

Along with Facts about Medications, Surgeries, and Self-Care Techniques to Manage Pain and Disability, Tips on Living with Arthritis, a Glossary of Related Terms, and Resources for Additional Help and Information

Edited by Amy L. Sutton. 600 pages. 2010. 978-0-7808-1077-8.

Asthma Sourcebook, 2nd Edition

Basic Consumer Health Information about the Causes, Symptoms, Diagnosis, and Treatment of Asthma in Infants, Children, Teenagers, and Adults, Including Facts about Different Types of Asthma, Common Co-Occurring Conditions, Asthma Management Plans, Triggers, Medications, and Medication Delivery Devices

Along with Asthma Statistics, Research Updates, a Glossary, a Directory of Asthma-Related Resources, and More

Edited by Karen Bellenir. 581 pages. 2006. 978-0-7808-0866-9.

SEE ALSO Lung Disorders Sourcebook; Respiratory Disorders Sourcebook, 2nd Edition

Attention Deficit Disorder Sourcebook

Basic Consumer Health Information about Attention Deficit/Hyperactivity Disorder in Children and Adults, Including Facts about Causes, Symptoms, Diagnostic Criteria, and Treatment Options Such as Medications, Behavior Therapy, Coaching, and Homeopathy

Along with Reports on Current Research Initiatives, Legal Issues, and Government Regulations, and Featuring a Glossary of Related Terms, Internet Resources, and a List of Additional Reading Material

Edited by Dawn D. Matthews. 447 pages. 2002. 978-0-7808-0624-5.

"Recommended reference source."
—Booklist, Jan '03

SEE ALSO Learning Disabilities Sourcebook, 3rd Edition

Autism and Pervasive Developmental Disorders Sourcebook

Basic Consumer Health Information about Autism Spectrum and Pervasive Developmental Disorders, Such as Classical Autism, Asperger Syndrome, Rett Syndrome, and Childhood Disintegrative Disorder, Including Information about Related Genetic Disorders and Medical Problems and Facts about Causes, Screening Methods, Diagnostic Criteria, Treatments and Interventions, and Family and Education Issues

Along with a Glossary of Related Terms, Tips for Evaluating the Validity of Health Claims, and a Directory of Resources for Additional Help and Information

Edited by Sandra J. Judd. 603 pages. 2007. 978-0-7808-0953-6.

"This book provides a current overview of disorders on the autism spectrum and information about various therapies, educational resources, and help for families with practical issues such as workplace adjustments, living arrangements, and estate planning. It is a useful resource for public and consumer health libraries."
—*American Reference Books Annual, 2009*

SEE ALSO *Learning Disabilities Sourcebook, 3rd Edition*

Back and Neck Disorders Sourcebook, 2nd Edition

Basic Consumer Health Information about Spinal Pain, Spinal Cord Injuries, and Related Disorders, Such as Degenerative Disk Disease, Osteoarthritis, Scoliosis, Sciatica, Spina Bifida, and Spinal Stenosis, and Featuring Facts about Maintaining Spinal Health, Self-Care, Pain Management, Rehabilitative Care, Chiropractic Care, Spinal Surgeries, and Complementary Therapies

Along with Suggestions for Preventing Back and Neck Pain, a Glossary of Related Terms, and a Directory of Resources

Edited by Amy L. Sutton. 607 pages. 2004. 978-0-7808-0738-9.

"Recommended... An easy to use, comprehensive medical reference book."
—*E-Streams, Sep '05*

"For anyone who has back or neck problems, this book is ideal. Its easy-to-understand language and variety of topics makes this sourcebook a worthwhile read. The price... is reasonable for the amount of information contained in the book"
—*Occupational Therapy in Health Care, 2007*

Blood & Circulatory Disorders Sourcebook, 3rd Edition

Basic Consumer Health Information about Blood and Circulatory System Disorders, Such as Anemia, Leukemia, Lymphoma, Rh Disease, Hemophilia, Thrombophilia, Other Bleeding and Clotting Deficiencies, and Artery, Vascular, and Venous Diseases, Including Facts about Blood Types, Blood Donation, Bone Marrow and Stem Cell Transplants, Tests and Medications, and Tips for Maintaining Circulatory Health

Along with a Glossary of Related Terms and a List of Resources for Additional Help and Information

Edited by Sandra J. Judd. 600 pages. 2010. 978-0-7808-1081-5.

SEE ALSO *Leukemia Sourcebook*

Brain Disorders Sourcebook, 3rd Edition

Basic Consumer Health Information about Acquired and Traumatic Brain Injuries, Brain Tumors, Cerebral Palsy and Other Genetic and Congenital Brain Disorders, Infections of the Brain, Epilepsy, and Degenerative Neurological Disorders Such as Dementia, Huntington Disease, and Amyotrophic Lateral Sclerosis (ALS)

Along with Information on Brain Structure and Function, Treatment and Rehabilitation Options, a Glossary of Terms Related to Brain Disorders, and a Directory of Resources for More Information

Edited by Joyce Brennfleck Shannon. 600 pages. 2010. 978-0-7808-1083-9.

SEE ALSO *Alzheimer Disease Sourcebook, 4th Edition*

Breast Cancer Sourcebook, 3rd Edition

Basic Consumer Health Information about Breast Health and Breast Cancer, Including Facts about Environmental, Genetic, and Other Risk Factors, Prevention Efforts, Screening and Diagnostic Methods, Surgical Treatment Options and Other Care Choices, Complementary and Alternative Therapies, and Post-Treatment Concerns

Along with Statistical Data, News about Research Advances, a Glossary of Related Terms, and Directories of Resources for Additional Information and Support

Edited by Karen Bellenir. 606 pages. 2009. 978-0-7808-1030-3.

"A very useful reference for people wanting to learn more about breast cancer and how to negotiate their care or the care of a loved one. The third edition is necessary as information/treatment options continue to evolve."
—Doody's Review Service, 2009

SEE ALSO Cancer Sourcebook for Women, 3rd Edition, Women's Health Concerns Sourcebook, 3rd Edition

Breastfeeding Sourcebook

Basic Consumer Health Information about the Benefits of Breastmilk, Preparing to Breastfeed, Breastfeeding as a Baby Grows, Nutrition, and More, Including Information on Special Situations and Concerns Such as Mastitis, Illness, Medications, Allergies, Multiple Births, Prematurity, Special Needs, and Adoption

Along with a Glossary and Resources for Additional Help and Information

Edited by Jenni Lynn Colson. 367 pages. 2002. 978-0-7808-0332-9.

SEE ALSO Pregnancy and Birth Sourcebook, 3rd Edition

Burns Sourcebook

Basic Consumer Health Information about Various Types of Burns and Scalds, Including Flame, Heat, Cold, Electrical, Chemical, and Sun Burns

Along with Information on Short-Term and Long-Term Treatments, Tissue Reconstruction, Plastic Surgery, Prevention Suggestions, and First Aid

Edited by Allan R. Cook. 604 pages. 1999. 978-0-7808-0204-9.

"This is an exceptional addition to the series and is highly recommended for all consumer health collections, hospital libraries, and academic medical centers."
—E-Streams, Mar '00

"This key reference guide is an invaluable addition to all health care and public libraries in confronting this ongoing health issue."
—American Reference Books Annual, 2000

SEE ALSO Dermatological Disorders Sourcebook, 2nd Edition

Cancer Sourcebook, 5th Edition

Basic Consumer Health Information about Major Forms and Stages of Cancer, Featuring Facts about Head and Neck Cancers, Lung Cancers, Gastrointestinal Cancers, Genitourinary Cancers, Lymphomas, Blood Cell Cancers, Endocrine Cancers, Skin Cancers, Bone Cancers, Metastatic Cancers, and More

Along with Facts about Cancer Treatments, Cancer Risks and Prevention, a Glossary of Related Terms, Statistical Data, and a Directory of Resources for Additional Information

Edited by Karen Bellenir. 1105 pages. 2007. 978-0-7808-0947-5.

"The 5th, updated edition of Cancer Sourcebook should be in every public and health lending library collection... An unparalleled discussion essential for any health collections considering an all-in-one basic general reference."
—California Bookwatch, Aug '07

SEE ALSO Breast Cancer Sourcebook, 3rd Edition, Cancer Survivorship Sourcebook, Leukemia Sourcebook

Cancer Sourcebook for Women, 4th Edition

Basic Consumer Health Information about Gynecologic Cancers and Other Cancers of Special Concern to Women, Including Cancers of the Breast, Cervix, Colon, Lung, Ovaries, Thyroid, and Uterus

Along with Facts about Benign Conditions of the Female Reproductive System, Cancer Risk

Factors, Diagnostic and Treatment Procedures, Side Effects of Cancer and Cancer Treatments, Women's Issues in Cancer Survivorship, a Glossary of Related Terms, and a Directory of Resources for Additional Help and Information

Edited by Karen Bellenir. 600 pages. 2010. 978-0-7808-1139-3.

SEE ALSO Breast Cancer Sourcebook, 3rd Edition, Women's Health Concerns Sourcebook, 3rd Edition

Cancer Survivorship Sourcebook

Basic Consumer Health Information about the Physical, Educational, Emotional, Social, and Financial Needs of Cancer Patients from Diagnosis, through Cancer Treatment, and Beyond, Including Facts about Researching Specific Types of Cancer and Learning about Clinical Trials and Treatment Options, and Featuring Tips for Coping with the Side Effects of Cancer Treatments and Adjusting to Life after Cancer Treatment Concludes

Along with Suggestions for Caregivers, Friends, and Family Members of Cancer Patients, a Glossary of Cancer Care Terms, and Directories of Related Resources

Edited by Karen Bellenir. 633 pages. 2007. 978-0-7808-0985-7.

"Well organized and comprehensive in coverage, the book speaks to issues encountered both during and after cancer treatment. Recommended for consumer health and public libraries."
—*Library Journal, Aug 1 '07*

"Cancer Survivorship Sourcebook will be useful to anyone who has a friend or loved one with a cancer diagnosis."
—*American Reference Books Annual, 2008*

SEE ALSO *Cancer Sourcebook, 5th Edition, Disease Management Sourcebook*

Cardiovascular Disorders Sourcebook, 4th Edition

Basic Consumer Health Information about Heart and Blood Vessel Diseases and Disorders, Such as Angina, Heart Attack, Heart Failure, Cardiomyopathy, Arrhythmias, Valve Disease, Atherosclerosis, Aneurysms, and

Congenital Heart Defects, Including Information about Cardiovascular Disease in Women, Men, Children, Adolescents, and Minorities

Along with Facts about Diagnosing, Managing, and Preventing Cardiovascular Disease, a Glossary of Related Medical Terms, and a Directory of Resources for Additional Information

Edited by Amy L. Sutton. 600 pages. 2010. 978-0-7808-1080-8.

Caregiving Sourcebook

Basic Consumer Health Information for Caregivers, Including a Profile of Caregivers, Caregiving Responsibilities and Concerns, Tips for Specific Conditions, Care Environments, and the Effects of Caregiving

Along with Facts about Legal Issues, Financial Information, and Future Planning, a Glossary, and a Listing of Additional Resources

Edited by Joyce Brennfleck Shannon. 583 pages. 2001. 978-0-7808-0331-2.

"Essential for most collections."
—*Library Journal, Apr 1 '02*

"An ideal addition to the reference collection of any public library. Health sciences information professionals may also want to acquire the Caregiving Sourcebook for their hospital or academic library for use as a ready reference tool by health care workers interested in aging and caregiving."
—*E-Streams, Jan '02*

Child Abuse Sourcebook, 2nd Edition

Basic Consumer Health Information about the Physical, Sexual, and Emotional Abuse of Children, Neglect, Münchhausen Syndrome by Proxy (MSBP), and Shaken Baby Syndrome, and Featuring Facts about Withholding Medical Care, Corporal Punishment, Child Maltreatment in Youth Sports, and Parental Substance Abuse

Along with Information about Child Protective Services, Foster Care, Adoption, Parenting Challenges, Abuse Prevention Programs, and Intervention, Treatment, and Recovery Guidelines, a Glossary of Related Terms, and Resources for Additional Help and Information

Edited by Joyce Brennfleck Shannon. 600 pages. 2009. 978-0-7808-1037-2.

SEE ALSO *Domestic Violence Sourcebook, 3rd Edition*

Childhood Diseases and Disorders Sourcebook, 2nd Edition

Basic Consumer Health Information about the Physical, Mental, and Developmental Health of Pre-Adolescent Children, Including Facts about Infectious Diseases, Asthma, Allergies, Diabetes, and Other Acute and Chronic Conditions Affecting the Gastrointestinal Tract, Ears, Nose, Throat, Liver, Kidneys, Heart, Blood, Brain, Muscles, Bones, and Skin

Along with Reports on Recommended Childhood Vaccinations, Wellness Guidelines, a Glossary of Related Medical Terms, and a List of Resources for Parents

Edited by Sandra J. Judd. 694 pages. 2009. 978-0-7808-1031-0.

"The strength of this source is the wide range of information given about childhood health issues... It is most appropriate for public libraries and academic libraries that field medical questions."
—*American Reference Books Annual, 2009*

SEE ALSO *Healthy Children Sourcebook*

Colds, Flu and Other Common Ailments Sourcebook

Basic Consumer Health Information about Common Ailments and Injuries, Including Colds, Coughs, the Flu, Sinus Problems, Headaches, Fever, Nausea and Vomiting, Menstrual Cramps, Diarrhea, Constipation, Hemorrhoids, Back Pain, Dandruff, Dry and Itchy Skin, Cuts, Scrapes, Sprains, Bruises, and More

Along with Information about Prevention, Self-Care, Choosing a Doctor, Over-the-Counter Medications, Folk Remedies, and Alternative Therapies, and Including a Glossary of Important Terms and a Directory of Resources for Further Help and Information

Edited by Chad T. Kimball. 622 pages. 2001. 978-0-7808-0435-7.

"A good starting point for research on common illnesses. It will be a useful addition to public and consumer health library collections."
—*American Reference Books Annual, 2002*

"Will prove valuable to any library seeking to maintain a current, comprehensive reference collection of health resources... Excellent reference."
—*The Bookwatch, Aug '01*

SEE ALSO *Contagious Diseases Sourcebook, 2nd Edition*

Communication Disorders Sourcebook

Basic Information about Deafness and Hearing Loss, Speech and Language Disorders, Voice Disorders, Balance and Vestibular Disorders, and Disorders of Smell, Taste, and Touch

Edited by Linda M. Ross. 533 pages. 1996. 978-0-7808-0077-9.

"This is skillfully edited and is a welcome resource for the layperson. It should be found in every public and medical library."
—*Booklist Health Sciences Supplement, Oct '97*

Complementary & Alternative Medicine Sourcebook, 4th Edition

Basic Consumer Health Information about Ayurveda, Acupuncture, Aromatherapy, Chiropractic Care, Diet-Based Therapies, Guided Imagery, Herbal and Vitamin Supplements, Homeopathy, Hypnosis, Massage, Meditation, Naturopathy, Pilates, Reflexology, Reiki, Shiatsu, Tai Chi, Traditional Chinese Medicine, Yoga, and Other Complementary and Alternative Medical Therapies

Along with Statistics, Tips for Selecting a Practitioner, Treatments for Specific Health Conditions, a Glossary of Related Terms, and a Directory of Resources for Additional Help and Information

Edited by Amy L. Sutton. 600 pages. 2010. 978-0-7808-1082-2.

Congenital Disorders Sourcebook, 2nd Edition

Basic Consumer Health Information about Nonhereditary Birth Defects and Disorders

Related to Prematurity, Gestational Injuries, Congenital Infections, and Birth Complications, Including Heart Defects, Hydrocephalus, Spina Bifida, Cleft Lip and Palate, Cerebral Palsy, and More

Along with Facts about the Prevention of Birth Defects, Fetal Surgery and Other Treatment Options, Research Initiatives, a Glossary of Related Terms, and Resources for Additional Information and Support

Edited by Sandra J. Judd. 619 pages. 2007. 978-0-7808-0945-1.

"Congenital Disorders Sourcebook provides an excellent, non-technical overview of many aspects of pregnancy with the focus on congenital disorders."
—American Reference Books Annual, 2008

"An excellent readable reference aimed at the lay public for difficult to understand medical problems. An excellent starting point for the interested parent or family member who may then be motivated to seek more information."
—Doody's Review Service, 2007

SEE ALSO Pregnancy and Birth Sourcebook, 3rd Edition

Contagious Diseases Sourcebook, 2nd Edition

Basic Consumer Health Information about Diseases Spread from Person to Person through Direct Physical Contact, Airborne Transmissions, Sexual Contact, or Contact with Blood or Other Body Fluids, Including Pneumococcal, Staphylococcal, and Streptococcal Diseases, Colds, Influenza, Lice, Measles, Mumps, Tuberculosis, and Others

Along with Facts about Self-Care and Over-the-Counter Medications, Antibiotics and Drug Resistance, Disease Prevention, Vaccines, and Bioterrorism, a Glossary, and a Directory of Resources for More Information

Edited by Joyce Brennfleck Shannon. 600 pages. 2010. 978-0-7808-1075-4.

SEE ALSO AIDS Sourcebook, 4th Edition, Hepatitis Sourcebook

Cosmetic and Reconstructive Surgery Sourcebook, 2nd Edition

Basic Consumer Information about Plastic Surgery and Non-Surgical Appearance-Enhancing Procedures, Including Facts about Botulinum Toxin, Collagen Replacement, Dermabrasion, Chemical Peels, Eyelid Surgery, Nose Reshaping, Lip Augmentation, Liposuction, Breast Enlargement and Reduction, Tummy Tucking, and Other Skin, Hair, Facial, and Body Shaping Procedures

Along with Information about Reconstructive Procedures for Congenital Disorders, Disfiguring Diseases, Burns, and Traumatic Injuries, a Glossary of Related Terms, and a Directory of Additional Resources

Edited by Karen Bellenir. 483 pages. 2007. 978-0-7808-0951-2.

"A comprehensive source for people considering cosmetic surgery... also recommended for medical students who will perform these procedures later in their careers; and public librarians and academic medical librarians who may assist patrons interested in this information."
—Medical Reference Services Quarterly, Fall '08

"A practical guide for health care consumers and health care workers... This easy-to-read reference guide would be useful for novice and veteran health care consumers, surgical technology students, nursing students, and perioperative nurses new to plastic and reconstructive surgery. It also may be helpful for medical-surgical nurses as a guide for patient teaching in their practices."
—AORN Journal, Aug '08

SEE ALSO Surgery Sourcebook, 2nd Edition

Death and Dying Sourcebook, 2nd Edition

Basic Consumer Health Information about End-of-Life Care and Related Perspectives and Ethical Issues, Including End-of-Life Symptoms and Treatments, Pain Management, Quality-of-Life Concerns, the Use of Life Support, Patients' Rights and Privacy Issues, Advance Directives, Physician-Assisted Suicide, Caregiving, Organ and Tissue Donation, Autopsies, Funeral Arrangements, and Grief

Along with Statistical Data, Information about the Leading Causes of Death, a Glossary, and Directories of Support Groups and Other Resources

Edited by Joyce Brennfleck Shannon. 626 pages. 2006. 978-0-7808-0871-3.

Dental Care and Oral Health Sourcebook, 3rd Edition

Basic Consumer Health Information about Dental Care and Oral Health Throughout the Lifespan, Including Facts about Cavities, Bad Breath, Cold and Canker Sores, Dry Mouth, Toothaches, Gum Disease, Malocclusion, Temporomandibular Joint and Muscle Disorders, Oral Cancers, and Dental Emergencies

Along with Information about Mouth Hygiene, Crowns, Bridges, Implants, and Fillings, Surgical, Orthodontic, and Cosmetic Dental Procedures, Pain Management, Health Conditions that Impact Oral Care, a Glossary of Related Terms, and a Directory of Additional Resources

Edited by Amy L. Sutton. 619 pages. 2008. 978-0-7808-1032-7.

"Could serve as turning point in the battle to educate consumers in issues concerning oral health. Tightly written in terms the average person can understand, yet comprehensive in scope and authoritative in tone, it is another excellent sourcebook in the Health Reference Series... Should be in the reference department of all public libraries, and in academic libraries that have a public constituency."
—American Reference Books Annual, 2009

Depression Sourcebook, 2nd Edition

Basic Consumer Health Information about Unipolar Depression, Bipolar Disorder, Dysthymia, Seasonal Affective Disorder, Postpartum Depression, and Other Depressive Disorders, Including Facts about Populations at Special Risk, Coexisting Medical Conditions, Symptoms, Treatment Options, and Suicide Prevention

Along with Statistical Data, a Glossary of Related Terms, and a Directory of Resources for Additional Help and Information

Edited by Sandra J. Judd. 646 pages. 2008. 978-0-7808-1003-7.

"Recommended for public libraries."
—American Reference Books Annual, 2009

SEE ALSO Mental Health Disorders Sourcebook, 4th Edition

Dermatological Disorders Sourcebook, 2nd Edition

Basic Consumer Health Information about Conditions and Disorders Affecting the Skin, Hair, and Nails, Such as Acne, Rosacea, Rashes, Dermatitis, Pigmentation Disorders, Birthmarks, Skin Cancer, Skin Injuries, Psoriasis, Scleroderma, and Hair Loss, Including Facts about Medications and Treatments for Dermatological Disorders and Tips for Maintaining Healthy Skin, Hair, and Nails

Along with Information about How Aging Affects the Skin, a Glossary of Related Terms, and a Directory of Resources for Additional Help and Information

Edited by Amy L. Sutton. 617 pages. 2006. 978-0-7808-0795-2.

"Well organized... presents a plethora of information in a manner that is appropriate in style and readability for the intended audience."
—Physical Therapy, Nov '06

"Helpfully brings together... sources in one convenient place, saving the user hours of research time."
—American Reference Books Annual, 2006

SEE ALSO Burns Sourcebook

Diabetes Sourcebook, 4th Edition

Basic Consumer Health Information about Type 1 and Type 2 Diabetes Mellitus, Gestational Diabetes, Monogenic Forms of Diabetes, and Insulin Resistance, with Guidelines for Lifestyle Modifications and the Medical Management of Diabetes, Including Facts about Insulin, Insulin Delivery Devices, Oral Diabetes Medications, Self-Monitoring of Blood Glucose, Meal Planning, Physical Activity Recommendations, Foot Care, and Treatment Options for People with Kidney Failure

Along with a Section about Diabetes Complications and Co-Occurring Conditions, a Glossary of Related Terms, and Directories of Re- sources for Additional Help and Information

Edited by Karen Bellenir. 627 pages. 2008. 978- 0-7808-1005-1.

"Completely and comprehensively covering almost everything a student or physician would need to know... well worth the invest- ment."
—Internet Bookwatch, Dec '08

SEE ALSO Endocrine and Metabolic Disorders Sourcebook, 2nd Edition

Diet and Nutrition Sourcebook, 3rd Edition

Basic Consumer Health Information about Dietary Guidelines and the Food Guidance System, Recommended Daily Nutrient In- takes, Serving Proportions, Weight Control, Vitamins and Supplements, Nutrition Issues for Different Life Stages and Lifestyles, and the Needs of People with Specific Medical Concerns, Including Cancer, Celiac Disease, Diabetes, Eating Disorders, Food Allergies, and Cardiovascular Disease

Along with Facts about Federal Nutrition Support Programs, a Glossary of Nutrition and Dietary Terms, and Directories of Addi- tional Resources for More Information about Nutrition

Edited by Joyce Brennfleck Shannon. 605 pages. 2006. 978-0-7808-0800-3.

"A valuable resource tool for any individual."
—Journal of Dental Hygiene, Apr '07

"From different recommended eating habits to reduce disease and common ailments to nutri- tion advice for those with specific conditions, Diet and Nutrition Sourcebook is especially important because so much is changing in this area, and so rapidly."
—California Bookwatch, Jun '06

SEE ALSO Eating Disorders Sourcebook, 2nd Edition, Vegetarian Sourcebook

Digestive Diseases and Disorders Sourcebook

Basic Consumer Health Information about Diseases and Disorders that Impact the Upper and Lower Digestive System, Including Celiac Disease, Constipation, Crohn's Disease, Cyclic Vomiting Syndrome, Diarrhea, Diverticulosis and Diverticulitis, Gallstones, Heartburn, Hemorrhoids, Hernias, Indigestion (Dyspep- sia), Irritable Bowel Syndrome, Lactose Intol- erance, Ulcers, and More

Along with Information about Medications and Other Treatments, Tips for Maintaining a Healthy Digestive Tract, a Glossary, and Di- rectory of Digestive Diseases Organizations

Edited by Karen Bellenir. 323 pages. 2000. 978- 0-7808-0327-5.

"An excellent addition to all public or patient- research libraries."
—American Reference Books Annual, 2001

"Recommended reference source."
—Booklist, May '00

SEE ALSO Gastrointestinal Diseases and Dis- orders Sourcebook, 2nd Edition

Disabilities Sourcebook

Basic Consumer Health Information about Physical and Psychiatric Disabilities, Including Descriptions of Major Causes of Disability, Assistive and Adaptive Aids, Workplace Is- sues, and Accessibility Concerns

Along with Information about the Americans with Disabilities Act, a Glossary, and Re- sources for Additional Help and Information

Edited by Dawn D. Matthews. 602 pages. 2000. 978-0-7808-0389-3.

"A must for libraries with a consumer health section."
—American Reference Books Annual, 2002

"A much needed addition to the Omnigraphics Health Reference Series. A current reference work to provide people with disabilities, their families, caregivers or those who work with them, a broad range of information in one vol- ume, has not been available until now... It is recommended for all public and academic li- brary reference collections."
—E-Streams, May '01

"An excellent source book in easy-to-read for- mat covering many current topics; highly rec- ommended for all libraries."
—CHOICE, Jan '01

Disease Management Sourcebook

Basic Consumer Health Information about Coping with Chronic and Serious Illnesses, Navigating the Health Care System, Communicating with Health Care Providers, Assessing Health Care Quality, and Making Informed Health Care Decisions, Including Facts about Second Opinions, Hospitalization, Surgery, and Medications

Along with a Section about Children with Chronic Conditions, Information about Legal, Financial, and Insurance Issues, a Glossary of Related Terms, and Directories of Additional Resources

Edited by Joyce Brennfleck Shannon. 621 pages. 2008. 978-0-7808-1002-0.

"Consumers need to know how to manage their health care the same way they manage anything else in their lives. The text is very readable and is written for the layperson and consumer. The cost is not prohibitive. This book should be in all collections of health care libraries and public libraries."
— *American Reference Books Annual, 2009*

"The information is very current, and the selection of font and layout make the book easy to read. A hardback that will stand up to much usage, this is an excellent resource for consumers... Recommended. General readers."
—*CHOICE, Nov '08*

"Intended for lay readers, this resource clarifies the many confusing and overwhelming details associated with chronic disease care. Meticulous and clearly explained, the book even includes diagrams intended to ease comprehension of over-the-counter medication labels. An essential guide to navigating the health-care rapids."
—*Library Journal, Aug '08*

Domestic Violence Sourcebook, 3rd Edition

Basic Consumer Health Information about Warning Signs, Risk Factors, and Health Consequences of Intimate Partner Violence, Sexual Violence and Rape, Stalking, Human Trafficking, Child Maltreatment, Teen Dating Violence, and Elder Abuse

Along with Facts about Victims and Perpetrators, Strategies for Violence Prevention, and Emergency Interventions, Safety Plans, and Financial and Legal Tips for Victims, a Glossary of Related Terms, and Directories of Resources for Additional Information and Support

Edited by Joyce Brennfleck Shannon. 634 pages. 2009. 978-0-7808-1038-9.

"A recommended pick for any library interested in consumer health and social issues... A 'must' for any serious health collection."
—*California Bookwatch, Jul '09*

SEE ALSO *Child Abuse Sourcebook, 2nd Edition*

Drug Abuse Sourcebook, 3rd Edition

Basic Consumer Health Information about the Abuse of Cocaine, Club Drugs, Hallucinogens, Heroin, Inhalants, Marijuana, and Other Illicit Substances, Prescription Medications, and Over-the-Counter Medicines

Along with Facts about Addiction and Related Health Effects, Drug Abuse Treatment and Recovery, Drug Testing, Prevention Programs, Glossaries of Drug-Related Terms, and Directories of Resources for More Information

Edited by Joyce Brennfleck Shannon. 600 pages. 2010. 978-0-7808-1079-2.

SEE ALSO *Alcoholism Sourcebook, 3rd Edition*

Ear, Nose, and Throat Disorders Sourcebook, 2nd Edition

Basic Consumer Health Information about Disorders of the Ears, Hearing Loss, Vestibular Disorders, Nasal and Sinus Problems, Throat and Vocal Cord Disorders, and Otolaryngologic Cancers, Including Facts about Ear Infections and Injuries, Genetic and Congenital Deafness, Sensorineural Hearing Disorders, Tinnitus, Vertigo, Ménière Disease, Rhinitis, Sinusitis, Snoring, Sore Throats, Hoarseness, and More

Along with Reports on Current Research Initiatives, a Glossary of Related Medical Terms, and a Directory of Sources for Further Help and Information

Edited by Sandra J. Judd. 631 pages. 2007. 978-0-7808-0872-0.

"A resource book for the general public that provides comprehensive coverage of basic up-to-date medical information about the causes, symptoms, diagnosis, and treatment of diseases and disorders that affect the ears, nose, sinuses, throat, and voice... The majority of information is presented in question and answer format, much like questions a patient might ask of a health care provider. An extensive index facilitates the reader's ability to easily access information on any specific topic."
—*Journal of Dental Hygiene, Oct '07*

"A handy compilation of information on common and some not so common ailments of the ears, nose, and throat."
—*Doody's Review Service, 2007*

Eating Disorders Sourcebook, 2nd Edition

Basic Consumer Health Information about Anorexia Nervosa, Bulimia, Binge Eating, Compulsive Exercise, Female Athlete Triad, and Other Eating Disorders, Including Facts about Body Image and Other Cultural and Age-Related Risk Factors, Prevention Efforts, Adverse Health Effects, Treatment Options, and the Recovery Process

Along with Guidelines for Healthy Weight Control, a Glossary, and Directories of Additional Resources

Edited by Joyce Brennfleck Shannon. 557 pages. 2007. 978-0-7808-0948-2.

"Recommended for the reference collection of large public libraries."
—*American Reference Books Annual, 2008*

"A basic health reference any health or general library needs."
—*Internet Bookwatch, Jun '07*

SEE ALSO Diet and Nutrition Sourcebook, 3rd Edition, Mental Health Disorders Sourcebook, 4th Edition

Emergency Medical Services Sourcebook

Basic Consumer Health Information about Preventing, Preparing for, and Managing Emergency Situations, When and Who to Call for Help, What to Expect in the Emergency Room, the Emergency Medical Team, Patient

Issues, and Current Topics in Emergency Medicine

Along with Statistical Data, a Glossary, and Sources of Additional Help and Information

Edited by Jenni Lynn Colson. 472 pages. 2002. 978-0-7808-0420-3.

"Handy and convenient for home, public, school, and college libraries. Recommended."
—*CHOICE, Apr '03*

"This reference can provide the consumer with answers to most questions about emergency care in the United States, or it will direct them to a resource where the answer can be found."
—*American Reference Books Annual, 2003*

SEE ALSO Injury and Trauma Sourcebook

Endocrine and Metabolic Disorders Sourcebook, 2nd Edition

Basic Consumer Health Information about Hormonal and Metabolic Disorders that Affect the Body's Growth, Development, and Functioning, Including Disorders of the Pancreas, Ovaries and Testes, and Pituitary, Thyroid, Parathyroid, and Adrenal Glands, with Facts about Growth Disorders, Addison Disease, Cushing Syndrome, Conn Syndrome, Diabetic Disorders, Multiple Endocrine Neoplasia, Inborn Errors of Metabolism, and More

Along with Information about Endocrine Functioning, Diagnostic and Screening Tests, a Glossary of Related Terms, and Directories of Additional Resources

Edited by Joyce Brennfleck Shannon. 597 pages. 2007. 978-0-7808-0952-9.

SEE ALSO Diabetes Sourcebook, 4th Edition

Environmental Health Sourcebook, 3rd Edition

Basic Consumer Health Information about the Environment and Its Effects on Human Health, Including Facts about Air, Water, and Soil Contamination, Hazardous Chemicals, Foodborne Hazards and Illnesses, Household Hazards Such as Radon, Mold, and Carbon Monoxide, Consumer Hazards from Toxic Products and Imported Goods, and Disorders

Linked to Environmental Causes, Including Chemical Sensitivity, Cancer, Allergies, and Asthma

Along with Information about the Impact of Environmental Hazards on Specific Populations, a Glossary of Related Terms, and Resources for Additional Help and Information.

Edited by Laura Larsen. 600 pages. 2010. 978-0-7808-1078-5

Ethnic Diseases Sourcebook

Basic Consumer Health Information for Ethnic and Racial Minority Groups in the United States, Including General Health Indicators and Behaviors, Ethnic Diseases, Genetic Testing, the Impact of Chronic Diseases, Women's Health, Mental Health Issues, and Preventive Health Care Services

Along with a Glossary and a Listing of Additional Resources

Edited by Joyce Brennfleck Shannon. 648 pages. 2001. 978-0-7808-0336-7.

"Not many books have been written on this topic to date, and the Ethnic Diseases Sourcebook is a strong addition to the list. It will be an important introductory resource for health consumers, students, health care personnel, and social scientists. It is recommended for public, academic, and large hospital libraries."
— *American Reference Books Annual, 2002*

"Will prove valuable to any library seeking to maintain a current, comprehensive reference collection of health resources... An excellent source of health information about genetic disorders which affect particular ethnic and racial minorities in the U.S."
—*The Bookwatch, Aug '01*

Eye Care Sourcebook, 3rd Edition

Basic Consumer Health Information about Eye Care and Eye Disorders, Including Facts about the Diagnosis, Prevention, and Treatment of Refractive Disorders, Cataracts, Glaucoma, Macular Degeneration, and Problems Affecting the Cornea, Retina, and Lacrimal Glands

Along with Advice about Preventing Eye Injuries and Tips for Living with Low Vision or

Blindness, a Glossary of Related Terms, and Directories of Resources for More Help and Information

Edited by Amy L. Sutton. 646 pages. 2008. 978-0-7808-1000-6.

"A solid reference tool for eye care and a valuable addition to a collection."
—*American Reference Books Annual, 2009*

Family Planning Sourcebook

Basic Consumer Health Information about Planning for Pregnancy and Contraception, Including Traditional Methods, Barrier Methods, Hormonal Methods, Permanent Methods, Future Methods, Emergency Contraception, and Birth Control Choices for Women at Each Stage of Life

Along with Statistics, a Glossary, and Sources of Additional Information

Edited by Amy Marcaccio Keyzer. 503 pages. 2001. 978-0-7808-0379-4.

"Recommended for public, health, and undergraduate libraries as part of the circulating collection."
—*E-Streams, Mar '02*

"Will prove valuable to any library seeking to maintain a current, comprehensive reference collection of health resources... Excellent reference."
—*The Bookwatch, Aug '01*

SEE ALSO *Pregnancy and Birth Sourcebook, 3rd Edition*

Fitness and Exercise Sourcebook, 3rd Edition

Basic Consumer Health Information about the Physical and Mental Benefits of Fitness, Including Cardiorespiratory Endurance, Muscular Strength, Muscular Endurance, and Flexibility, with Facts about Sports Nutrition and Exercise-Related Injuries and Tips about Physical Activity and Exercises for People of All Ages and for People with Health Concerns

Along with Advice on Selecting and Using Exercise Equipment, Maintaining Exercise Motivation, a Glossary of Related Terms, and a Directory of Resources for More Help and Information

Edited by Amy L. Sutton. 635 pages. 2007. 978-0-7808-0946-8.

"Updates the consumer information on the physical and mental benefits of physical activity throughout the lifespan offered in earlier editions... Recommended. All readers; all levels."
—CHOICE, Oct '07

"An exceptionally well-rounded coverage perfect for any concerned about developing and understanding a fitness program."
—California Bookwatch, Jun '07

SEE ALSO Sports Injuries Sourcebook, 3rd Edition

Food Safety Sourcebook

Basic Consumer Health Information about the Safe Handling of Meat, Poultry, Seafood, Eggs, Fruit Juices, and Other Food Items, and Facts about Pesticides, Drinking Water, Food Safety Overseas, and the Onset, Duration, and Symptoms of Foodborne Illnesses, Including Types of Pathogenic Bacteria, Parasitic Protozoa, Worms, Viruses, and Natural Toxins

Along with the Role of the Consumer, the Food Handler, and the Government in Food Safety, a Glossary, and Resources for Additional Help and Information

Edited by Dawn D. Matthews. 327 pages. 1999. 978-0-7808-0326-8.

"Recommended reference source."
—Booklist, May '00

"This book takes the complex issues of food safety and foodborne pathogens and presents them in an easily understood manner. [It does] an excellent job of covering a large and often confusing topic."
— American Reference Books Annual, 2000

Forensic Medicine Sourcebook

Basic Consumer Information for the Layperson about Forensic Medicine, Including Crime Scene Investigation, Evidence Collection and Analysis, Expert Testimony, Computer-Aided Criminal Identification, Digital Imaging in the Courtroom, DNA Profiling, Accident Reconstruction, Autopsies, Ballistics, Drugs and Explosives Detection, Latent Fingerprints, Product Tampering, and Questioned Document Examination

Along with Statistical Data, a Glossary of Forensics Terminology, and Listings of Sources for Further Help and Information

Edited by Annemarie S. Muth. 574 pages. 1999. 978-0-7808-0232-2.

"Given the expected widespread interest in its content and its easy to read style, this book is recommended for most public and all college and university libraries."
—E-Streams, Feb '01

"A wealth of information, useful statistics, references are up-to-date and extremely complete. This wonderful collection of data will help students who are interested in a career in any type of forensic field. It is a great resource for attorneys who need information about types of expert witnesses needed in a particular case. It also offers useful information for fiction and nonfiction writers whose work involves a crime. A fascinating compilation. All levels."
—CHOICE, Jan '00

"There are several items that make this book attractive to consumers who are seeking certain forensic data... This is a useful current source for those seeking general forensic medical answers."
—American Reference Books Annual, 2000

Gastrointestinal Diseases and Disorders Sourcebook, 2nd Edition

Basic Consumer Health Information about the Upper and Lower Gastrointestinal (GI) Tract, Including the Esophagus, Stomach, Intestines, Rectum, Liver, and Pancreas, with Facts about Gastroesophageal Reflux Disease, Gastritis, Hernias, Ulcers, Celiac Disease, Diverticulitis, Irritable Bowel Syndrome, Hemorrhoids, Gastrointestinal Cancers, and Other Diseases and Disorders Related to the Digestive Process

Along with Information about Commonly Used Diagnostic and Surgical Procedures, Statistics, Reports on Current Research Initiatives and Clinical Trials, a Glossary, and Resources for Additional Help and Information

Edited by Sandra J. Judd. 654 pages. 2006. 978-0-7808-0798-3.

"The text is designed for the general reader seeking information on prevention, disease warning signs, diagnostic and therapeutic questions... It is an excellent resource for the general reader to conveniently locate credible, coordinated and indexed information... The sourcebook will prove very helpful for patients, caregivers and should be available in every physician waiting room."

—*Doody's Review Service, 2006*

SEE ALSO *Diet and Nutrition Sourcebook, 3rd Edition, Digestive Diseases and Disorders Sourcebook*

Genetic Disorders Sourcebook, 4th Edition

Basic Consumer Health Information about Hereditary Diseases and Disorders, Including Facts about the Human Genome, Genetic Inheritance Patterns, Disorders Associated with Specific Genes, Such as Sickle Cell Disease, Hemophilia, and Cystic Fibrosis, Chromosome Disorders, Such as Down Syndrome, Fragile X Syndrome, and Turner Syndrome, and Complex Diseases and Disorders Resulting from the Interaction of Environmental and Genetic Factors, Such as Allergies, Cancer, and Obesity

Along with Facts about Genetic Testing, Suggestions for Parents of Children with Special Needs, Reports on Current Research Initiatives, a Glossary of Genetic Terminology, and Resources for Additional Help and Information

Edited by Sandra J. Judd. 600 pages. 2010. 978-0-7808-1076-1.

Head Trauma Sourcebook

Basic Information for the Layperson about Open-Head and Closed-Head Injuries, Treatment Advances, Recovery, and Rehabilitation

Along with Reports on Current Research Initiatives

Edited by Karen Bellenir. 414 pages. 1997. 978-0-7808-0208-7.

Headache Sourcebook

Basic Consumer Health Information about Migraine, Tension, Cluster, Rebound and Other Types of Headaches, with Facts about the Cause and Prevention of Headaches, the Effects of Stress and the Environment, Headaches during Pregnancy and Menopause, and Childhood Headaches

Along with a Glossary and Other Resources for Additional Help and Information

Edited by Dawn D. Matthews. 342 pages. 2002. 978-0-7808-0337-4.

"Highly recommended for academic and medical reference collections."

—*Library Bookwatch, Sep '02*

SEE ALSO *Pain Sourcebook, 3rd Edition*

Healthy Aging Sourcebook

Basic Consumer Health Information about Maintaining Health through the Aging Process, Including Advice on Nutrition, Exercise, and Sleep, Help in Making Decisions about Midlife Issues and Retirement, and Guidance Concerning Practical and Informed Choices in Health Consumerism

Along with Data Concerning the Theories of Aging, Different Experiences in Aging by Minority Groups, and Facts about Aging Now and Aging in the Future; and Featuring a Glossary, a Guide to Consumer Help, Additional Suggested Reading, and Practical Resource Directory

Edited by Jenifer Swanson. 537 pages. 1999. 978-0-7808-0390-9.

"Recommended reference source."

—*Booklist, Feb '00*

SEE ALSO *Adult Health Sourcebook, Physical and Mental Issues in Aging Sourcebook*

Healthy Children Sourcebook

Basic Consumer Health Information about the Physical and Mental Development of Children between the Ages of 3 and 12, Including Routine Health Care, Preventative Health Services, Safety and First Aid, Healthy Sleep, Dental Care, Nutrition, and Fitness, and Featuring Parenting Tips on Such Topics as Bedwetting, Choosing Day Care, Monitoring TV and Other Media, and Establishing a Foundation for Substance Abuse Prevention

Along with a Glossary of Commonly Used Pediatric Terms and Resources for Additional Help and Information.

Edited by Chad T. Kimball. 624 pages. 2003. 978-0-7808-0247-6.

"Should be required reading for parents and teachers."
—*E-Streams, Jun '04*

"It is hard to imagine that any other single resource exists that would provide such a comprehensive guide of timely information on health promotion and disease prevention for children aged 3 to 12."
—*American Reference Books Annual, 2004*

"This easy-to-read volume is a tremendous resource."
—*AORN Journal, May '05*

SEE ALSO Childhood Diseases and Disorders Sourcebook, 2nd Edition

Healthy Heart Sourcebook for Women

Basic Consumer Health Information about Cardiac Issues Specific to Women, Including Facts about Major Risk Factors and Prevention, Treatment and Control Strategies, and Important Dietary Issues

Along with a Special Section Regarding the Pros and Cons of Hormone Replacement Therapy and Its Impact on Heart Health, and Additional Help, Including Recipes, a Glossary, and a Directory of Resources

Edited by Dawn D. Matthews. 321 pages. 2000. 978-0-7808-0329-9.

"A good reference source and recommended for all public, academic, medical, and hospital libraries."
—*Medical Reference Services Quarterly, Summer '01*

"Contains very important information about coronary artery disease that all women should know. The information is current and presented in an easy-to-read format. The book will make a good addition to any library."
—*American Medical Writers Association Journal, Summer '00*

SEE ALSO Cardiovascular Diseases and Disorders Sourcebook, 4th Edition, Women's Health Concerns Sourcebook, 3rd Edition

Hepatitis Sourcebook

Basic Consumer Health Information about Hepatitis A, Hepatitis B, Hepatitis C, and Other Forms of Hepatitis, Including Autoimmune Hepatitis, Alcoholic Hepatitis, Nonalcoholic Steatohepatitis, and Toxic Hepatitis, with Facts about Risk Factors, Screening Methods, Diagnostic Tests, and Treatment Options

Along with Information on Liver Health, Tips for People Living with Chronic Hepatitis, Reports on Current Research Initiatives, a Glossary of Terms Related to Hepatitis, and a Directory of Sources for Further Help and Information

Edited by Sandra J. Judd. 570 pages. 2006. 978-0-7808-0749-5.

"The breadth of information found in this one book would not be readily found in another source. Highly recommended."
—*American Reference Books Annual, 2006*

SEE ALSO Contagious Diseases Sourcebook, 2nd Edition

Household Safety Sourcebook

Basic Consumer Health Information about Household Safety, Including Information about Poisons, Chemicals, Fire, and Water Hazards in the Home

Along with Advice about the Safe Use of Home Maintenance Equipment, Choosing Toys and Nursery Furniture, Holiday and Recreation Safety, a Glossary, and Resources for Further Help and Information

Edited by Dawn D. Matthews. 587 pages. 2002. 978-0-7808-0338-1.

"As a sourcebook on household safety this book meets its mark. It is encyclopedic in scope and covers a wide range of safety issues that are commonly seen in the home."
—*E-Streams, Jul '02*

Hypertension Sourcebook

Basic Consumer Health Information about the Causes, Diagnosis, and Treatment of High Blood Pressure, with Facts about Consequences, Complications, and Co-Occurring Disorders, Such as Coronary Heart Disease, Diabetes, Stroke, Kidney Disease, and Hypertensive Retinopathy, and Issues in Blood Pressure

683

Control, Including Dietary Choices, Stress Management, and Medications

Along with Reports on Current Research Initiatives and Clinical Trials, a Glossary, and Resources for Additional Help and Information

Edited by Dawn D. Matthews and Karen Bellenir. 588 pages. 2004. 978-0-7808-0674-0.

"Academic, public, and medical libraries will want to add the Hypertension Sourcebook to their collections."
—*E-Streams, Aug '05*

"The strength of this source is the wide range of information given about hypertension."
—*American Reference Books Annual, 2005*

SEE ALSO *Stroke Sourcebook, 2nd Edition*

Immune System Disorders Sourcebook, 2nd Edition

Basic Consumer Health Information about Disorders of the Immune System, Including Immune System Function and Response, Diagnosis of Immune Disorders, Information about Inherited Immune Disease, Acquired Immune Disease, and Autoimmune Diseases, Including Primary Immune Deficiency, Acquired Immunodeficiency Syndrome (AIDS), Lupus, Multiple Sclerosis, Type 1 Diabetes, Rheumatoid Arthritis, and Graves' Disease

Along with Treatments, Tips for Coping with Immune Disorders, a Glossary, and a Directory of Additional Resources

Edited by Joyce Brennfleck Shannon. 643 pages. 2005. 978-0-7808-0748-8.

"Highly recommended for academic and public libraries."
—*American Reference Books Annual, 2006*

"The updated second edition is a 'must' for any consumer health library seeking a solid resource covering the treatments, symptoms, and options for immune disorder sufferers... An excellent guide."
—*MBR Bookwatch, Jan '06*

SEE ALSO *AIDS Sourcebook, 4th Edition, Arthritis Sourcebook, 3rd Edition*

Infant and Toddler Health Sourcebook

Basic Consumer Health Information about the Physical and Mental Development of Newborns, Infants, and Toddlers, Including Neonatal Concerns, Nutrition Recommendations, Immunization Schedules, Common Pediatric Disorders, Assessments and Milestones, Safety Tips, and Advice for Parents and Other Caregivers

Along with a Glossary of Terms and Resource Listings for Additional Help

Edited by Jenifer Swanson. 570 pages. 2000. 978-0-7808-0246-9.

"As a reference for the general public, this would be useful in any library."
—*E-Streams, May '01*

"Recommended reference source."
—*Booklist, Feb '01*

Infectious Diseases Sourcebook

Basic Consumer Health Information about Non-Contagious Bacterial, Viral, Prion, Fungal, and Parasitic Diseases Spread by Food and Water, Insects and Animals, or Environmental Contact, Including Botulism, E. Coli, Encephalitis, Legionnaires' Disease, Lyme Disease, Malaria, Plague, Rabies, Salmonella, Tetanus, and Others, and Facts about Newly Emerging Diseases, Such as Hantavirus, Mad Cow Disease, Monkeypox, and West Nile Virus

Along with Information about Preventing Disease Transmission, the Threat of Bioterrorism, and Current Research Initiatives, with a Glossary and Directory of Resources for More Information

Edited by Karen Bellenir. 610 pages. 2004. 978-0-7808-0675-7.

"This reference continues the excellent tradition of the Health Reference Series in consolidating a wealth of information on a selected topic into a format that is easy to use and accessible to the general public."
—*American Reference Books Annual, 2005*

"Recommended for public and academic libraries."
—*E-Streams, Jan '05*

SEE ALSO *Environmental Health Sourcebook, 3rd Edition*

684

Injury and Trauma Sourcebook

Basic Consumer Health Information about the Impact of Injury, the Diagnosis and Treatment of Common and Traumatic Injuries, Emergency Care, and Specific Injuries Related to Home, Community, Workplace, Transportation, and Recreation

Along with Guidelines for Injury Prevention, a Glossary, and a Directory of Additional Resources

Edited by Joyce Brennfleck Shannon. 675 pages. 2002. 978-0-7808-0421-0.

"Practitioners should be aware of guides such as this in order to facilitate their use by patients and their families."
— *Doody's Health Sciences Book Review Journal, Sep-Oct '02*

"Recommended reference source."
— *Booklist, Sep '02*

"Highly recommended for academic and medical reference collections."
— *Library Bookwatch, Sep '02*

SEE ALSO *Emergency Medical Services Sourcebook, Sports Injuries Sourcebook, 3rd Edition*

Learning Disabilities Sourcebook, 3rd Edition

Basic Consumer Health Information about Dyslexia, Auditory and Visual Processing Disorders, Communication Disorders, Dyscalculia, Dysgraphia, and Other Conditions That Impede Learning, Including Attention Deficit/ Hyperactivity Disorder, Autism Spectrum Disorders, Hearing and Visual Impairments, Chromosome-Based Disorders, and Brain Injury

Along with Facts about Brain Function, Assessment, Therapy and Remediation, Accommodations, Assistive Technology, Legal Protections, and Tips about Family Life, School Transitions, and Employment Strategies, a Glossary of Related Terms, and Directories of Additional Resources

Edited by Joyce Brennfleck Shannon. 613 pages. 2009. 978-0-7808-1039-6.

"Intended to be a starting point for people who need to know about learning disabilities. Each chapter on a specific disability includes read-

able, well-organized descriptions... The book is well indexed and a glossary is included. Chapters on organizations and helpful websites will aid the reader who needs more information."
— *American Reference Books Annual, 2009*

"This book provides the necessary information to better understand learning disabilities and work with children who have them... It would be difficult to find another book that so comprehensively explains learning disabilities without becoming incomprehensible to the average parent who needs this information."
— *Doody's Review Service, 2009*

SEE ALSO *Attention Deficit Disorder Sourcebook, Autism and Pervasive Developmental Disorders Sourcebook*

Leukemia Sourcebook

Basic Consumer Health Information about Adult and Childhood Leukemias, Including Acute Lymphocytic Leukemia (ALL), Chronic Lymphocytic Leukemia (CLL), Acute Myelogenous Leukemia (AML), Chronic Myelogenous Leukemia (CML), and Hairy Cell Leukemia, and Treatments Such as Chemotherapy, Radiation Therapy, Peripheral Blood Stem Cell and Marrow Transplantation, and Immunotherapy

Along with Tips for Life During and After Treatment, a Glossary, and Directories of Additional Resources

Edited by Joyce Brennfleck Shannon. 564 pages. 2003. 978-0-7808-0627-6.

"Unlike other medical books for the layperson... the language does not talk down to the reader... This volume is highly recommended for all libraries."
— *American Reference Books Annual, 2004*

"A fine title which ranges from diagnosis to alternative treatments, staging, and tips for life during and after diagnosis."
— *The Bookwatch, Dec '03*

SEE ALSO *Blood & Circulatory Disorders Sourcebook, 3rd Edition, Cancer Sourcebook, 5th Edition*

Liver Disorders Sourcebook

Basic Consumer Health Information about the Liver and How It Works; Liver Diseases, Including Cancer, Cirrhosis, Hepatitis, and

Toxic and Drug Related Diseases; Tips for Maintaining a Healthy Liver; Laboratory Tests, Radiology Tests, and Facts about Liver Transplantation

Along with a Section on Support Groups, a Glossary, and Resource Listings

Edited by Joyce Brennfleck Shannon. 580 pages. 2000. 978-0-7808-0383-1.

"This title is recommended for health sciences and public libraries with consumer health collections."
—E-Streams, Oct '00

"Recommended reference source."
—Booklist, Jun '00

SEE ALSO Gastrointestinal Diseases and Disorders Sourcebook, 2nd Edition, Hepatitis Sourcebook

Lung Disorders Sourcebook

Basic Consumer Health Information about Emphysema, Pneumonia, Tuberculosis, Asthma, Cystic Fibrosis, and Other Lung Disorders, Including Facts about Diagnostic Procedures, Treatment Strategies, Disease Prevention Efforts, and Such Risk Factors as Smoking, Air Pollution, and Exposure to Asbestos, Radon, and Other Agents

Along with a Glossary and Resources for Additional Help and Information

Edited by Dawn D. Matthews. 657 pages. 2002. 978-0-7808-0339-8.

"Highly recommended for academic and medical reference collections."
—Library Bookwatch, Sep '02

SEE ALSO Asthma Sourcebook, 2nd Edition, Respiratory Disorders Sourcebook, 2nd Edition

Medical Tests Sourcebook, 3rd Edition

Basic Consumer Health Information about X-Rays, Blood Tests, Stool and Urine Tests, Biopsies, Mammography, Endoscopic Procedures, Ultrasound Exams, Computed Tomography, Magnetic Resonance Imaging (MRI), Nuclear Medicine, Genetic Testing, Home-Use Tests, and More

Along with Facts about Preventive Care and Screening Test Guidelines, Screening and

Assessment Tests Associated with Such Specific Concerns as Cancer, Heart Disease, Allergies, Diabetes, Thyroid Disfunction, and Infertility, a Glossary of Related Terms, and a Directory of Resources for Additional Help and Information

Edited by Karen Bellenir. 627 pages. 2008. 978-0-7808-1040-2

"This volume has a wide scope that makes it useful... Can be a valuable reference guide."
—American Reference Books Annual, 2009

"Would be a valuable contribution to any consumer health or public library."
—Doody's Book Review Service, 2009

Men's Health Concerns Sourcebook, 3rd Edition

Basic Consumer Health Information about Wellness in Men and Gender-Related Differences in Health, With Facts about Heart Disease, Cancer, Traumatic Injury, and Other Leading Causes of Death in Men, Reproductive Concerns, Sexual Dysfunction, Disorders of the Prostate, Penis, and Testes, Sex-Linked Genetic Disorders, and Other Medical and Mental Concerns of Men

Along with Statistical Data, a Glossary of Related Terms, and a Directory of Resources for Additional Information

Edited by Sandra J. Judd. 632 pages. 2009. 978-0-7808-1033-4.

"A good addition to any reference shelf in academic, consumer health, or hospital libraries."
—ARBAOnline, Oct '09

SEE ALSO Prostate and Urological Disorders Sourcebook

Mental Health Disorders Sourcebook, 4th Edition

Basic Consumer Health Information about the Causes and Symptoms of Mental Health Problems, Including Depression, Bipolar Disorder, Anxiety Disorders, Posttraumatic Stress Disorder, Obsessive-Compulsive Disorder, Eating Disorders, Addictions, and Personality and Psychotic Disorders

Along with Information about Medications and Treatments, Mental Health Concerns in

Children, Adolescents, and Adults, Tips on Living with Mental Health Disorders, a Glossary of Related Terms, and a Directory of Resources for Additional Help and Information

Edited by Amy L. Sutton. 680 pages. 2009. 978-0-7808-1041-9.

"Mental health concerns are presented in everyday language and intended for patients and their families as well as the general public... This resource is comprehensive and up to date... The easy-to-understand writing style helps to facilitate assimilation of needed facts and specifics on often challenging topics."
—*ARBAOnline, Oct '09*

"No health collection should be without this resource, which will reach into many a general lending library as well."
—*Internet Bookwatch, Oct '09*

SEE ALSO *Depression Sourcebook, 2nd Edition, Stress-Related Disorders Sourcebook, 2nd Edition*

Mental Retardation Sourcebook

Basic Consumer Health Information about Mental Retardation and Its Causes, Including Down Syndrome, Fetal Alcohol Syndrome, Fragile X Syndrome, Genetic Conditions, Injury, and Environmental Sources

Along with Preventive Strategies, Parenting Issues, Educational Implications, Health Care Needs, Employment and Economic Matters, Legal Issues, a Glossary, and a Resource Listing for Additional Help and Information

Edited by Joyce Brennfleck Shannon. 627 pages. 2000. 978-0-7808-0377-0.

"Public libraries will find the book useful for reference and as a beginning research point for students, parents, and caregivers."
—*American Reference Books Annual, 2001*

"The strength of this work is that it compiles many basic fact sheets and addresses for further information in one volume. It is intended and suitable for the general public."
—*E-Streams, Nov '00*

"An invaluable overview."
—*Reviewer's Bookwatch, Jul '00*

Movement Disorders Sourcebook, 2nd Edition

Basic Consumer Health Information about the Symptoms and Causes of Movement Disorders, Including Parkinson Disease, Amyotrophic Lateral Sclerosis, Cerebral Palsy, Muscular Dystrophy, Multiple Sclerosis, Myasthenia, Myoclonus, Spina Bifida, Dystonia, Essential Tremor, Choreatic Disorders, Huntington Disease, Tourette Syndrome, and Other Disorders That Cause Slowed, Absent, or Excessive Movements

Along with Information about Surgical and Nonsurgical Interventions, Physical Therapies, Strategies for Independent Living, a Glossary of Related Terms, and a Directory of Resources for Additional Help and Information

Edited by Amy L. Sutton. 618 pages. 2009. 978-0-7808-1034-1.

"The second updated edition of Movement Disorders Sourcebook is a winner, providing the latest research and health findings on all kinds of movement disorders in children and adults... a top pick for any health or general lending library's health reference collection."
—*California Bookwatch, Aug '09*

SEE ALSO *Muscular Dystrophy Sourcebook*

Multiple Sclerosis Sourcebook

Basic Consumer Health Information about Multiple Sclerosis (MS) and Its Effects on Mobility, Vision, Bladder Function, Speech, Swallowing, and Cognition, Including Facts about Risk Factors, Causes, Diagnostic Procedures, Pain Management, Drug Treatments, and Physical and Occupational Therapies

Along with Guidelines for Nutrition and Exercise, Tips on Choosing Assistive Equipment, Information about Disability, Work, Financial, and Legal Issues, a Glossary of Related Terms, and a Directory of Additional Resources

Edited by Joyce Brennfleck Shannon. 553 pages. 2007. 978-0-7808-0998-7.

Muscular Dystrophy Sourcebook

Basic Consumer Health Information about Congenital, Childhood-Onset, and Adult-Onset

687

Forms of Muscular Dystrophy, Such as Duchenne, Becker, Emery-Dreifuss, Distal, Limb-Girdle, Facioscapulohumeral (FSHD), Myotonic, and Ophthalmoplegic Muscular Dystrophies, Including Facts about Diagnostic Tests, Medical and Physical Therapies, Management of Co-Occurring Conditions, and Parenting Guidelines

Along with Practical Tips for Home Care, a Glossary, and Directories of Additional Resources

Edited by Joyce Brennfleck Shannon. 552 pages. 2004. 978-0-7808-0676-4.

"This book is highly recommended for public and academic libraries as well as health care offices that support the information needs of patients and their families."
—E-Streams, Apr '05

"Excellent reference."
—The Bookwatch, Jan '05

SEE ALSO Movement Disorders Sourcebook, 2nd Edition

Obesity Sourcebook

Basic Consumer Health Information about Diseases and Other Problems Associated with Obesity, and Including Facts about Risk Factors, Prevention Issues, and Management Approaches

Along with Statistical and Demographic Data, Information about Special Populations, Research Updates, a Glossary, and Source Listings for Further Help and Information

Edited by Wilma Caldwell and Chad T. Kimball. 360 pages. 2001. 978-0-7808-0333-6.

"The book synthesizes the reliable medical literature on obesity into one easy-to-read and useful resource for the general public."
—American Reference Books Annual, 2002

"Well suited for the health reference collection of a public library or an academic health science library that serves the general population."
—E-Streams, Sep '01

Osteoporosis Sourcebook

Basic Consumer Health Information about Primary and Secondary Osteoporosis and Juvenile Osteoporosis and Related Conditions, Including Fibrous Dysplasia, Gaucher Disease, Hyperthyroidism, Hypophosphatasia, Myeloma, Osteopetrosis, Osteogenesis Imperfecta, and Paget's Disease

Along with Information about Risk Factors, Treatments, Traditional and Non-Traditional Pain Management, a Glossary of Related Terms, and a Directory of Resources

Edited by Allan R. Cook. 568 pages. 2001. 978-0-7808-0239-1.

"This resource is recommended as a great reference source for public, health, and academic libraries, and is another triumph for the editors of Omnigraphics."
—American Reference Books Annual, 2002

"Will prove valuable to any library seeking to maintain a current, comprehensive reference collection of health resources... From prevention to treatment and associated conditions, this provides an excellent survey."
—The Bookwatch, Aug '01

SEE ALSO Healthy Aging Sourcebook, Women's Health Concerns Sourcebook, 3rd Edition

Pain Sourcebook, 3rd Edition

Basic Consumer Health Information about Acute and Chronic Pain, Including Nerve Pain, Bone Pain, Muscle Pain, Cancer Pain, and Disorders Characterized by Pain, Such as Arthritis, Temporomandibular Muscle and Joint (TMJ) Disorder, Carpal Tunnel Syndrome, Headaches, Heartburn, Sciatica, and Shingles, and Facts about Diagnostic Tests and Treatment Options for Pain, Including Over-the-Counter and Prescription Drugs, Physical Rehabilitation, Injection and Infusion Therapies, Implantable Technologies, and Complementary Medicine

Along with Tips for Living with Pain, a Glossary of Related Terms, and a Directory of Additional Resources

Edited by Joyce Brennfleck Shannon. 644 pages. 2008. 978-0-7808-1006-8.

"Excellent for ready-reference users and can be used for beginning students in health fields... appropriate for the consumer health collection in both public and academic libraries."
—American Reference Books Annual, 2009

SEE ALSO Arthritis Sourcebook, 3rd Edition; Back and Neck Sourcebook, 2nd Edition;

Headache Sourcebook; Sports Injuries Sourcebook, 3rd Edition

Pediatric Cancer Sourcebook

Basic Consumer Health Information about Leukemias, Brain Tumors, Sarcomas, Lymphomas, and Other Cancers in Infants, Children, and Adolescents, Including Descriptions of Cancers, Treatments, and Coping Strategies

Along with Suggestions for Parents, Caregivers, and Concerned Relatives, a Glossary of Cancer Terms, and Resource Listings

Edited by Edward J. Prucha. 575 pages. 1999. 978-0-7808-0245-2.

"An excellent source of information. Recommended for public, hospital, and health science libraries with consumer health collections."
—*E-Streams, Jun '00*

"A valuable addition to all libraries specializing in health services and many public libraries."
—*American Reference Books Annual, 2000*

SEE ALSO *Childhood Diseases and Disorders Sourcebook, 2nd Edition, Healthy Children Sourcebook*

Physical and Mental Issues in Aging Sourcebook

Basic Consumer Health Information on Physical and Mental Disorders Associated with the Aging Process, Including Concerns about Cardiovascular Disease, Pulmonary Disease, Oral Health, Digestive Disorders, Musculoskeletal and Skin Disorders, Metabolic Changes, Sexual and Reproductive Issues, and Changes in Vision, Hearing, and Other Senses

Along with Data about Longevity and Causes of Death, Information on Acute and Chronic Pain, Descriptions of Mental Concerns, a Glossary of Terms, and Resource Listings for Additional Help

Edited by Jenifer Swanson. 660 pages. 1999. 978-0-7808-0233-9.

"This is a treasure of health information for the layperson."
—*CHOICE Health Sciences Supplement, May '00*

"Recommended for public libraries."
—*American Reference Books Annual, 2000*

SEE ALSO *Healthy Aging Sourcebook*

Podiatry Sourcebook, 2nd Edition

Basic Consumer Health Information about Disorders, Diseases, and Deformities that Affect the Foot and Ankle, Including Sprains, Corns, Calluses, Bunions, Plantar Warts, Plantar Fasciitis, Neuromas, Clubfoot, Flat Feet, Achilles Tendonitis, and Much More

Along with Information about Selecting a Foot Care Specialist, Foot Fitness, Shoes and Socks, Diagnostic Tests and Corrective Procedures, Financial Assistance for Corrective Devices, a Glossary of Related Terms, and a Directory of Resources for Additional Help and Information

Edited by Ivy L. Alexander. 516 pages. 2007. 978-0-7808-0944-4.

"An excellent resource... Although there have been various types of 'foot books' published in the past, none are as comprehensive as this one. 5 Stars (out of 5)!"
—*Doody's Review Service, 2007*

"Perfect for both health libraries and general-interest lending collections."
—*Internet Bookwatch, Jul '07*

Pregnancy and Birth Sourcebook, 3rd Edition

Basic Consumer Health Information about Pregnancy and Fetal Development, Including Facts about Fertility and Conception, Physical and Emotional Changes during Pregnancy, Prenatal Care and Diagnostic Tests, High-Risk Pregnancies and Complications, Labor, Delivery, and the Postpartum Period

Along with Tips on Maintaining Health and Wellness during Pregnancy and Caring for Newborn Infants, a Glossary of Related Terms, and Directories of Resources for Additional Help and Information

Edited by Amy L. Sutton. 645 pages. 2009. 978-0-7808-1074-7.

SEE ALSO *Breastfeeding Sourcebook, Congenital Disorders Sourcebook, 2nd Edition, Family Planning Sourcebook, Women's Health Concerns Sourcebook, 3rd Edition*

689

Prostate and Urological Disorders Sourcebook

Basic Consumer Health Information about Urogenital and Sexual Disorders in Men, Including Prostate and Other Andrological Cancers, Prostatitis, Benign Prostatic Hyperplasia, Testicular and Penile Trauma, Cryptorchidism, Peyronie Disease, Erectile Dysfunction, and Male Factor Infertility, and Facts about Commonly Used Tests and Procedures, Such as Prostatectomy, Vasectomy, Vasectomy Reversal, Penile Implants, and Semen Analysis

Along with a Glossary of Andrological Terms and a Directory of Resources for Additional Information

Edited by Karen Bellenir. 604 pages. 2006. 978-0-7808-0797-6.

"Certain to be a popular pick among library reference holdings... No prior knowledge is assumed for any of the conditions or terms herein, making it a most accessible general-interest reference."
— *California Bookwatch, Apr '06*

SEE ALSO *Men's Health Concerns Sourcebook, 3rd Edition, Urinary Tract and Kidney Diseases and Disorders Sourcebook, 2nd Edition*

Prostate Cancer Sourcebook

Basic Consumer Health Information about Prostate Cancer, Including Information about the Associated Risk Factors, Detection, Diagnosis, and Treatment of Prostate Cancer

Along with Information on Non-Malignant Prostate Conditions, and Featuring a Section Listing Support and Treatment Centers and a Glossary of Related Terms

Edited by Dawn D. Matthews. 340 pages. 2001. 978-0-7808-0324-4.

"Recommended reference source."
— *Booklist, Jan '02*

"A valuable resource for health care consumers seeking information on the subject... All text is written in a clear, easy-to-understand language that avoids technical jargon. Any library that collects consumer health resources would strengthen their collection with the addition of the Prostate Cancer Sourcebook."
— *American Reference Books Annual, 2002*

SEE ALSO *Cancer Sourcebook, 5th Edition, Men's Health Concerns Sourcebook, 3rd Edition*

Rehabilitation Sourcebook

Basic Consumer Health Information about Rehabilitation for People Recovering from Heart Surgery, Spinal Cord Injury, Stroke, Orthopedic Impairments, Amputation, Pulmonary Impairments, Traumatic Injury, and More, Including Physical Therapy, Occupational Therapy, Speech/Language Therapy, Massage Therapy, Dance Therapy, Art Therapy, and Recreational Therapy

Along with Information on Assistive and Adaptive Devices, a Glossary, and Resources for Additional Help and Information

Edited by Dawn D. Matthews. 519 pages. 2000. 978-0-7808-0236-0.

"This is an excellent resource for public library reference and health collections."
— *American Reference Books Annual, 2001*

"Recommended reference source."
— *Booklist, May '00*

Respiratory Disorders Sourcebook, 2nd Edition

Basic Consumer Health Information about Infectious, Inflammatory, and Chronic Conditions Affecting the Lungs and Respiratory System, Including Pneumonia, Bronchitis, Influenza, Tuberculosis, Sarcoidosis, Asthma, Cystic Fibrosis, Chronic Obstructive Pulmonary Disease, Lung Abscesses, Pulmonary Embolism, Occupational Lung Diseases, and Other Bacterial, Viral, and Fungal Infections

Along with Facts about the Structure and Function of the Lungs and Airways, Methods of Diagnosing Respiratory Disorders, and Treatment and Rehabilitation Options, a Glossary of Related Terms, and a Directory of Resources for Additional Help and Information

Edited by Sandra L. Judd. 638 pages. 2008. 978-0-7808-1007-5.

"An excellent book for patients, their families, or for those who are just curious about respiratory disease. Public libraries and physician offices would find this a valuable resource as well. 4 Stars! (out of 5)"
— *Doody's Review Service, 2009*

"A great addition for public and school libraries because it provides concise health information... readers can start with this reference source and get satisfactory answers before proceeding to other medical reference tools for

more in depth information... A good guide for health education on lung disorders."
—*American Reference Books Annual, 2009*

SEE ALSO *Asthma Sourcebook, 2nd Edition, Lung Disorders Sourcebook*

Sexually Transmitted Diseases Sourcebook, 4th Edition

Basic Consumer Health Information about Chlamydial Infections, Gonorrhea, Hepatitis, Herpes, HIV/AIDS, Human Papillomavirus, Pubic Lice, Scabies, Syphilis, Trichomoniasis, Vaginal Infections, and Other Sexually Transmitted Diseases, Including Facts about Risk Factors, Symptoms, Diagnosis, Treatment, and the Prevention of Sexually Transmitted Infections

Along with Updates on Current Research Initiatives, a Glossary of Related Terms, and Resources for Additional Help and Information

Edited by Laura Larsen. 623 pages. 2009. 978-0-7808-1073-0.

"Extremely beneficial... The question-and-answer format along with the index and table of contents make this well-organized resource extremely easy to reference, read, and comprehend... an invaluable medical reference source for lay readers, and a highly appropriate addition for public library collections, health clinics, and any library with a consumer health collection"
—*ARBAOnline, Oct '09*

SEE ALSO *AIDS Sourcebook, 4th Edition, Contagious Diseases Sourcebook, 2nd Edition, Men's Health Concerns Sourcebook, 3rd Edition, Women's Health Concerns Sourcebook, 3rd Edition*

Sleep Disorders Sourcebook, 3rd Edition

Basic Consumer Health Information about Sleep Disorders, Including Insomnia, Sleep Apnea and Snoring, Jet Lag and Other Circadian Rhythm Disorders, Narcolepsy, and Parasomnias, Such as Sleep Walking and Sleep Talking, and Featuring Facts about Other Health Problems that Affect Sleep, Why Sleep Is Necessary, How Much Sleep Is Needed, the Physical and Mental Effects of Sleep Deprivation, and Pediatric Sleep Issues

Along with Tips for Diagnosing and Treating Sleep Disorders, a Glossary of Related Terms, and a List of Resources for Additional Help and Information

Edited by Sandra J. Judd. 600 pages. 2010. 978-0-7808-1084-6.

Smoking Concerns Sourcebook

Basic Consumer Health Information about Nicotine Addiction and Smoking Cessation, Featuring Facts about the Health Effects of Tobacco Use, Including Lung and Other Cancers, Heart Disease, Stroke, and Respiratory Disorders, Such as Emphysema and Chronic Bronchitis

Along with Information about Smoking Prevention Programs, Suggestions for Achieving and Maintaining a Smoke-Free Lifestyle, Statistics about Tobacco Use, Reports on Current Research Initiatives, a Glossary of Related Terms, and Directories of Resources for Additional Help and Information

Edited by Karen Bellenir. 595 pages. 2004. 978-0-7808-0323-7.

"Provides everything needed for the student or general reader seeking practical details on the effects of tobacco use."
—*The Bookwatch, Mar '05*

"Public libraries and consumer health care libraries will find this work useful."
—*American Reference Books Annual, 2005*

SEE ALSO *Respiratory Disorders Sourcebook, 2nd Edition*

Sports Injuries Sourcebook, 3rd Edition

Basic Consumer Health Information about Sprains and Strains, Fractures, Growth Plate Injuries, Overtraining Injuries, and Injuries to the Head, Face, Shoulders, Elbows, Hands, Spinal Column, Knees, Ankles, and Feet, and with Facts about Heat-Related Illness, Steroids and Sport Supplements, Protective Equipment, Diagnostic Procedures, Treatment Options, and Rehabilitation

Along with a Glossary of Related Terms and a Directory of Resources for Additional Help and Information

691

Edited by Sandra J. Judd. 623 pages. 2007. 978-0-7808-0949-9.

SEE ALSO *Fitness and Exercise Sourcebook, 3rd Edition, Podiatry Sourcebook, 2nd Edition*

Stress-Related Disorders Sourcebook, 2nd Edition

Basic Consumer Health Information about Stress and Stress-Related Disorders, Including Types of Stress, Sources of Acute and Chronic Stress, the Impact of Stress on the Body's Systems, and Mental and Emotional Health Problems Associated with Stress, Such as Depression, Anxiety Disorders, Substance Abuse, Posttraumatic Stress Disorder, and Suicide

Along with Advice about Getting Help for Stress-Related Disorders, Information about Stress Management Techniques, a Glossary of Stress-Related Terms, and a Directory of Resources for Additional Help and Information

Edited by Amy L. Sutton. 608 pages. 2007. 978-0-7808-0996-3.

"Accessible to the lay reader. Highly recommended for medical and psychiatric collections."
—*Library Journal, Mar '08*

"Well-written for a general readership, the 2nd Edition of Stress-Related Disorders Sourcebook is a useful addition to the health reference literature."
—*American Reference Books Annual, 2008*

SEE ALSO *Mental Health Disorders Sourcebook, 4th Edition*

Stroke Sourcebook, 2nd Edition

Basic Consumer Health Information about Stroke, Including Ischemic, Hemorrhagic, and Mini Strokes, as Well as Risk Factors, Prevention Guidelines, Diagnostic Tests, Medications and Surgical Treatments, and Complications of Stroke

Along with Rehabilitation Techniques and Innovations, Tips on Staying Healthy and Maintaining Independence after Stroke, a Glossary of Related Terms, and a Directory of Resources for Stroke Survivors and Their Families

Edited by Amy L. Sutton. 626 pages. 2008. 978-0-7808-1035-8.

"An encyclopedic handbook on stroke that is written in a language the layperson can understand... This is one of the most helpful, readable books on stroke. This volume is highly recommended and should be in every medical, hospital and public library; in addition, every family practitioner should have a copy in his or her office."
—*American Reference Books Annual, 2009*

SEE ALSO *Brain Disorders Sourcebook, 3rd Edition, Hypertension Sourcebook*

Surgery Sourcebook, 2nd Edition

Basic Consumer Health Information about Common Inpatient and Outpatient Surgeries, Including Critical Care and Trauma, Gastrointestinal, Gynecologic and Obstetric, Cardiac and Vascular, Neurologic, Ophthalmologic, Orthopedic, Reconstructive and Cosmetic, and Other Major and Minor Surgeries

Along with Information about Anesthesia and Pain Relief Options, Risks and Complications, Postoperative Recovery Concerns, and Innovative Surgical Techniques and Tools, a Glossary of Related Terms, and a Directory of Additional Resources

Edited by Amy L. Sutton. 645 pages. 2008. 978-0-7808-1004-4.

"Large public libraries and medical libraries would benefit from this material in their reference collections."
—*American Reference Books Annual, 2009*

SEE ALSO *Cosmetic and Reconstructive Surgery Sourcebook, 2nd Edition*

Thyroid Disorders Sourcebook

Basic Consumer Health Information about Disorders of the Thyroid and Parathyroid Glands, Including Hypothyroidism, Hyperthyroidism, Graves Disease, Hashimoto Thyroiditis, Thyroid Cancer, and Parathyroid Disorders, Featuring Facts about Symptoms, Risk Factors, Tests, and Treatments

Along with Information about the Effects of Thyroid Imbalance on Other Body Systems, Environmental Factors That Affect the Thyroid Gland, a Glossary, and a Directory of Additional Resources

Edited by Joyce Brennfleck Shannon. 573 pages. 2005. 978-0-7808-0745-7.

"Recommended for consumer health collections."
—American Reference Books Annual, 2006

"Highly recommended pick for Basic Consumer health reference holdings at all levels."
—The Bookwatch, Aug '05

SEE ALSO Endocrine and Metabolic Disorders Sourcebook, 2nd Edition

Transplantation Sourcebook

Basic Consumer Health Information about Organ and Tissue Transplantation, Including Physical and Financial Preparations, Procedures and Issues Relating to Specific Solid Organ and Tissue Transplants, Rehabilitation, Pediatric Transplant Information, the Future of Transplantation, and Organ and Tissue Donation

Along with a Glossary and Listings of Additional Resources

Edited by Joyce Brennfleck Shannon. 610 pages. 2002. 978-0-7808-0322-0.

"Recommended for libraries with an interest in offering consumer health information."
—E-Streams, Jul '02

"This is a unique and valuable resource for patients facing transplantation and their families."
—Doody's Review Service, Jun '02

Traveler's Health Sourcebook

Basic Consumer Health Information for Travelers, Including Physical and Medical Preparations, Transportation Health and Safety, Essential Information about Food and Water, Sun Exposure, Insect and Snake Bites, Camping and Wilderness Medicine, and Travel with Physical or Medical Disabilities

Along with International Travel Tips, Vaccination Recommendations, Geographical Health Issues, Disease Risks, a Glossary, and a Listing of Additional Resources

Edited by Joyce Brennfleck Shannon. 619 pages. 2000. 978-0-7808-0384-8.

"Recommended reference source."
—Booklist, Feb '01

"This book is recommended for any public library, any travel collection, and especially any collection for the physically disabled."
—American Reference Books Annual, 2001

SEE ALSO Worldwide Health Sourcebook

Urinary Tract and Kidney Diseases and Disorders Sourcebook, 2nd Edition

Basic Consumer Health Information about the Urinary System, Including the Bladder, Urethra, Ureters, and Kidneys, with Facts about Urinary Tract Infections, Incontinence, Congenital Disorders, Kidney Stones, Cancers of the Urinary Tract and Kidneys, Kidney Failure, Dialysis, and Kidney Transplantation

Along with Statistical and Demographic Information, Reports on Current Research in Kidney and Urologic Health, a Summary of Commonly Used Diagnostic Tests, a Glossary of Related Terms, and a Directory of Resources for Additional Help and Information

Edited by Ivy L. Alexander. 621 pages. 2005. 978-0-7808-0750-1.

"A good choice for a consumer health information library or for a medical library needing information to refer to their patients."
—American Reference Books Annual, 2006

SEE ALSO Prostate and Urological Disorders Sourcebook

Vegetarian Sourcebook

Basic Consumer Health Information about Vegetarian Diets, Lifestyle, and Philosophy, Including Definitions of Vegetarianism and Veganism, Tips about Adopting Vegetarianism, Creating a Vegetarian Pantry, and Meeting Nutritional Needs of Vegetarians, with Facts Regarding Vegetarianism's Effect on Pregnant and Lactating Women, Children, Athletes, and Senior Citizens

Along with a Glossary of Commonly Used Vegetarian Terms and Resources for Additional Help and Information

Edited by Chad T. Kimball. 337 pages. 2002. 978-0-7808-0439-5.

"Organizes into one concise volume the answers to the most common questions concerning vegetarian diets and lifestyles. This title is recommended for public and secondary school libraries."

—E-Streams, Apr '03

"**Invaluable reference for public and school library collections alike.**"

—Library Bookwatch, Apr '03

"**The articles in this volume are easy to read and come from authoritative sources. The book does not necessarily support the vegetarian diet but instead provides the pros and cons of this important decision... Recommended for public libraries and consumer health libraries.**"

—American Reference Books Annual, 2003

SEE ALSO *Diet and Nutrition Sourcebook, 3rd Edition*

Women's Health Concerns Sourcebook, 3rd Edition

Basic Consumer Health Information about Issues and Trends in Women's Health and Health Conditions of Special Concern to Women, Including Endometriosis, Uterine Fibroids, Menstrual Irregularities, Menopause, Sexual Dysfunction, Infertility, Cancer in Women, and Other Such Chronic Disorders as Lupus, Fibromyalgia, and Thyroid Disease

Along with Statistical Data, Tips for Maintaining Wellness, a Glossary, and a Directory of Resources for Further Help and Information

Edited by Sandra J. Judd. 679 pages. 2009. 978-0-7808-1036-5.

"**This useful resource provides information about a wide range of topics that will help women understand their bodies, prevent or treat disease, and maintain health... A detailed index helps readers locate information. This is a useful addition to public and consumer health library collections**"

—ARBAOnline, Jun '09

SEE ALSO *Breast Cancer Sourcebook, 3rd Edition, Cancer Sourcebook for Women, 4th Edition, Healthy Heart Sourcebook for Women*

Workplace Health and Safety Sourcebook

Basic Consumer Health Information about Workplace Health and Safety, Including the Effect of Workplace Hazards on the Lungs,

Skin, Heart, Ears, Eyes, Brain, Reproductive Organs, Musculoskeletal System, and Other Organs and Body Parts

Along with Information about Occupational Cancer, Personal Protective Equipment, Toxic and Hazardous Chemicals, Child Labor, Stress, and Workplace Violence

Edited by Chad T. Kimball. 610 pages. 2000. 978-0-7808-0231-5.

"**As a reference for the general public, this would be useful in any library.**"

—E-Streams, Jun '01

"**Provides helpful information for primary care physicians and other caregivers interested in occupational medicine... General readers; professionals.**"

—CHOICE, May '01

Worldwide Health Sourcebook

Basic Information about Global Health Issues, Including Malnutrition, Reproductive Health, Disease Dispersion and Prevention, Emerging Diseases, Risky Health Behaviors, and the Leading Causes of Death

Along with Global Health Concerns for Children, Women, and the Elderly, Mental Health Issues, Research and Technology Advancements, and Economic, Environmental, and Political Health Implications, a Glossary, and a Resource Listing for Additional Help and Information

Edited by Joyce Brennfleck Shannon. 597 pages. 2001. 978-0-7808-0330-5.

"**Named an Outstanding Academic Title.**"

—CHOICE, Jan '02

"**Yet another handy but also unique compilation in the extensive Health Reference Series, this is a useful work because many of the international publications reprinted or excerpted are not readily available. Highly recommended.**"

—CHOICE, Nov '01

SEE ALSO *Traveler's Health Sourcebook*

Teen Health Series

Complete Catalog

List price $69 per volume. School and library price $62 per volume.

Abuse and Violence Information for Teens

Health Tips about the Causes and Consequences of Abusive and Violent Behavior

Including Facts about the Types of Abuse and Violence, the Warning Signs of Abusive and Violent Behavior, Health Concerns of Victims, and Getting Help and Staying Safe

Edited by Sandra Augustyn Lawton. 411 pages. 2008. 978-0-7808-1008-2.

"A useful resource for schools and organizations providing services to teens and may also be a starting point in research projects."
—*Reference and Research Book News, Aug '08*

"Violence is a serious problem for teens... This resource gives teens the information they need to face potential threats and get help—either for themselves or for their friends."
—*American Reference Books Annual, 2009*

Accident and Safety Information for Teens

Health Tips about Medical Emergencies, Traumatic Injuries, and Disaster Preparedness

Including Facts about Motor Vehicle Accidents, Burns, Poisoning, Firearms, Natural Disasters, National Security Threats, and More

Edited by Karen Bellenir. 420 pages. 2008. 978-0-7808-1046-4.

"Aimed at teenage audiences, this guide provides practical information for handling a comprehensive list of emergencies, from sport injuries and auto accidents to alcohol poisoning and natural disasters."
—*Library Journal, Apr 1, '09*

"Useful in the young adult collections of public libraries as well as high school libraries."
—*American Reference Books Annual, 2009*

SEE ALSO *Sports Injuries Information for Teens, 2nd Edition*

Alcohol Information for Teens, 2nd Edition

Health Tips about Alcohol and Alcoholism

Including Facts about Alcohol's Effects on the Body, Brain, and Behavior, the Consequences of Underage Drinking, Alcohol Abuse Prevention and Treatment, and Coping with Alcoholic Parents

Edited by Lisa Bakewell. 410 pages. 2009. 978-0-7808-1043-3.

"This handbook, written for a teenage audience, provides information on the causes, effects, and preventive measures related to alcohol abuse among teens... The chapters are quick to make a connection to their teenage reading audience. The prose is straightforward and the book lends itself to spot reading. It should be useful both for practical information and for research, and it is suitable for public and school libraries."
—*ARBAOnline, Jun '09*

SEE ALSO *Drug Information for Teens, 2nd Edition*

Allergy Information for Teens

Health Tips about Allergic Reactions Such as Anaphylaxis, Respiratory Problems, and Rashes

Including Facts about Identifying and Managing Allergies to Food, Pollen, Mold, Animals, Chemicals, Drugs, and Other Substances

Edited by Karen Bellenir. 410 pages. 2006. 978-0-7808-0799-0.

"This is a comprehensive, readable text on the subject of allergic diseases in teenagers. 5 Stars (out of 5)!"
—*Doody's Review Service, Jun '06*

"This authoritative and useful self-help title is a solid addition to YA collections, whether for personal interest or reports."
—*School Library Journal, Jul '06*

Asthma Information for Teens, 2nd Ed.

Health Tips about Managing Asthma and Related Concerns

Including Facts about Asthma Causes, Triggers and Symptoms, Diagnosis, and Treatment

Edited by Kim Wohlenhaus. 400 pages. 2010. 978-0-7808-1086-0.

Body Information for Teens

Health Tips about Maintaining Well-Being for a Lifetime

Including Facts about the Development and Functioning of the Body's Systems, Organs, and Structures and the Health Impact of Lifestyle Choices

Edited by Sandra Augustyn Lawton. 458 pages. 2007. 978-0-7808-0443-2.

Cancer Information for Teens, 2nd Edition

Health Tips about Cancer Awareness, Symptoms, Prevention, Diagnosis, and Treatment

Including Facts about Common Cancers Affecting Teens, Causes, Detection, Coping Strategies, Clinical Trials, Nutrition and Exercise, Cancer in Friends or Family, and More

Edited by Karen Bellenir and Lisa Bakewell. 445 pages. 2010. 978-0-7808-1085-3.

Complementary and Alternative Medicine Information for Teens

Health Tips about Non-Traditional and Non-Western Medical Practices

Including Information about Acupuncture, Chiropractic Medicine, Dietary and Herbal Supplements, Hypnosis, Massage Therapy, Prayer and Spirituality, Reflexology, Yoga, and More

Edited by Sandra Augustyn Lawton. 407 pages. 2007. 978-0-7808-0966-6.

"This volume covers CAM specifically for teenagers but of general use also. It should be a welcome addition to both public and academic libraries."
—American Reference Books Annual, 2008

"This volume provides a solid foundation for further investigation of the subject, making it useful for both public and high school libraries."
—VOYA: Voice of Youth Advocates, Jun '07

Diabetes Information for Teens

Health Tips about Managing Diabetes and Preventing Related Complications

Including Information about Insulin, Glucose Control, Healthy Eating, Physical Activity, and Learning to Live with Diabetes

Edited by Sandra Augustyn Lawton. 410 pages. 2006. 978-0-7808-0811-9.

"A comprehensive instructional guide for teens... some of the material may also be directed towards parents or teachers. 5 stars (out of 5)!"
—Doody's Review Service, 2006

"Students dealing with their own diabetes or that of a friend or family member or those writing reports on the topic will find this a valuable resource."
—School Library Journal, Aug '06

"This text is directed to the teen population and would be an excellent library resource for a health class or for the teacher as a reference for class preparation. It can, however, serve a much wider audience. The clinical educator on diabetes may find it valuable to educate the newly diagnosed client regardless of age. It also would be an excellent reference and education tool for a preventive medicine seminar on diabetes."
—Physical Therapy, Mar '07

Diet Information for Teens, 2nd Edition

Health Tips about Diet and Nutrition

Including Facts about Dietary Guidelines, Food Groups, Nutrients, Healthy Meals, Snacks, Weight Control, Medical Concerns Related to Diet, and More

Edited by Karen Bellenir. 432 pages. 2006. 978-0-7808-0820-1.

"A very quick and pleasant read in spite of the fact that it is very detailed in the information it gives... A book for anyone concerned about diet and nutrition."
—American Reference Books Annual, 2007

SEE ALSO Eating Disorders Information for Teens, 2nd Edition

696

Drug Information for Teens, 2nd Edition

Health Tips about the Physical and Mental Effects of Substance Abuse

Including Information about Marijuana, Inhalants, Club Drugs, Stimulants, Hallucinogens, Opiates, Prescription and Over-the-Counter Drugs, Herbal Products, Tobacco, Alcohol, and More

Edited by Sandra Augustyn Lawton. 468 pages. 2006. 978-0-7808-0862-1.

"As with earlier installments in Omnigraphics' Teen Health Series, Drug Information for Teens is designed specifically to meet the needs and interests of middle and high school students... Strongly recommended for both academic and public libraries."
—*American Reference Books Annual, 2007*

"Solid thoughtful advice is given about how to handle peer pressure, drug-related health concerns, and treatment strategies."
—*School Library Journal, Dec '06*

SEE ALSO *Alcohol Information for Teens, 2nd Edition, Tobacco Information for Teens, 2nd Edition*

Eating Disorders Information for Teens, 2nd Edition

Health Tips about Anorexia, Bulimia, Binge Eating, And Other Eating Disorders

Including Information about Risk Factors, Diagnosis and Treatment, Prevention, Related Health Concerns, and Other Issues

Edited by Sandra Augustyn Lawton. 377 pages. 2009. 978-0-7808-1044-0.

"This handy reference offers basic information and addresses specific disorders, consequences, prevention, diagnosis and treatment, healthy eating, and more. It is written in a conversational style that is easy to understand... Will provide plenty of facts for reports as well as browsing potential for students with an interest in the topic."
—*School Library Journal, Jun '09*

"Written in a straightforward style that will appeal to its teenage audience. The author does not play down the danger of living with an eating disorder and urges those struggling with this problem to seek professional help.

This work, as well as others in this series, will be a welcome addition to high school and undergraduate libraries."
—*American Reference Books Annual, 2009*

SEE ALSO *Diet Information for Teens, 2nd Edition*

Fitness Information for Teens, 2nd Edition

Health Tips about Exercise, Physical Well-Being, and Health Maintenance

Including Facts about Conditioning, Stretching, Strength Training, Body Shape and Body Image, Sports Nutrition, and Specific Activities for Athletes and Non-Athletes

Edited by Lisa Bakewell. 432 pages. 2009. 978-0-7808-1045-7.

"This no-nonsense guide packs a great deal into its pages... This is a helpful reference for basic diet and exercise information for health reports or personal use."
—*School Library Journal, April 2009*

"An excellent source for general information on why teens should be active, making time to exercise, the equipment people might need, various types of activities to try, how to maintain health and wellness, and how to avoid barriers to becoming healthier... This would still be an excellent addition to a public library ready-reference collection or a high school health library collection."
—*American Reference Books Annual, 2009*

"This easy to read, well-written, up-to-date overview of fitness for teenagers provides excellent wellness and exercise tips, information, and directions... It is a useful tool for them to obtain a base knowledge in fitness topics and different sports."
—*Doody's Review Service, 2009*

SEE ALSO *Diet Information for Teens, 2nd Edition, Sports Injuries Information for Teens, 2nd Edition*

Learning Disabilities Information for Teens

Health Tips about Academic Skills Disorders and Other Disabilities That Affect Learning

Including Information about Common Signs of Learning Disabilities, School Issues, Learning to Live with a Learning Disability, and Other Related Issues

Edited by Sandra Augustyn Lawton. 400 pages. 2006. 978-0-7808-0796-9.

"This book provides a wealth of information for any reader interested in the signs, causes, and consequences of learning disabilities, as well as related legal rights and educational interventions... Public and academic libraries should want this title for both students and general readers."
—*American Reference Books Annual, 2006*

Mental Health Information for Teens, 3rd Edition

Health Tips about Mental Wellness and Mental Illness

Including Facts about Mental and Emotional Health, Depression and Other Mood Disorders, Anxiety Disorders, Behavior Disorders, Self-Injury, Psychosis, Schizophrenia, and More

Edited by Karen Bellenir. 400 pages. 2010. 978-0-7808-1087-7.

SEE ALSO *Stress Information for Teens, Suicide Information for Teens, 2nd Edition*

Pregnancy Information for Teens

Health Tips about Teen Pregnancy and Teen Parenting

Including Facts about Prenatal Care, Pregnancy Complications, Labor and Delivery, Postpartum Care, Pregnancy-Related Lifestyle Concerns, and More

Edited by Sandra Augustyn Lawton. 434 pages. 2007. 978-0-7808-0984-0.

Sexual Health Information for Teens, 2nd Edition

Health Tips about Sexual Development, Reproduction, Contraception, and Sexually Transmitted Infections

Including Facts about Puberty, Sexuality, Birth Control, Chlamydia, Gonorrhea, Herpes, Human Papillomavirus, Syphilis, and More

Edited by Sandra Augustyn Lawton. 430 pages. 2008. 978-0-7808-1010-5.

"This offering represents the most up-to-date information available on an array of topics including abstinence-only sexual education and pregnancy-prevention methods... The range of coverage—from puberty and anatomy to sexually transmitted diseases—is thorough and extensive. Each chapter includes a bibliographic citation, and the three back sections containing additional resources, further reading, and the index are all first-rate... This volume will be well used by students in need of the facts, whether for educational or personal reasons."
—*School Library Journal, Nov '08*

"Presents information related to the emotional, physical, and biological development of both males and females that occurs during puberty. It also strives to address some of the issues and questions that may arise... The text is easy to read and understand for young readers, with satisfactory definitions within the text to explain new terms."
—*American Reference Books Annual, 2009*

Skin Health Information for Teens, 2nd Edition

Health Tips about Dermatological Concerns and Skin Cancer Risks

Including Facts about Acne, Warts, Hives, and Other Conditions and Lifestyle Choices, Such as Tanning, Tattooing, and Piercing, That Affect the Skin, Nails, Scalp, and Hair

Edited by Edited by Kim Wohlenhaus. 418 pages. 2009. 978-0-7808-1042-6.

"The material in this work will be easily understood by teenagers and young adults. The publisher has liberally used bulleted lists and sidebars to keep the reader's attention... A useful addition to school and public library collections."
—*ARBAOnline, Oct '09*

Sleep Information for Teens

Health Tips about Adolescent Sleep Requirements, Sleep Disorders, and the Effects of Sleep Deprivation

Including Facts about Why People Need Sleep, Sleep Patterns, Circadian Rhythms, Dreaming, Insomnia, Sleep Apnea, Narcolepsy, and More

Edited by Karen Bellenir. 355 pages. 2008. 978-0-7808-1009-9.

"Clear, concise, and very readable and would be a good source of sleep information for anyone—not just teenagers. This work is highly recommended for medical libraries, public school libraries, and public libraries."
—*American Reference Books Annual, 2009*

SEE ALSO Body Information for Teens

Sports Injuries Information for Teens, 2nd Edition
Health Tips about Acute, Traumatic, and Chronic Injuries in Adolescent Athletes
Including Facts about Sprains, Fractures, and Overuse Injuries, Treatment, Rehabilitation, Sport-Specific Safety Guidelines, Fitness Suggestions, and More

Edited by Karen Bellenir. 429 pages. 2008. 978-0-7808-1011-2.

"An engaging selection of informative articles about the prevention and treatment of sports injuries... The value of this book is that the articles have been vetted and are often augmented with inserts of useful facts, definitions of technical terms, and quick tips. Sensitive topics like injuries to genitalia are discussed openly and responsibly. This revised edition contains updated articles and defines sport more broadly than the first edition."
—*School Library Journal, Nov '08*

"This work will be useful in the young adult collections of public libraries as well as high school libraries... A useful resource for student research."
—*American Reference Books Annual, 2009*

SEE ALSO Accident and Safety Information for Teens

Stress Information for Teens
Health Tips about the Mental and Physical Consequences of Stress
Including Information about the Different Kinds of Stress, Symptoms of Stress, Frequent Causes of Stress, Stress Management Techniques, and More

Edited by Sandra Augustyn Lawton. 392 pages. 2008. 978-0-7808-1012-9.

"Understanding what stress is, what causes it, how the body and the mind are impacted by it, and what teens can do are the general categories addressed here... The chapters are brief but informative, and the list of community-help organizations is exhaustive. Report writers will find information quickly and easily, as will those who have personal concerns. The print is clear and the format is readable, making this an accessible resource for struggling readers and researchers."
—*School Library Journal, Dec '08*

"The articles selected will specifically appeal to young adults and are designed to answer their most common questions."
— *American Reference Books Annual, 2009*

SEE ALSO Mental Health Information for Teens, 3rd Edition

Suicide Information for Teens, 2nd Edition
Health Tips about Suicide Causes and Prevention
Including Facts about Depression, Risk Factors, Getting Help, Survivor Support, and More

Edited by Kim Wohlenhaus. 400 pages. 2010. 978-0-7808-1088-4.

SEE ALSO Mental Health Information for Teens, 3rd Edition

Tobacco Information for Teens, 2nd Edition
Health Tips about the Hazards of Using Cigarettes, Smokeless Tobacco, and Other Nicotine Products
Including Facts about Nicotine Addiction, Nicotine Delivery Systems, Secondhand Smoke, Health Consequences of Tobacco Use, Related Cancers, Smoking Cessation, and Tobacco Use Statistics

Edited by Karen Bellenir. 400 pages. 2010. 978-0-7808-1153-9.

SEE ALSO Drug Information for Teens, 2nd Edition

Health Reference Series

Adolescent Health Sourcebook, 3rd Edition

Adult Health Concerns Sourcebook

AIDS Sourcebook, 4th Edition

Alcoholism Sourcebook, 3rd Edition

Allergies Sourcebook, 3rd Edition

Alzheimer Disease Sourcebook, 4th Edition

Arthritis Sourcebook, 3rd Edition

Asthma Sourcebook, 2nd Edition

Attention Deficit Disorder Sourcebook

Autism & Pervasive Developmental Disorders Sourcebook

Back & Neck Sourcebook, 2nd Edition

Blood & Circulatory Disorders Sourcebook, 3rd Edition

Brain Disorders Sourcebook, 3rd Edition

Breast Cancer Sourcebook, 3rd Edition

Breastfeeding Sourcebook

Burns Sourcebook

Cancer Sourcebook for Women, 4th Edition

Cancer Sourcebook, 5th Edition

Cancer Survivorship Sourcebook

Cardiovascular Disorders Sourcebook, 4th Edition

Caregiving Sourcebook

Child Abuse Sourcebook

Childhood Diseases & Disorders Sourcebook, 2nd Edition

Colds, Flu & Other Common Ailments Sourcebook

Communication Disorders Sourcebook

Complementary & Alternative Medicine Sourcebook, 4th Edition

Congenital Disorders Sourcebook, 2nd Edition

Contagious Diseases Sourcebook

Cosmetic & Reconstructive Surgery Sourcebook, 2nd Edition

Death & Dying Sourcebook, 2nd Edition

Dental Care & Oral Health Sourcebook, 3rd Edition

Depression Sourcebook, 2nd Edition

Dermatological Disorders Sourcebook, 2nd Edition

Diabetes Sourcebook, 4th Edition

Diet & Nutrition Sourcebook, 3rd Edition

Digestive Diseases & Disorder Sourcebook

Disabilities Sourcebook

Disease Management Sourcebook

Domestic Violence Sourcebook, 3rd Edition

Drug Abuse Sourcebook, 3rd Edition

Ear, Nose & Throat Disorders Sourcebook, 2nd Edition

Eating Disorders Sourcebook, 3rd Edition

Emergency Medical Services Sourcebook

Endocrine & Metabolic Disorders Sourcebook, 2nd Edition

Environmental Health Sourcebook, 3rd Edition

Ethnic Diseases Sourcebook

Eye Care Sourcebook, 3rd Edition

Family Planning Sourcebook

Fitness & Exercise Sourcebook, 4th Edition

Food Safety Sourcebook

Forensic Medicine Sourcebook

Gastrointestinal Diseases & Disorders Sourcebook, 2nd Edition

Genetic Disorders Sourcebook, 3rd Edition

Head Trauma Sourcebook

Headache Sourcebook

Health Insurance Sourcebook

Healthy Aging Sourcebook

Healthy Children Sourcebook

Healthy Heart Sourcebook for Women

Hepatitis Sourcebook

Household Safety Sourcebook

Hypertension Sourcebook

Immune System Disorders Sourcebook, 2nd Edition

Infant & Toddler Health Sourcebook

Infectious Diseases Sourcebook

Injury & Trauma Sourcebook